Online Recovery Module/Bonus(es)* Online Redemption   1-220907-10

. Visit https://www.DrLamCoaching.com. New users click "Register" at top right and complete information required. Current users please sign in.

. At the main menu, click the blue "Redeem Bonus(es)*" button and follow the on-screen instructions (such as entering purchase type, PIN, order number, etc.) and click "I Agree, Submit". Your gift(s) will be in your Private Library.

Scratch off to reveal your PIN number

* Online Recovery Module/Bonus promotional gift(s) provided with your purchase of this product is redeemable online only at DrLam.com based on your nontransferable and personal use at your private library limited to a single user per valid PIN number. Corporate or library use and access, as well as any direct or indirect sharing is strictly prohibited and will invalidate your access and/or PIN number. Access may not be shared, resold, or otherwise circulated. Access to the Bonus item(s) available in your Private Library will terminate 1 year after redemption. Content in the Online Recovery Module may change without prior notice to you. Access is subject to your acceptance of detailed terms and conditions upon registration/redemption. Limit 1 PIN per customer. Offer good while supplies last. Access to the Online Recovery Module and Bonus item(s) will terminate on publication of the next edition of this product. Other conditions may apply on additional gifts and coupons.

Adrenal Fatigue Syndrome sufferers are talking about Dr. Lam ...

When we found Dr. Lam, I was what he called the living dead. I literally was on death's doorstep. Not one person associated with Western Medicine could find anything wrong with me, and my health was declining rapidly. I have been to over thirty doctors and not one of them has helped me in the slightest. Dr. Lam saved my life and set me on the road to recovery. Thank you for saving my life!

— Dena H., Colorado

I just wanted to thank you for bringing life back to me. I was so sick and now I am feeling as good as I did 20 years ago! It has been a long battle: no energy, aches and pains going from one doctor to the next. They told me it was anything from arthritis to depression; they had me on steroids for three years... All behind me now!

I just don't know how to thank you. I think it would be wonderful if you could just be everywhere with your caring heart, your information and the real reason behind all of the bad, sick days that so many of us have had.

— Jessica, Washington

Dr. Lam has given Bret his life back and me my husband back. I am forever grateful to him because without his knowledge of adrenal fatigue we may still be fighting a "non-existent" disease by the medical establishment. I am happy to report that he is not on any medication and is not depressed! It means the world when your Doctor knows what you are currently experiencing. Without Dr. Lam, I don't where I would be.

— Brandy and Bret, Wife, N. Carolina

Thank you kindly for this speedy and clear response. I can't thank you enough and wish there were more doctors like you. It's people like you who prove that medicine still remains the noblest of professions. Thank you again for your comprehensive explanation and a game plan—deeply appreciated.

— N.S., Singapore

Thank you so very, very much for all of your good advice and help. Your detailed analysis and in-depth articles have been extremely useful and have helped my Doctors to understand what is happening within my system. Now I know that I need to support my body and be very careful of pushing it. I also know what type of things will help support my body and what type of signs I need to look for. Keep up the great work you are doing and thanks so much once again!

— Marcia S., Nambia

May I thank you for such speedy and efficient service in responding to my inquiries. I live in the UK and, to be honest, never thought you would offer to help from such a distance.

I am very much looking forward to talking to your dietician, Dorine. You offer a wonderful service and I feel hope for the first time that a recovery is possible. Thank you, I wish more doctors in the UK would read your website and have open minds!!

– Alys, United Kingdom

Thanks Dr. Lam—I really do appreciate your clear and quick reply. I can finally talk intelligently to my young son about this.

– Glenn S., Brazil

Thank you so very much for the help you have given me with my health. Not only is your knowledge amazing, but you are able to counsel with clear, easy to understand explanations and the directions I received were simple.

– Brenda A., British Columbia

Thank you so very much for all your help. Not only have you helped me tremendously with my Adrenal Fatigue, but you have helped me lower my cholesterol. In only three and a half months on your protocol (natural and no drugs) my total cholesterol has gone down 53 points, Triglycerides down 53 points, HDL up four points, LDL down 46 points, and VLDL down 11 points.

– Dallas W., Iowa

Thank you so much for all your in-depth information and guidance ... I am truly thankful ... you are really changing other people's lives by your spirit to give freely of your knowledge and sharing it with others selflessly ... that is truly an inspiration to work with such an admirable person, especially these days ... I applaud you as a guide and as an example to others. Again, thank you ... you are a very special person ... here on this earth with a great purpose that you are fulfilling.

– JC Rose, Georgia

I am able to handle stress better, function fairly normally around the house while taking rests throughout the day. I am no longer bedridden as I was before. I now sleep though the night consistently for the first time in many years, and my mind is once again able to think clearly. Though I will occasionally have an adrenal crash, it is unlike my earlier recurring dizzy symptoms, and I recover within a few days and not weeks or months.

– Diane M, Tennessee

Thank you for showing me how to significantly reduce my cardiovascular risk. Through your coaching, I have been able to reduce my LP (a) level by 50 percent. Thank you for the great work.

– Kent C., California

I contacted Dr. Lam the first week in May and he told me in 3 to 4 weeks I would begin to feel better, 6 to 8 good, and 10 to 12 great. He was right on the money. He brought my adrenal gland back slowly and I never suffered a crash. Thank you Dr. Lam, for getting me back on track and feeling better than ever! You are a pioneer for women. Keep doing research to help women stay in balance naturally.

– Lisa O., Pennsylvania

I have come to the conclusion that you do not need to speak/call with me in regards to my now non-existent adrenal disorder. When I was hospitalized they did a battery of tests and three of the results proved that your therapy worked and I am as healthy as I can be.
   1) My adrenal gland is functioning properly.
   2) My cortisol levels are normal.
   3) My potassium/sodium levels are normal and balanced.
Again, thanks for all your advice—I have never felt better.

– Rich M., Pennsylvania

I am feeling well—taking the supplements you suggested. Thank you for your help. You gave me the energy at 84 years to move from a condo to a large modular home— I enjoy doing housework again and walking without a cane around this mobile home park. I'm also driving a car again. Thanks to you, I feel much younger.

– Vivian

I wanna thank you. Your advice to me was one of my keys to recovery from Lymes Disease and handling it as well as my fibromyalgia. you said "JERRY YOU'RE TRYING TO DO THE 'RIGHT THING AT THE WRONG TIME'" and you were very right. I stopped trying to force feed my unready highly sensitive body with vitamins and went back to the basics. Although the vitamin pushers still tried to insist, I knew we are individuals and our body knows. Thank you Dr. Lam, you were part of my recovery.

– Jerry H.

Thank you greatly for your book, Estrogen Dominance—it helped me diagnose my condition having gone from one doctor to another for 6 months to no effect. This book is amazing and has been an eye opener. You are a true doctor and educator!

– N., Book Buyer

Thank you and God bless you for your compassion, patience, time and un-selfishness! You are a very caring and loving person! Such an excellent doctor! There are a lot of doctors who could learn true integrity by your fine example—including the unselfish time you make for people who aren't even your patients! I'm simply too moved for words—your sacrifice is a blessing to me.

– Cindy

It has now been 12 months of recovery. Almost all of my symptoms have largely subsided. Most significantly, my sleep has been deep and restful, and my ability to tolerate stress has increased. I have more energy and my body is stronger. Yoga in particular helped almost all by itself to restore my sleeping patterns and give me a deep sleep.

Eight months ago when I came home with groceries, I could only carry two bags at a time up the stairs. After carrying all the bags, I would suffer an adrenal crash. I felt like sleeping immediately. It took one week just to recover! Now I can carry eight bags in one hand with no ill-effects or fatigue!

Ten months ago, I could not read more than five pages of a book due to fatigue. Now, I read 320 pages in three days with no ill-effects!

– Yours Sincerely,
David B., Australia

Professionials Are Talking about Dr. Lam ...

I did not know at first I had Adrenal Fatigue. After many visits to specialists, a friend suggested I may have this. I was debilitated. Even my dear Naturopath helped all she could but I was drained completely! I am a Dentist and even my thriving practice started to suffer. I just couldn't find the energy I used to have. At my lowest point, I would be in bed for nearly 15 hours straight. Even my little children were worried about me.

After reading Dr. Lam's website, I knew this Doctor understood what I was going through. Western medicine offered me nothing—his program was outstanding. All through his wonderful program, I was so happy, working with him for 9 months. I hate to even think of how I felt before. When he said I would be able to start running again, all I could think is, 'I've heard that before.' Well, slowly but surely, I came back and just began running again.

It was a slow recovery from my advanced stage of Adrenal Fatigue to be sure. But yes, I am 100% now. This Doctor knows his stuff! I am so grateful to Dr. Lam, I can hardly find the words. When I walk and run, I feel thankful for his knowledge. He saved my life, my practice and my family. If you are serious about healing, he can guide you there.

– Dr. Samantha K., Dentist

I'm an Anatomy Instructor at one of our nation's most prestigious medical institutions. I wanted to write and let you know that I truly have found your recommendations effective for me personally. I am a testimonial to your work!

– Shelley, Professor

I am a Gynecologist who now lectures and teaches Holistic Medicine and Natural Remedies to other health care providers throughout the United States. I can't thank you enough for putting your knowledge out there for the good of mankind.

– M. Green, M.D.

I'm a licensed Naturopath practicing in Nova Scotia, Canada. I want to commend you on the wonderful information on your site. I refer many clients to it for references regarding Adrenal disorders, reproductive hormone imbalances and much more. One client contacted you with her adrenal questions and was excited to hear back from you. I want to thank you for taking the time to listen to her questions and for responding.

– Dr. Scott W., Naturopath

I am a Registered Dietitian. I am writing to compliment you on your fantastic write-up on Estrogen Dominance. Also, I am much involved in educating doctors that wish to incorporate more nutrition into their practices. Your knowledge is very impressive. I am trying to get more doctors up to speed like you are, especially in the area of causes of disease and natural treatments.

– Linda L, R.D., C.D.N.

Your website is a huge help and I refer people to it all the time. I am a drug and alcohol counselor and always encourage people to do things with their diet and exercise. I have given many your web address and talked about your programs in groups and individual sessions.

– Drug and Alcohol Counselor

They Use the *DrLam.com* Website ...

About 8 years ago, I noticed that flour and dairy products caused me to be congested. No matter how much work I put in the gym, I just could not eliminate fat. I found your site last year and started your recommended blood type diet. In six months, I dropped 20 pounds of fat, from wearing a 36 pants size to a 28. I am able to work out harder and longer than I ever thought possible and I owe it all to your research. Thank you for everything.

– Arnold G.

What an excellent compilation of information on skin aging! Thanks so much for providing comprehensive yet understandable information on-line and free to boot.

– Elan

This is the absolute best site on the Internet for Adrenal Fatigue.

– John O.

Thanks for your quick response. I appreciate it very, very much—it's helpful and comforting to me. It's very kind of you to take the time to email me.

– George

Just wanted to say that I've been following your guideline diet completely word-by-word and I have lost weight rapidly, from 85 kg to 68 kg.

– Roony

I just wanted to thank you for your info. I have had 4 episodes of atrial fibrillation in 12 years, the last happening in January of this year. I've added Hawthorn Berry and Magnesium to my diet along with Armour Thyroid for my hypothyroidism. I play golf 3 times a week and walked every hole. Thanks, Dr. Lam!

– J. D.

Thank you so much for all of the prompt replies! I have read all of the information and watched your videos as well. Over the years, I have extensively read adrenal information on the web. I don't remember how I found your site, but everything there is EXCEPTIONAL! It put all of the pieces together that I have read elsewhere and I now understand it.

– Charlene

Your work has benefited millions of sufferers including myself …. Thank you for this information.

– HC Lee, Malaysia

To read the latest testimonials and accolades, visit *www.DrLam.com*

Adrenal Fatigue Syndrome

Reclaim Your Energy and Vitality with Clinically Proven Natural Programs

Other publications by Michael Lam, M.D., M.P.H.

Books

5 Proven Secrets to Longevity

How to Stay Young and Live Longer

Beating Cancer with Natural Medicine

Estrogen Dominance – The 21st Century Hormonal Imbalance

CDs

Adrenal Breathing™ Exercise

Mind-Body and Adrenal Fatigue

Adrenal Fatigue in a Complex World

Adrenal Health and Anti-aging

DVDs

Adrenal Yoga™ Exercise Vols. 1-4

For more information, visit *www.DrLam.com*

Adrenal Fatigue Syndrome

Reclaim Your Energy and Vitality with Clinically Proven Natural Programs

Michael Lam, M.D., M.P.H.
Dorine Lam, R.D., M.S., M.P.H.

Adrenal Fatigue Syndrome: Reclaim Your Energy and Vitality with Clinically Proven Natural Programs
by Michael Lam, M.D., M.P.H. and Dorine Lam, R.D., M.S., M.P.H.

© Copyright 2012 by Michael Lam, M.D.

Published in the United States by:

Adrenal Institute Press, Loma Linda, CA 92354
www.AdrenalInstitute.org

Cover and Interior Design: Nick Zelinger, NZ Graphics
Editing: John Maling (Editing By John), Virginia McCullough
Book Shepherding: Judith Briles

ISBN (Soft Cover, with Flaps): 978-1-937930-00-4
Library of Congress Control Number (Soft Cover, with Flaps): 2012931272

ISBN (Soft Cover, without Flaps): 978-1-937930-01-1
Library of Congress Control Number (Soft Cover, without Flaps): 2012931272

ISBN (e-Book): 978-1-937930-02-8
Library of Congress Control Number (e-Book): 2012931272

Adrenal Fatigue Syndrome: Reclaim Your Energy and Vitality with Clinically Proven Natural Programs /
Michael Lam, Dorine Lam. First edition, 2012; Includes Index

10 9 8 7 6 5

1. Health   2. Adrenal glands—Disease.   3. Fatigue   4. Stress (Physiology)   5. neuroendocrine

First Edition

Printed in the United States of America

To our Creator, with awe, humility, dedication, and love.

In loving memory of our mother who exemplifies self-sacrifice.

To our children Daren, Justin, Carrie, and Jeremy, for now and always.

To our clients who taught us more than we can ever hope to teach them.

To all the doctors who dare to think for themselves.

About *DrLam.com*

DrLam.com is a free public educational website offering cutting edge information on natural medicine. Founded in 2001 by Michael Lam, M.D., nutritional medicine expert and board certified anti-aging medicine specialist, the site features the world's most comprehensive scientific, evidenced-based information on Adrenal Fatigue Syndrome.

Dr. Lam's mission is to educate and empower others to take control of their health. You can ask questions about your health concerns online. Because of his willingness to answer specific questions, Dr. Lam has helped legions of individuals learn how to use safe, effective and clinically proven natural protocols for self-healing. This educational service is provided free.

Other resources on the website include:

- Quick 3 minute Adrenal Fatigue Test to assess your adrenal function.

- Sign up for free email Adrenal Fatigue Newsletter to stay up on the latest AFS research. Get the latest information presented in easy-to-understand language.

- Hundreds of cutting-edge original special reports and videos by Dr. Lam on everything related to Adrenal Fatigue Syndrome.

- An extensive and archive-rich library of answers to questions previously asked by others that are certain to help you in your recovery from Adrenal Fatigue Syndrome.

- Over 30 conditioned based health centers with specific clinically proven natural protocols ranging from heart health to cancer.

Dr. Lam offers a worldwide, telephone-based, one-on-one, nutritional coaching service. Personalizing the natural principles discussed in this book, his coaching service has successfully helped countless Adrenal Fatigue Syndrome sufferers recover and reclaim their vitality.

For more information, visit
www.DrLam.com

Contents

Figures and Tables

Figures

Tables

Authors' Note

For well over half a century, we have devoted our clinical nutrition careers to educating others about the importance of preventive medicine and the power of nutrition as a healing tool. Nothing is as satisfying as seeing individuals rise from an almost bedridden state of fatigue and returning to their normal and productive lives. For the most part, these men and women had been abandoned by conventional medicine after being told there was nothing wrong with them.

When extensive medical workups fail to detect the cause of fatigue and lethargy, these symptoms are often dismissed as psychogenic in origin. However, we have now found out that they can actually be traced to a condition called Adrenal Fatigue Syndrome (AFS), which in advanced stages can be incapacitating.

The host of concurrent complaints can include hypoglycemia, low blood pressure, brain fog, heart palpitation, anxiety, difficulty losing weight, insomnia, PMS, crashes, salt cravings, low thyroid function, depression, intolerance to medication and supplementation, low libido, and so forth. The many signs and symptoms complicate the clinical picture and defy traditional medical logic. Adrenal Fatigue Syndrome is even more confusing and overwhelming in advanced stages. Conventionally trained physicians are universally under-educated in Adrenal Fatigue Syndrome and they eventually give up. This is why those who suffer are often left to self-navigate as they jump from one practitioner to another in search of help.

If this description sounds like you, we know what you are going through. Many of you come to us for help, often in desperation. We know Adrenal Fatigue Syndrome is real, and you need to know that you are not alone. You also need to know that recovery is possible, and help is available. Right here. Right now. *Guiding you in your recovery is the primary focus of Adrenal Fatigue Syndrome.*

We are compelled to write this book because you need to know the full scientific basis, particularly from a neuroendocrine perspective, of this condition and its clinical relevance to your specific experience. Until you and your doctor know the root cause of your suffering, long term successful recovery is almost impossible. The reason is simple—you cannot fix something when you don't know what is wrong with it. Trying to "patch" symptoms, as most do, only worsens Adrenal Fatigue Syndrome over time. It is one of the most common reasons of recovery failure.

If you or a loved one has unrelenting fatigue and nowhere to turn, this book is for you. If your physician told you there is nothing left to try to reverse lethargy, this book is for you. If family members and friends want to know why you are tired all the time, this book is for you and for them. If you look good on the outside but believe you're falling apart inside, this book is for you. If you feel you are among the self-described living dead, this book is a must read. Finally, this book is for anyone wishing to avoid this potentially debilitating condition that has now reached epidemic proportion. Whether you are tired occasionally because of a stressful event, or experience fatigue all the time, you can only benefit by knowing more about Adrenal Fatigue Syndrome.

Note: When physicians write books about health problems and conditions, there exists a temptation to water down the information presented, diluting it at every turn, in order to make the information as simple as possible. However, we don't believe this is the best way to address those who suffer from Adrenal Fatigue Syndrome. It may sell short readers and AFS sufferers who want more complete information even if it is complex. In short, we believe you are entitled to our comprehensive approach that attempts to explain the physiology and chemistry involved in this potentially devastating and life-changing condition. In our experience, patients are eager for answers, and they are surely smart enough to take in the scientific information that explains what is going in their bodies. In addition, it is our hope that physicians and other clinicians will use this book to educate themselves about this common but misunderstood situation that affects, at one time or another, nearly all the patients they will see over a lifetime of medical practice!

How to Use *Adrenal Fatigue Syndrome*

Part I of this book focuses on the problem, Adrenal Fatigue Syndrome: how to identify it, the terminology we use, the symptoms, the physiology behind the condition, the staging, the phases, the natural progression, the crashes and recovery, and the consequences if unattended. We also present a complete case history at the end to help summarize the problem.

Part II of this book focuses on the solution. It contains specific information about what comprehensive recovery programs should look like, and things you can do to restore your vitality. We go through a total body approach, detailing a supplementation plan, hormones you may need, nontoxic and nurturing diets, adrenal-specific exercises, and mind-body lifestyle modifications, drawing from experiences in our everyday practice that have helped countless others regain their health.

We've also included short descriptions of symptoms in the words of the men and women who experienced them and struggled to find answers, plus one full chapter that is the story of one woman's struggle and recovery. Of course, we've changed their names and other details to protect their privacy, but we want you to see the way Adrenal Fatigue Syndrome affects the lives of individuals on a daily basis. You may see yourself in these stories, and we trust they will give you hope. We guided each person through a personalized recovery program using the tools presented in this book. Because each case is unique, we can't describe every single recovery plan, but we can assure you that with the right professional approach, a path to recovery exists, even for those who are severely afflicted and incapacitated.

In addition, our expanded Appendices contain a resource guide to help you look for the right practitioner, and a 3 Minute Adrenal Fatigue Syndrome test to help you decide if the information in this book applies to you. .

We recommend reading the book in sequence because the concepts progressively build on each other.

Finally, understand that Adrenal Fatigue Syndrome affects virtually every adult at one time or another to varying degrees. You aren't to blame for developing it, but you can take responsibility for finding and following advice that will help you recover. That advice is what you will find in this book.

Michael Lam, M.D., M.P.H.
Dorine Lam, R.D., M.S., M.P.H.

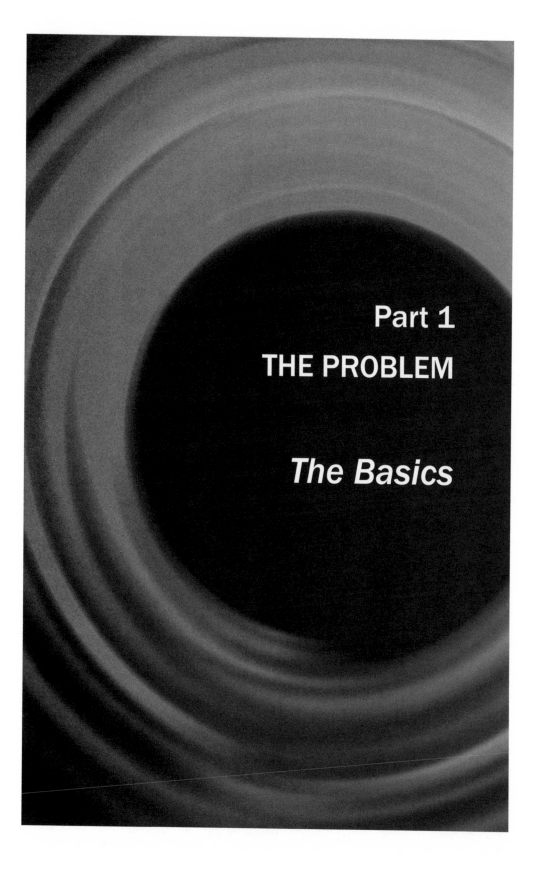

Part 1
THE PROBLEM

The Basics

Chapter 1

The Adrenal Fatigue Syndrome

If you are seeking information found in this book, then it's likely that you or a loved one has experienced symptoms or changes in your health status that you can't explain. Perhaps the symptoms or changes came on slowly over time. For example, you don't feel quite as energetic as you once did, and you can't figure out why. Until recently you maintained your weight with a balanced diet and a couple of walks or bike rides or trips to the health club each week. You seldom complained about insomnia or fitful sleep, but now you can't seem to get a good night's sleep. You've told your doctor that you've been feeling down and tired and now you have to force yourself to get through the day.

Today's physicians commonly hear these kinds of statements. In fact, fatigue and anxiety are two of the most common complaints doctors hear from their adult patients, both of which are symptoms of a silent epidemic condition known as Adrenal Fatigue Syndrome (AFS). This condition is as old as humankind, but its incidence has skyrocketed as our society and our lifestyles have become increasingly complex and high pressured.

The Many Symptoms of Adrenal Fatigue Syndrome

From a sufferer's point of view, Adrenal Fatigue Syndrome is confusing and frustrating. It's difficult to grasp that so many symptoms, often associated with a host of other conditions, could point to AFS. We can see the everyday consequences of Adrenal Fatigue Syndrome in the following statements:

- I'm tired all the time—I manage to keep going on my job, but I drink coffee every few hours to get through the day.

- I used to merely gripe and complain about feeling tired, but now the fatigue is so overwhelming and debilitating, I'm underperforming on my job.

- I'm anxious and fearful much of the time.

- I seem to catch every cold or flu that comes around.

- My joints ache, and my doctor said I probably have arthritis, even though I just turned forty.

- I'm depressed and can't think straight—I feel like I walk around with brain fog.

- I've tried every diet in the book, but I can't lose weight.

- Last year I lost my job, and shortly after those emotional and financial blows, I've been chronically tired and depressed.

- I wake up at 3:00 AM and toss and turn for hours and cannot fall asleep again.

- I used to have great energy, but now a short walk wears me out.

These statements personalize some of the typical—and persistent—signs and symptoms of Adrenal Fatigue Syndrome, most likely Stage 3 (discussed later). You might have described these same things to your doctor, or you may have noted these changes in your health or know someone who has these complaints, but you don't know what to make of them. If you're over age forty-five or fifty, you might even be told to attribute your symptoms to "normal" aging!

Below, you'll find an expanded list of the signs and symptoms of Adrenal Fatigue Syndrome. As you can see, many of these symptoms are also related to other conditions, and they match the statements listed above:

- Progressively increasing lethargy and lack of energy

- Increased effort needed just to perform daily tasks

- Decreased ability to handle stress

- Tendency to gain weight, coupled with an inability to lose it, especially settling around the waist

- Frequent bouts of influenza and other respiratory diseases, with symptoms lasting longer than usual

- Trembling under pressure

- Reduced sex drive

- Tendency to feel lightheaded especially when rising from a horizontal position

- Inability to remember things

- Lack of energy in the morning and in the afternoon between 3:00 and 5:00 PM

- Tendency to feel better suddenly for a brief period after a meal

- Often feels tired between 9:00 and 10:00 PM, but resists going to bed

- Difficulty getting out of bed in the morning

- Once out of bed, needs coffee or other stimulants to get going

- Cravings for salty, fatty, and high protein food such as meat and cheese

- For women, increased symptoms of PMS and irregular menstrual bleeding, with days of heavy flow that stops (or nearly stops) on day 4, only to resume on days 5 or 6 of the menstrual cycle

- Pain in the upper back or neck with no apparent reason

- Tendency to feel better on vacation and when stress is relieved

- Mild depression

- Food and or inhalant (air borne) allergies

- Dry and thin skin

- Hypoglycemia

- Low body temperature

- Nervousness

- Heart palpitations

- Unexplained hair loss

- Alternating constipation and diarrhea

- Dyspepsia (indigestion)

As you can see, Adrenal Fatigue Syndrome has a broad spectrum of symptoms, many of which seem nonspecific, and, therefore, are often reframed as psychological in origin, such as anxiety or depression. Sometimes patients are told that these symptoms are "nothing that some rest won't cure." However, it is clear that Adrenal Fatigue Syndrome is not that simple.

> **As you will learn, this condition from a scientific perspective represents the body's normal neuroendocrine stress response when under threat. (Neuroendocrinology is the study of the extensive interactions between the nervous system and the endocrine system.)**

This book is about Adrenal Fatigue Syndrome, not *adrenal fatigue*, a term the public may be familiar with. Key differences exist, which may be important for your overall understanding and recovery. We start with the basics.

Syndrome vs. Disease

A disease is an actual diagnosed health impairment or a condition of abnormal functioning. With a disease we see a defined cause: genetic, toxicological, bacterial, viral, and so forth. Mercury poisoning, for example, is a disease caused by excessive heavy metal in the body. Blood tests are available to guide us about acceptable levels; beyond those levels, toxicity is common. Addison's disease (also called adrenal insufficiency) is a rare, endocrine disorder where the adrenal glands do not produce sufficient steroid hormones. To qualify for diagnosis of this disease, endocrinologists have agreed on a set of specific clinical and laboratory parameters that has to be met. Once diagnosed, patients embark on a predefined set of protocols commonly accepted as standard within the medical community. In order to be treated for the disease, patients must be under a physician's care.

In medicine, a syndrome is a group of signs and symptoms that together are characteristic of a specific condition, disorder, disease, or the like. A syndrome is usually associated with several clinically recognizable features: signs (observed by a physician), symptoms (reported by the patient), and phenomena or characteristics; all of which often occur together. The presence of one or more features alerts the physician to the possible presence of the others.

Syndromes tend to have a range of possible causes that could create a particular set of circumstances rather than specific etiology. In other words, a syndrome connotes multiple causes, some of which may be unknown. For example, Parkinson's disease is a specific illness, while Parkinsonian syndrome tends to be nonspecific. The latter could be caused by the former, but also by other conditions such as progressive supranuclear palsy (a rare brain disorder that destroys nerve cells) or multiple system atrophy (a degenerative condition originating in parts of the brain).

The description of a syndrome usually includes a number of *essential characteristics,* which, when appearing together, lead to the diagnosis of the condition. These often are classified as a combination of typical major symptoms and signs—essential to the diagnosis—together with minor findings, of which some or all can be absent. A formal description may specify the minimum number of major and minor findings respectively that are required for the diagnosis.

For example, metabolic syndrome is a combination of medical disorders. When they occur together, we see an increase in the risk of developing adult onset diabetes and cardiovascular disease. This syndrome affects one in five people in the United States and its prevalence increases with age. To qualify for this diagnosis, central obesity is a major required finding, along with any two other minor findings from a list of other symptoms or disorders ranging from Type II diabetes, low HDL (high density lipoproteins, the so-called good cholesterol), hypertension, and so forth.

More about Syndromes

Syndromes are important, because they alert us that we have dysfunction going on in the body that may not have a clear cut cause-and-effect relationship. Premenstrual syndrome (PMS), for example, is simply a descriptive term for a set of symptoms associated with the onset of the menstrual cycle. It does not tell us the cause.

Syndromes also serve as important clinical lighthouses, directing our focus on the big picture when needed. For example, those who have polycystic ovarian syndrome (PCOS) should be on the lookout for increased chances of insulin resistance and adult onset diabetes. In fact, diabetic medications are commonly used to treat PCOS.

In recent years, we've seen the word syndrome used rather loosely. For example, SARS (severe acute respiratory syndrome) is caused by a virus but is still called a syndrome. Similarly, AIDS (acquired immune deficiency syndrome) is still used, despite the identification of HIV (human immunodeficiency virus) as the culprit. Technically, HIV infection is the disease, and AIDS is the syndrome—the set of symptoms—caused by it; one can have the HIV infection without having AIDS. Individuals can carry the HIV infection for years before symptoms appeared. (Today, those with HIV are being treated before symptoms appear.) The terms HIV and AIDS overlap substantially, and sometimes you can only tell what a particular person (even a medical person) means by the context of the use. AIDS acquired the label of syndrome before the cause was known, and it has stuck.

As a general principle, a syndrome is a set of symptoms or conditions that occur together and suggest the presence of a certain disease or an increased chance of developing the disease. However, the syndrome itself may not be a disease as defined by conventional medical standards. A syndrome can indicate a disease, but not necessarily. In addition, several different diseases can all cause the same syndrome.

> **To be clear, Adrenal Fatigue Syndrome is not a disease under current conventional medicine definitions.**

Why all the Confusion?

Newly discovered syndromes eventually evolve into accepted medical condition, but this usually takes decades of scientific research and scrutiny, and rightfully so. Modern medical advances have shortened this process. In recent years, we started labeling certain syndromes as diseases once diagnostic standards were set. For example, chronic fatigue syndrome (CFS) is now a recognized disorder and so is irritable bowel syndrome (IBS). Both names describe symptoms once considered elusive not too long ago. Over time, we've seen factors that are direct causes for CFS and IBS, such as infection. The exact etiology, or the ultimate cause of both these syndromes, however, is still far from clear. In addition, it's likely many factors are involved in these two syndromes. *Unfortunately, when symptoms are treated as disease, too many physicians are then led down a clinical path that focuses on relieving symptoms and often miss healing the root causes that trigger the symptoms in the first place.*

Terminology and Important Distinctions

Given the variation in labeling syndromes and diseases, it's not surprising to see confusion about the right terminology to describe symptoms associated with stress-induced neuroendocrine and adrenal response. This is a relatively new concept in modern medicine. For example, many in the alternative medicine circles use the terms *adrenal fatigue, adrenal burnout, adrenal exhaustion,* and *hypoadrenia* interchangeably, leaving us with a lack of consistency in our terms and therefore confusion in our understanding of the broad picture. For our purposes in this book, we use *Adrenal Fatigue Syndrome* (AFS) as the overall name for the condition, and for good reasons.

The term *adrenal fatigue* is most widely used, but it doesn't shed much light on the root cause of the condition. Instead, this name implies structural abnormality of the adrenal glands as the etiology, with resulting low output of the main anti-stress adrenal hormone, cortisol. However, we know many causes that can lead to similar symptoms with clinical presentation consistent with low cortisol output. They range from metabolic imbalances and infections, to psychogenic issues and genetic factors. Furthermore, many symptoms of advanced AFS are primarily due to a dysregulated neuroendocrine system, with cortisol playing a minor role. In other words, low cortisol output is not the only dominant clinical presentation in advanced stages of this condition. Invariably, the adrenal glands remain structurally intact, and traditional laboratory test results are normal (according to standards set by conventional endocrinologists) at all times.

In addition, adrenal fatigue implies that the adrenal glands themselves are dysfunctional and therefore responsible for cortisol dysregulation. This is not necessarily true. For example, low cortisol output has been strongly associated with Post-Traumatic Stress Disorder (PTSD), a condition that originates in the brain. The adrenal glands are structurally intact in AFS pathologically under current medical standards. In many ways, therefore, the term *adrenal fatigue* leaves much to be desired in terms of accuracy and clarity, although it may be a simple and easy concept to grasp for the public at large.

The more scientifically accurate term for this condition is *Adrenal Fatigue Syndrome* (AFS). Using the word *syndrome* implies that the symptoms may or may not arise from the adrenal glands, and in addition, that the cause may not be completely known. This term removes the assumption that a pathological problem with the adrenal glands exists. It also allows a more liberal interpretation of what conventional doctors consider the threshold of a low or high cortisol level. Finally, it allows the physician to determine which out of the long list of signs and symptoms are appropriate for the syndrome. In other words, it allows for the recognition and validation of the neurological and endocrinological basis of this condition, and the many associated hormonal dysregulations that may or may not be adrenal related, without violating the current definition of adrenal dysfunction used in conventional medicine.

As you will learn in this book, AFS could be called many things. For example, many symptoms of AFS, especially in advanced stages, are associated with dysfunction of the *hypothalamic-pituitary-adrenal (HPA) axis.* This hormone axis dysregulation originates in the brain. Those in neuroscience may prefer the term *HPA Axis Dysregulation* to reflect their perspective of brain involvement. Medical historians may be more comfortable with simply calling this a severe form of general adaptation syndrome (a theory of stress advanced by the late researcher, Dr. Hans Selye, who first described the three main stages of general stress response decades ago). On the other hand, modern endocrinologists may find the terminology of non-adrenal illness syndrome (NAIS) more palatable. This term recognizes the symptoms of high cortisol when AFS is in early stages, and low cortisol associated with advanced AFS, while acknowledging that the glands are structurally normal and that the cause may lie outside the adrenal glands.

The use of such terminology is not new. In non-thyroid illness syndrome (NTIS), severe starvation or advanced illness can produce symptoms of low thyroid function, but the thyroid gland itself is structurally sound. It does not, however, point us to the root cause of the problem. None of the alternative nomenclature therefore is comprehensive. Remember that from a conventional endocrinologist's perspective, no adrenal *illness* exists as long as laboratory values of abnormal adrenal function have not been breached.

Modern medical science and research has now shown that our body's stress response is, for the most part, regulated by both our neurological and endocrine components working hand-in-hand. Looking from afar, AFS is a part of the body's overall continuum of neuroendocrine response to stress. Therefore, perhaps the most suitable name for this condition is *stress-induced neuroendocrine syndrome* (SINS). This name alerts us to the cause of the condition as being stress-induced. It also points to the neuroendocrine system's response to stress as the mechanism of the resulting pathophysiology. It validates this condition as one characteristic of a syndrome and not a specific disease. It allows the inclusion of adrenal related signs and symptoms, and does not exclude non-adrenal related symptoms as part of the overall clinical presentation.

For simplicity and practicality, we use the term *Adrenal Fatigue Syndrome* (AFS) as the overall name of this condition. This validates the physiological basis of the loss of energy and other symptoms commonly seen in this condition, but recognizes that we can't fully explain the cause and it may lie outside the adrenal glands. Furthermore, this terminology does not conflict with the only current definition of low adrenal output accepted by conventional medicine, *adrenal insufficiency*.

Addison's Disease and Adrenal Fatigue Syndrome

Addison's disease, also called *adrenal insufficiency* or *hypocortisolism,* is a rare, but recognized disease in which the adrenal hormonal output falls below a level that meets established clinical parameters. It affects about four out of 100,000 people and is diagnosed with blood testing. In this case, if blood tests results are abnormal we know the adrenal glands are structurally dysfunctional and the patient needs lifelong *steroid* replacement.

Addison's disease is often caused by an autoimmune dysfunction, whereas stress and a host of other factors are the primary culprits of Adrenal Fatigue Syndrome. The symptoms of Addison's disease include low energy, joint and abdominal pain, weight loss, diarrhea, fever, and electrolyte imbalances. Some Adrenal Fatigue Syndrome sufferers report these symptoms too, but they are usually much less intense.

Addison's disease therefore refers specifically to *primary adrenal insufficiency*, in which the adrenal glands themselves malfunction. *Secondary adrenal insufficiency*, which is not considered Addison's disease, occurs when the anterior pituitary gland does not produce enough adrenocorticotropic hormone (ACTH) to adequately stimulate the adrenal glands. Both lead to low cortisol output. Currently, conventional medicine recognizes only these two as legitimate diseases of low cortisol secretion. If, for example, you ask your doctor if your symptoms could point to Adrenal Fatigue Syndrome, you may learn that he or she has not heard of AFS or may deny its existence.

Do not confuse this with Cushing's syndrome or primary hypercortisolism, where the opposite occurs, with chronic over-secretion of cortisol. That is not our concern in this book.

More Clarification on AFS

Adrenal Fatigue Syndrome (AFS) consists of four broad and overlapping clinical stages, from mild to severe. We call Stage 3 of AFS, *Adrenal Exhaustion (or Neuroendocrine Exhaustion for those technically minded)*, in order to distinguish it from the less severe Stages 1 and 2. The most serious, Stage 4, we call *Adrenal Failure (or Neuroendocrine Failure)*.

> **AFS is confusing in large part because most people have gone into Stage 1 and even Stage 2, but never knew it.**

Like early stages of cancer, cardiovascular disease, or diabetes, early AFS is hardly noticeable. Besides, AFS can be brought on by almost any situation or life event. For example, a day or two of intense work or travel, jetlag, staying up late, a long hike in the mountains or an unusually hard workout, an argument at home or at the office, are all stressful events. As far as the body is concerned, any or all of them may have left you tired and worn out. You consciously experienced this unusual fatigue, a symptom of Stage 1, but you took the weekend off and relaxed, made your next workout lighter, or had a peaceful night's sleep and your body recovered fully.

If the stress lasted longer, or intensified, or perhaps another stressor was added, i.e., you caught a cold before your work load lightened, then on a short term basis you experienced additional symptoms. You may have reached Stage 2 AFS, but still, you recovered without knowing that your adrenals were affected.

As the body reaches Stage 3 AFS, symptoms are difficult to ignore, but they are usually attributed to some other condition. As you read and absorb knowledge about AFS, you'll understand why much of our discussion and advice relates to Stage 3, a critical crossroad in the health of any sufferer.

Adrenal Fatigue Syndrome and You

Many adults are puzzled when they first hear about adrenal fatigue (which from here on out we call Adrenal Fatigue Syndrome), because they generally have little knowledge of the adrenal glands and their function. They simply never considered that their adrenal glands could be linked to a cascade of symptoms, such as mild to extreme fatigue, lowered immunity, thyroid disease, low libido, menstrual disorders, metabolic disorders, mild to moderate depression, and so on. Yet, AFS is neither rare nor mysterious. Research suggests 11.9 percent of adult population in the United States suffer from severe fatigue, extreme tiredness, or exhaustion lasting more than one month. Many times more of the population suffer mild to moderate fatigue, with less debilitating symptoms. This number is growing exponentially as stress of living in the modern world takes its toll on our body.

> AFS is therefore one of the most prevalent health conditions, afflicting most adults at one time or another at varying degrees. It is a silent epidemic. Who hasn't experienced stressful events or even periods of prolonged stress? However, the situation is seldom seen as a serious threat to health and is therefore seldom identified.

Even when identified, many healthcare professionals believe that no recovery protocols exist and perhaps tell their patients to relax and manage their stress. Often, AFS is thought of as a condition of the mind only, and doctors prescribe antidepressants. AFS also is commonly tied to thyroid gland disease and many doctors order thyroid replacement drugs. Unfortunately, these treatments often leave the root causes unresolved. As a result, the condition worsens over time, sometimes for months but often over years and even decades. With the complex and often convoluted progression of AFS, which admittedly defies conventional medical logic, it's no wonder that AFS is so often the "victim" of misidentification.

When considering Adrenal Fatigue Syndrome, it's important to keep in mind the following principles:

- AFS exists on a continuum of severity, with individually defined stages and phases. The more advanced the stage, the more severe the condition. Stages 1 and 2 are considered mild, and Stages 3 and 4 are considered advanced and increasingly severe in terms of symptoms.

- Adrenal Fatigue Syndrome, particularly in Stage 3 (Adrenal Exhaustion), is related to many *recognized* diseases, such as hypothyroidism, polycystic ovary syndrome (PCOS), fibroids, hypoglycemia, depression, Lyme disease, irritable bowel syndrome (IBS), autoimmune diseases, and many other defined and regularly diagnosed and treated medical conditions.

- AFS, even in advanced stages, is often elusive. We can't rely on laboratory tests to provide a definitive diagnosis. The multiple symptoms are not in question, but they can be attributed to other conditions and not AFS. Structurally, the adrenal glands are intact as defined by conventional medicine.

- It's critical to understand that therapies that may benefit those with mild AFS may actually have the opposite effect on those with severe AFS and make their symptoms worse.

- AFS recovery needs to be individualized—a one-size-fits-all approach is ineffective and wastes time and money. It also leaves sufferers disappointed and confused, and often worse off.

- Recovery takes time, patience, and commitment on the sufferer's part.

The vague nature of AFS explanations can be attributed to the often slow onset of the condition. In addition, when sufferers learn their condition is stress related, they may feel relief on one hand, but panic on the other. Many people are afraid of stress and fear they will develop hypertension (high blood pressure) or heart disease if they don't get a handle on what's going on in their lives. Meanwhile, the unidentified AFS goes unattended and sufferers feel worse and worse. So, telling sufferers that they need to learn to relax and manage stress may be true to a certain degree, but that alone is incomplete. It can also intensify AFS if these individuals aren't also guided in other recovery tools.

Stressors that Can Lead to Adrenal Fatigue Syndrome

When we add the pressures we face at work to the pressures at home, it's no wonder that chronic stress is very common in western society. Of course, at any given time, we may need to tend to an ill loved one or mourn the death of a family member or friend. Problems and conflicts with spouses or children represent major causes of stress in modern life. Balance between work and home responsibilities has become a monumental task for many already stressed to the limit.

Illness itself is also a stressor, and millions of men and women cope with chronic conditions such as diabetes, arthritis, depression, and so forth. Adrenal Fatigue Syndrome occurs when the amount of physical or emotional stress overextends the body's capacity to compensate and recover. Because one of the main stress control centers of the body resides in the adrenal glands, these glands can become damaged and dysfunction when overtaxed during the stress response.

Stressors can be physical, chemical, emotional, or mental, as you can see from the list of common stressors below:

- Anger, depression, fear, or guilt

- Chronic fatigue, other illnesses, or infection

- Chronic pain

- Excessive exercise

- Gluten intolerance

- Low blood sugar

- Malabsorption and/or mal-digestion

- Over-exposure to toxins and heavy metals

- Severe or chronic stress, including toxic relationships

- Surgery

- Overwork and keeping late hours

- Sleep deprivation

- Excessive sugar consumption and/or excessive caffeine intake

- Chronically infected root canal or poor oral health

- Stealth viruses and chronic subclinical infections

Stressors come in many forms and intensity, and the body's response to stress is mediated largely by hormones. In the next chapter, we offer a primer on stress and the adrenal glands that will help you understand these hormones and other critical information presented in this book.

Key Points to Remember

- If you are under stress or constantly fatigued and your doctor cannot figure out what is wrong, consider Adrenal Fatigue Syndrome (AFS). AFS represents the body's neuroendocrine response to stress and threat.

- Adrenal Fatigue Syndrome is the overall name. There are 4 stages. Stages 1 and 2 are considered mild. Stages 3 and 4 are advanced. We call Stage 3 Adrenal Exhaustion. Stage 4 is most serious and is called Adrenal Failure.

- AFS is the most accurate scientific term to describe this condition. The cause of AFS is not fully known, but chronic stress plays a large part.

- Do not confuse AFS with Addison's disease, a medical condition requiring steroidal medication for treatment. AFS is not a disease. It is the subclinical non-Addison's form of adrenal dysfunction characterized by low cortisol output along with dysregulated neuroendocrine response often caused by stress and other factors.

- AFS is comprised of many seemingly unrelated symptoms: fatigue, lethargy, mild depression, reduced sex drive, insomnia, salt craving, heart palpitations, hypoglycemia, low blood pressure, constipation, low thyroid function, and difficulty in losing weight.

- Do not be surprised if your doctor is unfamiliar with AFS.

Chapter 2

Stress, Hormone Basics, and the "Forgotten" Adrenals

The very word *stress* can elicit fear. That's because most adults—and many young people too—talk about coping with the daily pressures or problems in their lives but do not understand the role of stress in either maintaining or deteriorating health. Stress can be physical, emotional, or both. We discuss stress and the body's response to it throughout this book. To start, it's enough to understand that we have multiple, built in stress management systems.

How Stress Enters the Body

Emotional stress enters the body through the brain via our senses. Once the emotion is perceived as stress and an unwelcomed threat, an area of the brain stem called the locus ceruleus (LC) is activated. This nucleus is also the origin of most norepinephrine pathways in the brain. Norepinephrine is the principal neurotransmitter involved in the way the central nervous system handles stress. It is part of a massive system of chemical communication between neurons (brain cells) and other cells in the body.

Norepinephrine belongs to a family of biological compounds called catecholamines, along with epinephrine (popularly known as adrenaline) and dopamine. Norepinephrine has many functions. In the brain, it influences the amygdala (a part of the brain that helps regulate mood and emotional response, such as fear and anxiety), leading to alertness and arousal. Once the locus ceruleus is activated, neurons carrying norepinephrine send signals to both sides of the brain along distinct pathways and to many locations within the neurotransmitter network. These locations include the cerebral cortex, hippocampus, limbic system, amygdala, hypothalamus, and the spinal cord. Large areas of the brain are affected. Without norepinephrine, the body would be helpless and totally unprepared.

The following diagram illustrates how our brain deals with stress from a neuroendocrine perspective:

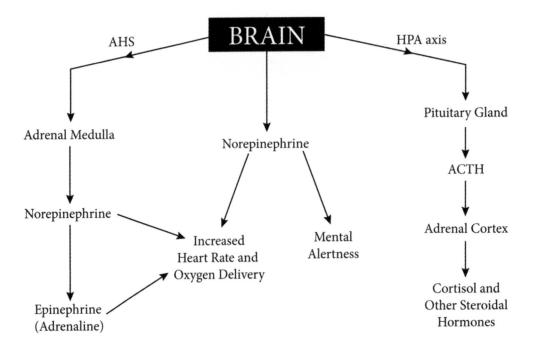

Figure 1. Neuroendocrine Basis of AFS

We can think of norepinephrine as an important "first responder" from the neurological system. It acts locally in the brain as a neurotransmitter of arousal, as well as peripherally as a hormone to handle minor stresses of daily living, such as standing up and moderate exercise. Our overall anti-stress preparation is thus activated by norepinephrine through its duo function.

In addition to putting the brain on alert, norepinephrine activates the hypothalamus. The hypothalamic-pituitary-adrenal (HPA) hormonal axis is called into action. Physiologists and endocrinologists use the term axis to describe the effect of various endocrine glands as if they were collectively grouped into a single entity. This term is appropriate because the glands involved often behave in cooperation. Various axes exist, such as the hypothalamic-pituitary-gonadal (HPG) axis, and hypothalamic-pituitary-adrenal (HPA) axis.

The HPA axis is a major part of the neuroendocrine system that controls reactions to stress and regulates many body processes, including digestion, the immune system, mood and emotions, sexuality, and energy storage and metabolism. We will have much more to say about this in Chapter 5, *Early Adrenal Fatigue Syndrome: Stages 1 and 2.*

Upon activation by norepinephrine from the LC, the hypothalamus releases corticotropin-releasing hormone (CRH), which is both a hormone and a neurotransmitter. CRH acts as a bridge between the body's neurological and endocrine system. Upon arrival to the pituitary gland, CRH triggers the release of adrenocorticotropic hormone (ACTH) that travels downstream and acts on the adrenal glands, the end organ of this axis. The adrenal glands produce an entire class of anti-stress hormones including cortisol. The neurological and endocrinological systems, therefore, work hand-in-hand to ensure we are able to handle the stressors of daily living. In addition, these two systems equip us to handle physical and emotional stress resulting from emergencies and illness, and then return us to balance and good health when the extra stress is over. Much of this is regulated through norepinephrine and the HPA axis as you can see from the diagram above and as you will learn more about in this book.

If stress becomes acute, severe, or chronic, a final stress response system, one of last resort, is activated. This provides the more powerful hormone, *epinephrine,* also called adrenaline, to the rescue. Epinephrine is produced in the adrenal medulla and released directly into the blood stream modulated by the adrenomedullary hormonal system (AHS) (discussed later in Chapter 9, *Stage 3C Disequilibrium*). Epinephrine increases heart rate, constricts blood vessels, dilates air passages, and is the main conductor of the fight-or-flight response. Being more potent than norepinephrine, the more intense the stress, the more likely epinephrine production will increase. Both norepinephrine and epinephrine, therefore, play critical roles in the body's anti-stress response, with norepinephrine called upon to do the day-to-day work, and epinephrine called upon as responder of last resort. (See Appendix D for a detailed scientific discussion on the neuroendocrine basis of AFS.) While the central stress control center rests with the brain, the field control anti-stress management system for the most part falls on the adrenal glands. Activation of this is via the HPA axis discussed above. To deal with stress, the adrenal glands make *steroids,* a class of anti-stress hormones of which cortisol is the most "famous." Problems in regulating steroid production are linked to many symptoms of AFS.

The Basics of Steroidal Hormones

The roles steroidal hormones play differ markedly in the various chemical factories of our bodies.

A steroid is a chemical substance with a specific and unique chemical structure (for the technically minded, four carbon ring structures attached to each other). Cortisol, DHEA, testosterone, progesterone, and estrogen are all steroid based hormones whose basic molecular structures are chemically similar to each other. In addition, these hormones are made in the adrenals using cholesterol as the raw material. Synthesized in sequence, when all the hormones are working well and performing their critical roles, they are like an orchestra that plays in harmony.

In addition, we need to understand that certain hormones also act as *pro-hormones*, such as *pregnenolone* and *DHEA*. They are placed at the top of the hormonal synthesis cascade. In addition to having their own weak hormonal properties, they also act as *precursors*, meaning they are necessary to produce other substances. In this case, the precursors allow the adrenals to make downstream hormones, such as testosterone and cortisol. As such, pro-hormones are gentler than the downstream hormones and are the least potent. On the other hand, cortisol is the most potent, with the greatest potential side effects.

The simplified diagram below shows the way the key adrenal hormones are made.

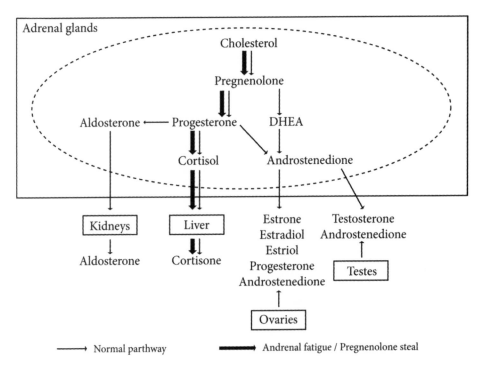

Figure 2. Steroid Hormone Synthesis Pathways

It may not seem obvious, but the above hormones are related to the progression, symptoms, and effects of Adrenal Fatigue Syndrome. In addition, you likely can see that these hormones are among the most common steroidal *hormone replacements*, which also have clinical implications in AFS. These hormones include: cortisol, pregnenolone, DHEA, testosterone, estrogen, and progesterone. We will discuss thyroid hormone function and the role of thyroid replacement in Chapter 8, *Stage 3B—Hormonal Axis Imbalances*. You also will come to see that we use these hormones in AFS recovery (Chapter 22, *Tools of Last Resort*).

The "Forgotten" Adrenals

Situated on top of each kidney, the two adrenal glands are small, about the size of walnuts. Their purpose is to help the body cope with and survive stress. Each adrenal gland has two compartments:

- The adrenal medulla secretes epinephrine which is responsible for the body's emergency fight or flight response.

- The outer adrenal cortex comprises 80 percent of the adrenal gland and is responsible for producing over fifty different types of hormones in three major classes: glucocorticoids, mineralocorticoids, and androgens.

Cortisol is the most important *glucocorticoid*, and when cortisol is low the body is unable to deal with stress, which is what happens with advanced AFS.

Aldosterone is an example of *mineralocortocoids*. Aldosterone modulates the delicate balance of minerals in the cell, especially sodium and potassium. Therefore, aldosterone plays a role in regulating blood pressure and the body's fluid balance. Stress increases the release of aldosterone, causing sodium retention, which in turns leads to water retention and elevated blood pressure. However, the situation is not always straightforward, and as AFS advances, blood pressure may be low.

The *adrenal cortex* also produces sex hormones, although in small amounts. One exception is DHEA, a weak androgenic hormone that both sexes produce in large amounts. DHEA, together with testosterone and estrogen, are made from pregnenolone.

These relationships are important because pregnenolone is needed to produce progesterone and is involved in making cortisol. Pregnenolone is one of the most important pro-hormones. In advanced AFS, we can see prolonged deficiencies in pregnenolone, which in turn lead to reduced overall production and levels of glucocorticosteroids, such as cortisol, and mineralocortocoids, such as aldosterone.

The Stress Hormone: Cortisol

Produced in the adrenal cortex, cortisol is the most important anti-stress hormone in the body. Too much cortisol leads to Cushing's syndrome, with symptoms like weight gain, stretch marks, extra hair growth, irregular menses, loss of muscle, depression, and insomnia. Too little cortisol leads to Addison's disease.

If the adrenals make insufficient cortisol, the pituitary gland automatically compensates by releasing ACTH, a hormone that travels to the adrenals and increases cortisol production. We can diagnose Addison's disease by observing low blood cortisol and high ACTH level. If the pituitary gland is not functioning properly, then both ACTH and cortisol levels may be low.

Cortisol protects the body from excessive stress in the following ways:

- *Cortisol normalizes blood sugar:* Cortisol provides the body with the energy needed to physically escape the threat of injury and survive. Cortisol works in tandem with insulin, which is released from the pancreas, to provide adequate glucose to the cells for energy, especially when the body is under stress. In AFS, more cortisol is secreted during the early stages, but in later stages (when the adrenal glands become exhausted) cortisol output is reduced.

- *Anti-inflammation Response:* Cortisol is a powerful anti-inflammatory agent. When we have a minor injury or muscle strain, the body initiates its inflammatory cascade which leads to the swelling and redness we see with a sprained ankle or an insect bite. Cortisol is secreted as part of this anti-inflammatory response, with the objective to remove and prevent swelling and redness in nearly all tissues. These anti-inflammatory responses prevent mosquito bites from getting bigger, counteract bronchial stress, and prevent the eyes from swelling shut due to allergies.

- *Immune System Suppression:* Those with *high* cortisol levels are weakened immunologically. Cortisol influences most cells that participate in the body's immune reaction, but especially white blood cells, natural killer cells, monocytes, macrophages, and mast cells.

- *Vasoconstriction:* Cortisol contracts midsize arteries. Those with low cortisol levels, a hallmark of advanced stages of Adrenal Fatigue Syndrome, experience low blood pressure, plus they have a blunted response to other agents within the body that constrict blood vessels.

Stress Tolerance Physiology

Individuals with Adrenal Fatigue Syndrome cannot tolerate stress, especially severe stress. As the stress level increases, the body needs progressively higher levels of cortisol. When the cortisol level cannot rise in response to stress, it is impossible to maintain the body in its optimum stress response condition. As mentioned earlier, cortisol production in the adrenal glands is controlled via the hypothalamic-pituitary-adrenal (HPA) axis. A feedback loop governs the amount of adrenal hormones secreted under normal circumstances in normal people. When more cortisol is needed, more CRH and ACTH are released. When ACTH binds to the walls of the adrenal gland cells, a chain reaction occurs within the cells leading to the release of cholesterol. This is then manufactured into pregnenolone, the first hormone in the adrenal cascade. After this, cortisol is released into the blood stream where it travels in the circulatory system to all parts of the body and back to the hypothalamus.

Cortisol production in the adrenal glands inhibits both the hypothalamus and pituitary gland, which reduces CRH secretion and thus ACTH secretion. This negative feedback loop ensures that the body is able to shut down anti-stress hormones once they are no longer needed.

On the other hand, norepinephrine is in a positive feedback loop with CRH. This ensures that the body is on full alert during stressful times and continually stays alert if stress remains. Fortunately, this loop is interrupted by cortisol signaling. Otherwise, once we are exposed to stress, we would be "wired" much of the time.

Maintaining the delicate balance between these various anti-stress hormones and feedback loops is an automatic process in healthy bodies. It goes on in the background 24/7 without our conscious awareness. It allows our body to face stress quickly and properly when needed, and to relax when stressors have dissipated.

In AFS, we see many symptoms that are the direct result of the body's anti-stress effort mediated through these systems. This is why it's so important that you have a basic understanding of the way these systems work

Cortisol Rhythm and Breakdown

Cortisol and ACTH are not secreted uniformly throughout the day. They follow a diurnal (daily) pattern: The highest level is secreted at around 8:00 AM, after which there is a gradual decline throughout the day. We can experience spikes in these hormones during the day, particularly when the body is stressed.

Cortisol levels are at their lowest between midnight and 4:00 AM, at which point it begins to rise, resulting in the peak of output in the morning when we wake up and start our day. The pattern is depicted in the graph below:

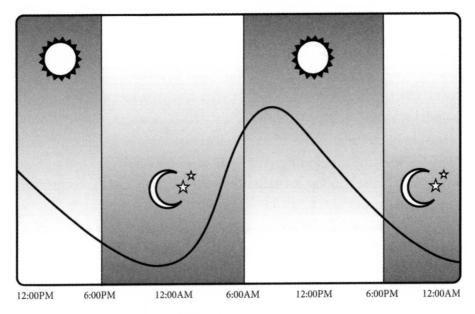

Figure 3. Circadian Release of Cortisol

In Stages 1 and 2 of Adrenal Fatigue Syndrome, morning cortisol levels remain characteristically high; however, the adrenals are put on overdrive to produce more cortisol to neutralize stress. As AFS progresses, cortisol output will eventually peak and then start to decline. Those in Stage 3 AFS often face a low cortisol level in the morning. After this, the body's cortisol output remains low for the rest of the day. In advanced phases of Stage 3, cortisol output tends to stay low throughout the day. We will have much more to say about this in a later chapter.

We also must consider how these adrenal hormones are broken down and metabolized because compromised breakdown and excessive metabolites can cause havoc within the body. To a great degree, steroidal hormones are broken down or metabolized by the liver. Generally we see that the more advanced the

Adrenal Fatigue Syndrome, the more compromised the liver function, although laboratory tests may be normal. The body's overall ability to clear metabolites, meaning the efficiency of the body to get rid of the byproducts, is an important consideration in addition to the absolute level of hormones. Proper balancing of hormones in a damaged body is therefore a complicated process.

The Body and Stress

In the language of stress, we might say we're "under stress"—a general term. When asked to elaborate, however, we very likely would name individual events or circumstances, such as going through a divorce or other family crisis, losing a job, taking care of an ill loved one, or too much pressure at work.

During the stress response, the body arms itself to face what it perceives of as danger. As described before, the brain secretes norepinephrine, and the adrenal medulla secretes epinephrine and norepinephrine. The HPA axis is called into action with CRH and ACTH release, resulting in increased cortisol output from the adrenal glands.

When a person experiences continued unresolved stress, the cortisol level may rise to such a high level that its production is compromised, ultimately being reduced as the adrenal glands become increasingly taxed. This is the cycle or process that leads to adrenal exhaustion. At the same time, DHEA production begins to decrease. Unlike cortisol, DHEA does not "rev up" production and hit a peak. Rather, chronic stress causes reduced production of DHEA. As a result, the ratio of cortisol to DHEA increases as can be seen in the diagram below:

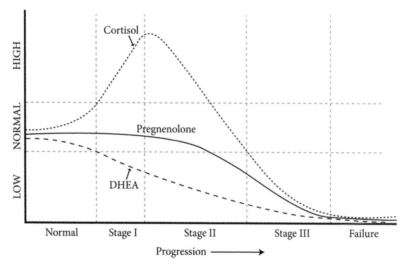

Figure 4. Production of Cortisol and DHEA at
Each Stage is Highly Variable

As with most endocrine systems, a negative feedback system exists in the body that is designed to limit the production of each hormone. This is true with cortisol as discussed earlier, with one exception. During prolonged or acute stress, when the body perceives that its survival is at stake, the excessive cortisol output can actually blunt the negative feedback response. In other words, cortisol is on the side of survival. Instead of the negative feedback system slowing down or shutting down cortisol production when the total cortisol is high, the body reacts in a positive feedback system, meaning the body senses the high cortisol level and allows more cortisol to be produced. The more advanced the AFS, the more prominent this phenomenon can be. This is the body's way of saying that it needs all the tools it can get to cope with ongoing stress and impending danger.

Pregnenolone: The Mother of All Steroidal Hormones

You now understand that pregnenolone is a pro-hormone. Made from cholesterol, it's called the mother of all steroid hormones because it sits on the top of the hormonal production cascade and is the precursor in the synthesis of female hormones such as estrogen and progesterone. It also is needed to produce other chemicals including mineralocortocoids, such as aldosterone; glucocorticoids, such as cortisol that suppress inflammation and help to reduce stress; and androgens (male hormones, such as testosterone). The cells of the adrenal glands, as well as the central nervous system, synthesize pregnenolone.

Researchers began experimenting with pregnenolone in the 1940s and soon realized it had the ability to alleviate stress and increase energy in those reporting fatigue. This information receded to the background as data about the newly discovered and more potent hormone, cortisol, stole the limelight. For example, when individuals with rheumatoid arthritis or other inflammatory conditions were given cortisol, patients reported significant short term improvements

During periods of stress, the output of adrenal steroids, such as cortisol, increases. This, in turn, puts greater demand on pregnenolone production. Over time, the increase in cortisol can lead to pregnenolone deficiency, with a cascading effect that can ultimately lead to reduced glucocorticosteroids and mineralocortocoids such as cortisol and aldosterone respectively. Pregnenolone levels usually remain high during early stages of AFS, but tend to be low as adrenal weakness progresses. This is due to a phenomenon known as *pregnenolone steal*. This means that pregnenolone levels drop because the body bypasses pregnenolone production in favor of producing more downstream hormones such as DHEA and cortisol. We see this similar type phenomenon with progesterone clinically, although research studies have not been conclusive.

Over time, numerous pregnenolone studies have shown that the hormone boosts energy, elevates mood, and improves memory and mental performance, along with creating a sense of well-being and improving the ability to tolerate stress. Overall, pregnenolone influences numerous body systems, from mental functioning to inflammation to sleep patterns, and many more.

Pregnenolone also has rejuvenating properties and we can consider it a complex tool in the AFS recovery toolkit. That said, as you will see later, using pregnenolone for Adrenal Fatigue Syndrome is a complex undertaking.

DHEA

DHEA (dehydroepiandrosterone), the biological daughter of pregnenolone, is a weak androgenic hormone made in large amounts in the adrenal glands of both sexes. DHEA is a precursor of testosterone, estrogen, and other corticosteroids. Although their actions are similar, DHEA is generally more potent than pregnenolone. Think of DHEA as a potent pregnenolone analogically.

> You may have noted that DHEA is found in some health food stores, is advertised to enhance energy, and is sometimes recommended in anti-aging efforts. Commercial supplements of 25-50 mgs of DHEA, along with 15-25 mg of pregnenolone, can improve well-being, energy levels, moods, and libido for normal healthy people, particularly women. Men are less hormonally sensitive and the results may not be as evident.
> Note: *We don't recommend that AFS sufferers self-navigate with DHEA, but it can be used judiciously in a professionally guided recovery program for Adrenal Fatigue Syndrome.*

Testosterone

Both men and women produce testosterone, but the amount produced by women is much smaller and the production comes from the adrenal glands. A decline in the testosterone level is associated with a decrease in sex drive and libido in both sexes, and we commonly see this condition is in those with Adrenal Fatigue Syndrome. Testosterone replacement therapy (TRT) reenergizes the entire body, increases lean muscle mass, and reverses the fat accumulation and muscular atrophy characteristic of aging in normal people. Unfortunately, aggressive use of testosterone in Adrenal Fatigue Syndrome can lead to over-stimulation and eventually to adrenal crashes.

Estrogen, Progesterone, and Estrogen Dominance

Estrogen and progesterone are the two main sex hormones in women, although both are produced in both men and women in different quantities. Estrogen and progesterone work in synchronization with each other. They oppose each other in their actions and work as checks and balances to achieve hormonal harmony in both sexes.

Estrogen is produced in the ovaries and also by adrenal and fat tissues. It's responsible for regulating the menstrual cycle and promotes cell division. During puberty, estrogen is largely responsible for the development of secondary female characteristics. During menopause, the amount of estrogen in the body declines but not as extremely as progesterone. Production, however, is augmented in the adrenals and in the fat cells.

Estrogen is actually a family of female-related hormones consisting of three primary components: E1 (estrone), E2 (estradial), and E3 (estriol). E1 is the most potent and is also known to be carcinogenic; E3 is the most gentle and known to have anti-cancer properties. When naturally in proportional balance, E3 is the highest and E1 is the lowest. Because estrogen is manufactured in the fat cells in addition to the ovaries and the adrenal glands, chances of having too much circulating estrogen increases in those who are overweight as well as those with Adrenal Fatigue Syndrome.

Progesterone, made from pregnenolone, is produced primarily in the ovaries just prior to ovulation and increases rapidly after ovulation. Progesterone is the precursor to estrogen, testosterone, and cortisol. The adrenal glands also produce progesterone in both sexes. During chronic stress, progesterone production may be reduced as the body favors cortisol production.

In women of reproductive age, progesterone levels are highest during ovulation (days 13 to 15 of the menstrual cycle). If fertilization does not take place, progesterone decreases and menstruation occurs. If fertilization occurs, progesterone is secreted during pregnancy by the placenta, acts to prevent spontaneous abortion, and promotes survival and development of the embryo and fetus. About 20-25 mg of progesterone is produced per day during a woman's monthly cycle. Up to 300-400 mg are produced daily during pregnancy. During menopause, the total amount of progesterone produced declines drastically as compared to the premenopausal level.

Progesterone acts primarily as an antagonist (in opposition) to estrogen in our body. We will have more say about this in Chapter 22, *Tools of Last Resort.*

Estrogen Dominance (*Progesterone Deficiency*)

Estrogen and progesterone work in synchrony to achieve harmony in the hormonal orchestra. In Adrenal Fatigue Syndrome, absolute deficiencies of estrogen and progesterone are not the primary issues; rather, the main culprit is the relative dominance of estrogen and relative deficiency of progesterone. When the amount of progesterone needed to balance estrogen is insufficient, a condition known as estrogen dominance develops.

The Problem with Estrogen Dominance

As you will see later, estrogen dominance has numerous adverse effects, from fibrocystic breast changes to disturbances in blood sugar to uterine fibroids. The many symptoms that come from a host of conditions take a toll on millions of women worldwide.

We discuss estrogen dominance in this book because it is closely related to Adrenal Fatigue Syndrome. The presence of estrogen dominance is one of the hallmarks of Adrenal Fatigue Syndrome Stage 3B (Chapter 8, *Stage 3B—Hormonal Axis Imbalances*). Aside from progesterone imbalance during stress, other dysfunctions can also trigger estrogen dominance. We can see this in thin women who are not particularly stressed, but still experience symptoms of estrogen dominance.

Stress Response from a Hormonal Perspective

As you have seen so far, we have multiple excellent stress defense mechanisms already in place, mediated by various hormonal systems. These systems are automatically activated when needed without our knowing, 24/7. From a hormonal perspective, when the body is exposed to stress we see a series of responses:

- The brain first perceives stress as a threat.

- Norepinephrine is the key signaling agent and one of the first responders called to action.

- The body is aroused and put on alert (from norepinephrine in the brain).

- Blood pressure and heart rate increase (from norepinephrine outside the central nervous system).

- The HPA axis is stimulated as central norepinephrine is released from the brain, leading to ACTH released from the pituitary gland.

- ACTH stimulates the adrenal cortex to secrete cortisol and others such as pregnenolone, DHEA, and aldosterone.

- Cortisol levels increase and convert more stored glycogen into blood sugar for energy.

- Energy is increased.

- The sympathetic nervous system is activated and helps us deal with stress concurrently. As a last resort, the adrenal medulla is also activated, putting out epinephrine as a fight-or-flight hormone.

- The heart rate increases (from the epinephrine and norepinephrine).

- Muscle tension increases (from the cortisol and catecholamines).

- The menstrual cycle may be affected (from estrogen and progesterone imbalance).

- Digestion slows down as blood is diverted away to more important tissues (from Autonomic Nervous System [ANS] modulation).

- Your bladder and rectum muscles may relax (from ANS modulation).

- Increased physical energy and mental alertness allow the person to overcome stress.

- When stress subsides, all systems return to baseline and normal function resumes.

This stress response system can reach its limit if stressors are not reduced over time, or if we fail to support the adrenals and the various stress response systems. When these systems are overworked or break down, Adrenal Fatigue Syndrome may ensue. We do not exaggerate when we warn that, indeed, stress can kill.

Looking Ahead

By now, we hope you can see why a full understanding of stress related hormonal systems are relevant and why an understanding of them is necessary to fully grasp AFS and its implications. Your knowledge will allow you to comprehend the advanced concepts we are about to present and will allow what appears to be a clinically convoluted picture of AFS to fall into place.

Key Points to Remember

- Stress enters the body through the brain, and the body activates its first responders. This is a built-in system designed to protect the body and promote survival. Norepinephrine is the key neurotransmitter and hormone involved in our stress response.

- The potent hormone epinephrine (adrenaline), secreted by the adrenal glands, is most responsible for the emergency fight-or-flight response. The adrenal glands also produce many hormones that help the anti-stress response, the most important of which is called cortisol.

- Cortisol levels rise and fall throughout the day and during stressful times. They eventually drop as AFS advances, and tend to be low throughout the day at advanced stages of AFS.

- Pregnenolone tends to be low as AFS progresses.

- Aldosterone, a hormone made in the adrenal glands, is responsible for regulating salt balance in the body and, thus, blood pressure.

- Estrogen and progesterone are opposing hormones, and both are made in the adrenal glands. Estrogen also is made in the ovaries and the fat cells. AFS tends to trigger a state of estrogen dominance or relative progesterone deficiency, which is responsible for a continuum of illnesses ranging from endometriosis, PMS, irregular menses, and fibroids. Estrogen dominance is implicated in breast cancer.

Chapter 3

Defining Our Terms

Throughout *Adrenal Fatigue Syndrome*, you will come upon certain terms and words that might or might not be familiar to you. Some terms come up in the text frequently, while others appear only once or twice. Rather than include a glossary at the end of the book, we decided to use this chapter to offer some easy, working definitions of commonly used terms. That way you can refresh your memory as they appear within the book. For example, throughout the text we refer to the components of the body's nervous system, and the definitions below will serve as a convenient reference. In other cases, we've defined terms we didn't define thoroughly when first seen in the text because they were used less often and we didn't want to stop the flow of information. Therefore, we added them to the list below. We also combined definitions of terms that logically fit together, rather than maintaining a strict glossary-style alphabetical order.

Acute/Chronic: When symptoms appear suddenly, we consider it an ***acute*** condition. For example, some common infections, such as colds, influenza, and pneumonia, come on quickly. The symptoms run their course and disappear as the body heals. Anaphylaxis shock is an acute allergic reaction to an allergen, and may be a life-threatening episode in an allergy considered to be ***chronic***, that is, an ongoing condition. Many conditions have both acute and chronic components.

Diabetes is a chronic condition with long term implications, but acute episodes of blood sugar/insulin dysregulation can bring on symptoms, such as fainting or severe weakness, serious enough to require emergency room visits. Rheumatoid arthritis and cardiovascular disease have both acute and chronic components. Avoiding acute episodes is one goal of managing chronic diseases.

Adaptogen: The ability to modulate and adjust to conditions as they change, whether or not these conditions are optimal. In the context of herbs, the term usually refers to the ability to bring the biochemical function back to normal, no matter if it is too high or too low.

Anabolic/Catabolic: Anabolic—The buildup phase of metabolism, in that our tissues are synthesized from the proteins and other substances we provide. *Catabolic*—The breakdown phase of metabolism, in which the body supplies energy from the materials we have provided.

Autoimmune disorders: Many conditions, from rheumatoid arthritis to lupus to common allergies, result from the body's complex immune system. This system normally reacts to and works toward eradicating substances it perceives as "invaders." An autoimmune response occurs when the normal response is interrupted or disturbed and the immune system reacts to the body's tissues as invaders.

Challenge: Specific tests or protocols designed to prove or disprove a hypothesis.

Clearance: A measure of kidney and liver function. This refers to clearing a unit of a specific compound from a specific volume of plasma. The lower the clearance, the more compromised the function.

Crash: An abrupt state of reduced energy output and severe fatigue as the body reverts back to a simplistic form of function to conserve existing energy.

Decompensation: In medicine, when a previously working organ system or structure deteriorates, we call this decompensation. It can occur because of illness, stress, or aging. *Compensating* means the organ still tries to function despite the stressors. As Adrenal Fatigue Syndrome advances, the adrenals and other organ systems eventually begin to decompensate, potentially bringing on many confusing symptoms and organ system disorders.

Dysfunction: Impairment of a physiological function.

Dysregulation: Impairment of a physiological regulatory mechanism.

Metabolism: The overall term for the physical and chemical processes by which we produce, maintain, or breakdown the body's material substances.

Metabolites: The byproducts or results of metabolism. In addition, a metabolite is a product of metabolism that is more or less toxic to the organism producing it.

The nervous system: The central nervous system (CNS)—The portion of the nervous system that consists of the brain and spinal cord. The CNS gathers, stores, and controls information and is involved in all bodily and psychological functions, from breathing and walking to experiencing sadness and joy. *The peripheral nervous system*—Consists of nerves and ganglia outside the CNS. It is divided into two parts: the somatic nervous system, which regulates musculoskeletal functions that help us deal with the outside world, and the *autonomic nervous system (ANS)*, which regulates functions of the smooth muscles and glands within the body as described below.

Autonomic nervous system (ANS): The component of the nervous system that regulates involuntary actions, meaning we don't consciously control them, including heart and glandular activity. Multiple branches exist, the key ones being the **sympathetic nervous system (SNS),** the **parasympathetic nervous system (PNS),** and the **adrenomedullary hormonal system (AHS).**

Recovery cycle: When pertaining to Adrenal Fatigue Syndrome, recovery is the period immediately following a crash. Individuals will likely experience many cycles as they recover.

Stress: Put simply, stress is an individual's response to physical challenges, exertion, and events that create internal emotional pressure. We sometimes refer to the external events or circumstances as stressors, but our reactions are the source of stress, not the event itself.

Subclinical: Some conditions stay below the threshold at which we can detect and measure clinical signs and symptoms. For example, diabetes, hypertension, and hypothyroidism often produce symptoms, but clinical tests often show results in the normal range. We refer to this as a subclinical state. However, if left unattended, the condition can eventually worsen and abnormalities can appear on tests, hence, providing *clinical* evidence of their presence.

Unfortunately, subclinical states often occur but are ignored because the conditions are allowed to advance untreated until testing "proves" that the symptoms are real. In Adrenal Fatigue Syndrome, current testing techniques may produce results that look like there is normal adrenal function all the way up to adrenal failure. Therefore, we don't recommend relying on lab results as the final answer in diagnosing complex medical conditions and, in particular, AFS.

We hope these definitions will help you get the most from this book. Now, we begin discussing other issues related to AFS, as well as the stages of Adrenal Fatigue Syndrome.

Chapter 4

Adrenal Fatigue Syndrome in a Complex World

Why is Adrenal Fatigue Syndrome a major health issue today? We need to look no further than our day-to-day lives. As touched on earlier, surviving well in our complex, modern world is a monumental task. We see the proof all around us.

Individuals are struggling with low energy and stamina—signs of premature aging. As clinicians, we see these signs showing up in individuals at increasingly younger ages. We also see large numbers of people who are hooked on coffee and have to start each day with a jolt of caffeine just to wake up. Some either skip breakfast or grab pastries or donuts on the fly, and then, because they are hungry by midmorning, they consume more of these sugary foods during coffee breaks.

During the last century and into this one, physical work (farming, manual factory labor, and so forth) has decreased as sedentary and/or automated labor has increased. When we combine the relative lack of physical activity with the unhealthy, simple carbohydrate foods we see in office vending machines, schools, and on menus at typical restaurants, it's not surprising that many men and women experience a high degree of sluggishness (food coma) following lunch and through the afternoon. Many typically follow this pattern through the evening with a heavy dinner and an oversized dessert and snacking until bedtime (and for many, fitful sleep follows). Meanwhile, combined with stress and poor health habits, family issues await attention, and spouses and kids might be irritable and tired. What a bleak picture.

It's not bad enough that we overeat well beyond the calories we need, with each generation consuming more food than the last, but so many of the calories are empty, meaning they have little to no nutritional value. Some among us tend to binge on sugar, or drink alcohol to excess, thus suffering oxidative stress. In addition, our bodies are continually exposed to environmental toxins, including potentially carcinogenic synthetic hormones and genetically modified foods whose consequences remain poorly understood.

If we take an honest look, we can see that we're literally eating and working ourselves down a path of premature death, expecting to be rescued by modern medicine. Rather than using today's complex medical knowledge and technology to our advantage, some of us have developed an unhealthy dependency on medical advances. We see too many individuals counting on medical technology and the next "miracle" surgery or drug to save them from destructive behaviors and perpetually bad habits that cause or contribute to most common health problems. Mounting evidence shows that our society has unknowingly embarked on a course of self-destruction.

Consider the story of the boiling frog. Toss a frog into a pot of boiling water and it instinctively jumps out to protect itself. Place the frog into a pot of cool water and heat the water up very gradually and what does the frog do? Instead of getting out, it acclimates to untenable circumstances—and slowly cooks. The frog doesn't notice what's happening to him until it's too late. How are we different?

The Rise of Complexity

Throughout human civilization, we can trace a trend toward higher levels of complexity and specialization. As our societies have evolved from simple to highly complex, our approach to problem-solving has also become more complex. Facing ever more demands, complexity, and uncertainty, our initial response is to push ourselves harder and more relentlessly, without taking account of the costs we're incurring. We march toward more complex endeavors in every area of human life. We build bigger and more complex dams, planes, stadiums, buildings, governments, and computers. Equally complex are the rules, regulations, and protocols that manage and govern organizations and workers. This complexity increases and requires an ever greater quantity of energy, information, and research to sustain.

Medical researchers, for example, once considered the body as a whole, insepara-ble unit, but current research now reduces the body into its component parts. We have learned how to connect each body part and make the connections work with medications or surgeries. Not too long ago, few would have imagined that certain kinds of body part replacements would become routine. Not only do we remove hips and knees, we transplant vital organs such as the heart, liver, and kidneys. Modern medicine truly is spectacular. A surgeon removes a gall bladder with three simple holes in the abdomen, and a robot, controlled some distance away, can perform cardiac surgery.

The rise of complexity in medical science, and our reliance on it, has created over-confidence in our belief that we can maintain the body like we maintain the machines we invent and control. Some express a false sense of complacency that medicine has triumphed over Mother Nature. Is that so? Do we really have an upper hand on Mother Nature? We must ask if we've actually solved problems at the root level. Or, do our complex maneuvers and patches simply suppress the symptoms at the surface, thus passing off our fixes as a cure for the many chronic diseases and painful conditions associated with wear and tear of the body.

Medicine in a Complex World

Taking the long view, modern western medicine of the last 200 years is a recent development. Human civilization, far older than modern medicine, carries cumulative medical wisdom passed from one generation to the next, often verbally. Some are valid protocols, some are only ritual. Just because we can't list scientific documentation that adheres to today's scientific research protocols, it doesn't render the centuries of accumulated wisdom useless. The accomplishments of modern medicine are astounding, but many follow it blindly and fail to ask important questions. It is imperfect and certainly doesn't have a monopoly on the global-collective medical know-how.

In reality, as modern medicine continues to advance, its clinicians and researchers create a complicated system of near mechanized protocols, specialties, and subspecialties. As we endeavor to dissect, isolate, and compartmentalize every malfunction into its smaller components, we create an ever larger pool of diagnoses. This in turn leads to additional investigative tests designed to validate and justify each diagnosis, resulting in further reliance on complex and often imperfect tests. Test results are not absolute, and their relevance depends on correct interpretation and correlation with clinical findings. This points to the importance of finding capable clinicians to manage the complexity.

We run the risk of overreliance on tests. For example, in addressing many chronic conditions, experienced clinicians can often come up with a detailed narrative history for a patient that yields more information than laboratory testing. Unfortunately, many patients and clinicians tend to put great faith in tests, even viewing them as infallible.

> Ironically, over-reliance on test results creates confusion because multiple tests sometimes produce conflicting information.

Over the last century, we've seen a great increase in life expectancy, an outcome worth the energy expended in medical research. A century ago, life expectancy was a mere forty-three years in the U.S. Today, we see our grandparents and parents living well into their late seventies, eighties, and beyond. Progress is not guaranteed to last, however. Looking forward, for the first time in the developed world, the current generation is at risk of having a shorter life expectancy than their parents. This trend is due to the *early and massive* onslaught of what used to be age-related diseases such as atherosclerosis and adult-onset diabetes. Much of this downward trend is known to be lifestyle related.

Pay Attention to Complexity

Sooner or later, we all must function within this complexity of life and face the warning signs that threaten the basic health of individuals, families, communities, and even countries. We've observed many adults who are driven to perform in careers and relationships in ways that may be well beyond the capabilities of their individual bodies. Being unaware of these limitations, either through lack of knowledge or by ignoring the warning signs, they may not take the time to listen to their bodies and learn to recognize the internal signals telling them they're approaching the maximum capacity to handle all they've taken on. To truly excel within our complex environment, it's imperative to study what the body needs and wants and not give all our attention to the desires of the conscious mind, let alone what society demands.

Maximum Complexity-Handling Threshold

Science has repeatedly demonstrated that when the body has exceeded its pre-defined capacity to handle any given emotional or physical load, the consequence is internal breakdown. This is common sense, but still we often ignore the warning signs. Intellectually we're aware of our mortality, but we behave as if we'll live forever. This is why we push ourselves to engage in high pressure relationships and jobs as if we've evolved into superhumans who don't need time for proper rest and recuperation.

Our biological ability to handle complexities of life varies. Some ability to handle complexity is needed for normal and ordinary daily function, such as going to work, shopping, and taking a bath. Our overall capacity to handle complexity and stress of life is limited by our body's unique threshold. Some of us can handle multiple complex tasks with ease, while others can't. The drive to achieve complexity starts with our mind and is executed by our body. Therefore, knowing oneself is the key to successfully tackling complexities of life without damaging the body. Those who don't pursue self-knowledge will pay a hefty price for this over time. Unfortunately, for many of us, accepting ourselves as we are is not a socially positive or admired experience. Society's pressure to perform may be too great and we succumb. Most with strong career paths end up sacrificing the body. It takes a backseat while we drive ourselves and ignore the internal signals telling us that the maximum threshold has been reached.

Adrenal Fatigue Syndrome: Ignoring Signs of Complexity for Too Long

At its core, Adrenal Fatigue Syndrome, especially in advanced stages, is a sign of accelerated decline after the body has reached the maximum threshold for handling the complexity of life as described here. In this situation, we see a dysregulation of the body's internal homeostasis. That is, we see imbalance in neurotransmitter and hormone production, regulation, and suboptimal organ function. In other words, we see dysregulation of the neuroendocrine system.

> The most prominent physical symptom of early AFS, fatigue, is a sign of reduced energy output. Simply put, at the cellular level the internal nutritional reserve is insufficient to be converted into energy that allows the body to perform its normal functions. It's as if the body's gasoline tank is nearly empty and the warning light is on.

In its wisdom, when the body is low on fuel it slows down all *non-essential* functions in order to preserve its remaining fuel. Adrenal Fatigue Syndrome, through its symptoms, shows us the slowing-down process. As AFS progresses beyond Stages 1 and 2, it warns of impending doom in the absence of corrective action.

People often ask what brings on AFS, and they may be surprised to learn that the condition can be triggered by something as simple as a common cold, over-exercising, or a minor car accident. The triggering incident could also be something profound, such as a surgical procedure or the death of a loved one. Under normal conditions, the body may experience AFS, but it recovers and we never knew that AFS was an issue.

Internally, however, the body has experienced pressure and stress for a long time, usually decades. These pressures could be a complex combination of weak constitution, poor dietary habits, troubled relationships, changes in financial status, a demanding career, and so forth, including those of psychological origin.

The final breakdown of the body can be fast and furious and can come as a surprise. Yet in retrospect, most Adrenal Fatigue Syndrome (in the later stages) sufferers eventually say if only they'd looked closely, they would have seen it coming for years.

A Tale of the Species: Survival and Marginal Return

To achieve optimum performance, the body needs to be adequately nourished every day. If we fail to provide proper nutrition, and perhaps supplementation, then each time we face stress we draw on our internal reserve at the cellular level. Over time, when the output is greater than the input, we deplete energy which is our most valued nutritional resource. If resources are not constantly replenished as we age, when a greater demand is placed on the body, this leads to fatigue, then exhaustion, and finally, failure.

Common sense would tell us to choose carefully the pursuits in which we expend energy, much like doing a cost-benefit analysis. For example, animal predators are smarter than humans in that they know not to engage in a quest whose energy expenditure is high but offers only a marginal return. They instinctively know to preserve their nutritional store, the precursor to energy, and instead follow the principle of cost versus return. They stay in environments where food is plentiful, and when unable to do so, they conserve in other ways. For example, during winter, polar bears (and others species) simplify their lives by hibernating, thereby restricting energy output. Pursuing a path of declining marginal return leads to weakening, which ultimately leads to extinction.

We humans tend to do the opposite: We try to solve problems by *increasing* the complexity in our quest towards higher productivity. At first, this works, but eventually this kind of scheme backfires. As schoolchildren we learned that if farmers plant the same crops in the same soil year after year, vital minerals are depleted. Some farmers try to increase production in the short term by adding fertilizers to the soil, or they take the long view and rotate crops to replenish the soil. As for domestic animals, we now use medications and hormones to enhance rapid maturation, rather than allowing animals to roam and exercise. When those methods fail to speed up production, we turn to genetically modified corn, sugar, and even fish as alternatives for feed. All this adds up to declining marginal returns.

Those with intense Type A personalities, the aggressive go-getters among us, are particularly vulnerable to trading off a long term survival strategy for success (by society's standards of success). In these individuals, we might see marginal and subclinical obsessive-compulsive behavior, often regarded as a positive attribute for success and a model to emulate. After all, doesn't society want us to solve the big problems of the world, work harder, make more money, build bigger houses, and drive bigger cars, and on and on?

Aggressively pursuing success, however defined, is ingrained in childhood, and many forget that the body has a gentler side that also needs nurturing. Certain people tend to be at higher risk of ignoring the gentler side, including those considered the most successful and brilliant. We've observed that brilliance and complexity can lead to a lack of wisdom. Therefore, when not accompanied by practical wisdom, brilliance can be devastating.

The most capable are particularly at risk, because without realizing it they tend to take on more than they can physically and emotionally handle. Brilliant lawyers, corporate executives, teachers, secretaries, writers, athletes, and physicians are all vulnerable. No occupation is spared.

The brilliant and capable often expend too much energy for too long in their pursuit of endeavors with low marginal return. For example, many men and women pay a hefty price for successful careers. They might fight with competitors over trivial details or succumb to greed. They might drink too much alcohol, sugary drinks, or coffee, failing to see how these habits undermine long term survival and marginalize their return on investment. In other words, these brilliant, capable people do not heed the simplest warning signs that their habits are not in line with how nature intended life to be.

Resource Depletion and the Adrenals

The later stages of Adrenal Fatigue Syndrome serve as a major warning that survival is in jeopardy. During times of perceived danger, AFS is perhaps the body's most appropriate neuroendocrine response. In situations of declining margin return, AFS is the only way the body knows how to take back control of itself rather than allowing the conscious mind to continue destroying it. The worst is yet to come for those who ignore this yellow flashing light, showing us once again that the body really does know best.

As explained earlier, the adrenal glands are primary conductors within this orchestrated collapse because they function as the body's stress control center. However, they are by no means the only player, and no organ system is spared. In Chapter 1, we provided a list of common symptoms which, as you likely noted, are numerous and convoluted, and as a result seem to defy conventional medical logic.

The clinical picture also can be clouded by a wide range of possible or concurrent clinical conditions, including heavy metal toxicity, infection, fibromyalgia, chronic fatigue syndrome (CFS), and long standing hormonal imbalance. Laboratory tests often offer little help and clinical correlation is imperfect. These are a few reasons that AFS is so difficult to comprehend.

A Symphony, Not a Solo

We cannot fully understand AFS until we first appreciate that the body works as one unit, not as a group of independent parts acting as competing soloists in the orchestra. A part-by-part approach which grew out of the complexity of modern medicine, led to specialties and numerous sub-specialties. However, the body cannot be compartmentalized. As a total unit it is subject to resource depletion, similar to that of a country that overspends and eventually faces a treasury drained of capital reserve. The fall of the Roman Empire is one such example.

The body has a nutrient store inside each cell. We derive energy, the body's currency, from this nutrient reserve, which is why it's vitally important to keep the nutrient reservoir full. When nutritional stores are deficient, the body is unable to pursue new endeavors requiring additional energy expenditure. This deficiency affects all organ systems, not just one. Although one organ may be more severely affected than others, few organs are ever spared completely.

If the body has undergone depletion of its nutrient stores for years or decades, it's unlikely that the body can mount an effective defense against stress, such as an infection or an emotionally charged event. When the body goes into Adrenal Fatigue Syndrome, the internal structures that provide support services to ensure homeostasis start to lose their capability. In advanced stages of AFS, the body crashes as fatigue becomes overwhelming, and many other disturbing clinical symptoms can steadily worsen over time. These include hypoglycemia, low blood pressure, fluid and electrolyte imbalance, anxiety, insomnia, and irregular heart rate.

This crash is the body's cry to replenish our reserves at the cellular level, because it has been automatically reduced to the lowest physiologically sustainable levels. The more advanced the Adrenal Fatigue Syndrome, the lower the level of functioning. In advanced stages, as the body moves closer to Adrenal Failure, some individuals remain bedridden for days, others require ambulatory help just to perform normal daily activities. The body's natural recovery efforts dictate that all nonessential functions, such as reproduction or exercise, temporarily shut down. Metabolism slows to reduce energy expenditure, which in turn forces the individual to decrease activity, thereby conserving energy.

The Hidden Gift

No one welcomes Adrenal Fatigue Syndrome, but it's not a fatal condition unless we do nothing to address it. Indeed, it can be a precious gift in the form of a wakeup call that sends the signal that the body has reached its maximum capacity for complexity in life, and the law of diminishing returns applies. In other words, as the amount of energy needed goes up, the productivity gained per unit of expended energy diminishes.

How do these facts about depleted energy apply to daily life? In short, we no longer accomplish as much from the same energy expended. A trip to the supermarket can be exhausting. We might manage at the office, but have no energy for family and friends, let alone hobbies and exercise. We may comment that we just don't have the energy we used to. It's not the imagination working overtime; we have, in fact, depleted our energy reserve.

> **No individual can escape the general limits of his or her internal nutritional resources. This physical law cannot be violated without significant damage and, ultimately, death. Yet this is what many of us try to do—literally defy the physical laws that sustain life.**

AFS can be misleading because we can look normal on the outside and still be nutritionally depleted and hormonally dysregulated inside. Some have a misconception about what nutritional deficiencies look like. We see TV images of undernourished and malnourished populations that are dangerously thin, and then we erroneously conclude that this is the picture of depletion. However, we need to correct that misconception.

Malnourishment is a pathological clinical disease state, but because backup internal reserves are at play, nutritional deficiencies have been present well before one reaches a malnourished state. The absence of outward signs of recognized disease is not the same as having optimal nutritional reserves. The body goes through a long period of transition from good health to becoming ill, a process that can last for years and sometimes decades. This is usually the case for Adrenal Fatigue Syndrome, hormonal imbalances, cancer, and heart disease.

Once ill, efforts to initiate a planned, logical recovery program, along with enhancing longevity and preventing further disease, must start with replenishing internal nutritional resources on the cellular level, while concurrently reducing energy expenditure. The key rests in understanding that each of us handles complexity differently. Ultimately, our capacity is determined by a combination of our constitution, age, body makeup, emotional well-being, and nutritional reserve.

Before we move on to more detailed discussions of Adrenal Fatigue Syndrome, keep in mind the information contained in this chapter. Use it to evaluate your life and your health. The take home lesson is simple:

> *Once Adrenal Fatigue Syndrome arrives on our doorstep, whatever energy we expend to continue our current quest and our dreams will cost us dearly in terms of our health. No longer can we expend the energy required without incurring internal damage.*

Finally, we need to address some preconceived ideas you may bring to this book. We understand that misconceptions about AFS abound. Although many of these issues come up throughout the book, we can dispel a few myths right now.

Myths and Common Misconceptions about Adrenal Fatigue Syndrome

We've come up with the list below after listening to sufferers talk about what they had heard about AFS, along with what they believe caused their symptoms. You might encounter terms and conditions that are unfamiliar to you, but rest assured we explain them as they become relevant throughout the book.

- **Adrenal Fatigue Syndrome is a psychological condition.** In AFS, we see a condition in which stress causes the activation, overstimulation, and subsequent breakdown of the neuroendocrine system as AFS progresses. This continuum manifests itself in a wide variety of symptoms. The stressors can be physical, emotional, or mental, and resulting symptoms have both physical and psychological components which are biochemically mediated through hormones and neurotransmitters starting from the brain. For this reason, recovery incorporates a mind-body approach which ultimately allows sufferers to concurrently heal emotional issues and rebuild body chemistry.

- **Adrenal Fatigue Syndrome occurs only in those with high stress jobs and hectic lifestyles.** Stress is a trigger for AFS, as is a lifestyle with no provision for rest. Stress affects people differently and affects those in both low and high stress jobs and of varying income and educational levels. No one is totally immune.

- **Adrenal Fatigue Syndrome comes on slowly over a period measured in years.** AFS usually takes decades to surface, except if a person is constitutionally weak or experiences an acutely stressful event. Emotional traumas and toxic relationships occurring in rapid succession can trigger Adrenal Fatigue Syndrome. Whether one goes into AFS as a result of an illness, accident, divorce, overwork, or other stressors depends very much on one's intrinsic ability to handle stress, which is a function of individual constitution.

- **Those with Adrenal Fatigue Syndrome have no energy and cannot work at all.** On the contrary, most adults with Adrenal Fatigue Syndrome hold fulltime jobs and lead active lives. They may struggle to keep up appearances in their work and social lives, and take off the mask of well-being only at home. Those in Stages 1 and 2 often compensate with a sugar fix, rest, or coffee. Those in Stage 3 feel physically drained, but many continue to hold down jobs, though with difficulty. Only those in late Stages 3 and 4 are incapacitated.

- **Adrenal Fatigue Syndrome occurs mainly in men.** This is a pervasive myth, yet women comprise the vast majority of Adrenal Fatigue Syndrome sufferers. Today, many women hold down the equivalent of three jobs— their paid jobs/careers, their work in their homes, and motherhood. The hormonal system is particularly stressed by this kind of overload.

- **Adrenal Fatigue Syndrome can be determined by imaging tests (i.e. CT scans) or blood tests.** *X-rays and even our most sophisticated imaging technology cannot diagnose Adrenal Fatigue Syndrome.* Patients who describe AFS symptoms to their doctors are generally told they need routine blood tests, but no blood tests sensitive enough to definitively diagnose AFS currently exist. Saliva tests are not foolproof and can be misleading as well. The best way to determine if you have Adrenal Fatigue Syndrome is through a detailed history by a health professional trained and experienced in this area.

- **Fatigue is due to low thyroid function and has nothing to do with the adrenals.** Hypothyroidism and Adrenal Fatigue Syndrome can have similar symptoms. They are easily confused because symptoms of one condition often mimic the other. Simply increasing thyroid medication may make fatigue worse and mask the root cause—Adrenal Fatigue Syndrome. This situation is very common. If you are on thyroid medication and not improving, AFS should be considered.

- **Steroid drugs are fast and effective treatments for Adrenal Fatigue Syndrome.** While the use of steroids (such as hydrocortisone) can be useful under proper circumstances, we see many drawbacks using powerful hormones for Adrenal Fatigue Syndrome, which include their many well known side effects. Many people recover from AFS without steroids by using appropriate and gentle nutrients that nurture the body and allow it to heal itself.

- **If left to nature, most people recover from Adrenal Fatigue Syndrome.** This applies to those in Stage 1 or early Stage 2, but not to advanced stages when sufferers often become worse when they are left on their own to self navigate. Few seek help until the adrenals are quite damaged and weak, and they are then often led down a treatment path that is incorrect. The body heals itself significantly better when the correct and proper natural tools are used. Unless stressors are removed and adrenals supported, the natural progression of AFS is one of gradual deterioration.

- **Natural nutrients are always beneficial.** Unfortunately, the right nutrients for one person can be toxic for another. This occurs frequently in the more advanced stages of Adrenal Fatigue Syndrome. In fact, failing to recover from AFS can often be attributed to misuse of certain nutrients.

- **Taking herbs and glandulars for Adrenal Fatigue Syndrome over long periods of time can't hurt, because, after all, these are natural products.** Certain herbs and glandulars can be beneficial for adrenal function during early stages of AFS, but they can backfire and make the condition worse over time if a knowledgeable healthcare professional does not modulate and adjust the amounts taken. Those who are in advanced stages are particularly vulnerable.

- **Eliminating carbohydrates will help Adrenal Fatigue Syndrome.** While refined carbohydrates tend to affect the metabolism and often contribute to worsening Adrenal Fatigue Syndrome, you need some carbohydrates to maintain a normal blood sugar balance. To restore adrenal health, it's important to follow a customized diet guided by an experienced professional.

- **Fasting and detoxification will help Adrenal Fatigue Syndrome.** Accumulation of toxins in the body can trigger or worsen AFS. However, self guided fasting and detoxification programs can backfire, not only because the body is already drained of energy, but because these programs can potentially release more toxins into the body, which is already unable to efficiently excrete and clear them. A gentle program that completely rebuilds and nourishes the body is better, especially in advanced stages. As adrenal function returns, toxin elimination will proceed on its own.

- **Vigorous exercise is good for Adrenal Fatigue Syndrome.** For those in Stages 1 and 2, when the body's reserve is still ample, vigorous exercise helps increase energy and may be beneficial. However, excessive exercise can trigger adrenal crashes, so the intensity of exercise is a complicating factor. Those in Stage 3 AFS should be careful to avoid vigorous exercise because it can drain the body of valuable energy reserves and make matters worse. Those in late Stage 3 onwards should reduce exercise to a minimum during the initial healing phases and follow a customized program described later in this book. However, Adrenal Breathing Exercises (See Chapter 27, *Adrenal Fatigue Syndrome and Healing Exercise*) can benefit those in all stages of Adrenal Fatigue Syndrome.

- **Only rest is needed to recover from Adrenal Fatigue Syndrome.** In early AFS, rest is a good way to help restore some adrenal function. However, rest is seldom enough to bring about complete healing for those with advanced Adrenal Fatigue Syndrome (Stages 3 or 4), who have multiple organ dysfunctions and nutrient depletion. In these stages, rest alone often cannot lead to full recovery without the help of personalized nutrition, lifestyle, and diet protocols.

- **Adrenal Fatigue Syndrome only affects one generation at a time.** Unfortunately, burned-out parents usually give birth to children who are nutritionally and constitutionally weaker and thus prone to Adrenal Fatigue Syndrome. We now often see Adrenal Fatigue Syndrome in multiple generations in a family, and pairs of mothers and daughters with AFS are particularly common. Young people who are high achievers, perfectionists, athletes, and those with toxic family relationships are more prone to developing Adrenal Fatigue Syndrome, even in their teen years.

Finally, when we first talk with sufferers, many of whom have sought help from numerous physicians, we often hear hopelessness: *I'm afraid I'll never recover; I've have tried everything and nothing works.* Please believe us when we say that this simply isn't true. Many women and men achieve full recovery *if they receive proper help.*

Key Points to Remember

- We live in a complex and stressful world which is getting more complex as society advances. Most of us have to balance between our spouse, children, parents, work, health, and spiritual and social lives.

- Our body has the built-in ability to help us cope with stress. When this stress capability is overwhelmed, the body enters a state of dysregulation, with imbalances and impaired hormone production, resulting in suboptimal organ function.

- Fatigue is the most prominent symptom of the body's decompensation. Energy is the universal currency of the body. A low energy state is the body's way of forcing us to slow down and rest to survive.

- Continued exposure to stress when we cannot withstand it forces us to live in an environment of declining marginal return. More energy is expended by the body in order to stay at the same state. This is not an efficient use of energy and leads to resource depletion; AFS advances as resource depletion progresses.

- AFS can be Mother Nature's gift to alert us of danger within.

- Myths and misconceptions about AFS abound because of lack of formal research.

Facts: Adrenal weakness has been around for over a century. It has a strong physiological component as well as a psychological component in advanced stages. It can come on slowly or quickly. Most sufferers are working women. AFS cannot be diagnosed by conventional testing, and conventionally trained physicians are universally undereducated in this area. Rest can help AFS recovery, but it is seldom sufficient if AFS is in advanced stages. Natural compounds are beneficial only if used properly.

Chapter 5

Early Adrenal Fatigue Syndrome: Stages 1 and 2

Without question, Adrenal Fatigue Syndrome, with its myriad manifestations, is both confusing and perplexing, a situation made worse by the lack of consistency in the way we refer to the condition. As we've said, for our purposes in this book we use Adrenal Fatigue Syndrome as the overall name. Stages 3 and 4 refer to advanced AFS, and we call Stage 3 and its phases, Adrenal Exhaustion. Stage 4 is referred to as Adrenal Failure. *To avoid confusion, except for providing the basic definitions, we use the term Adrenal Exhaustion only when referring to Stage 3.*

Bear in mind that the stages and phases of AFS overlap greatly. The boundaries are indistinct. They are presented here to help us clinically get a feel for the broad perspective as it is very easy to be overwhelmed and miss the big picture. These definitions should not be used as tools for diagnosis.

Stage 1: Alarm Reaction

In this stage, which can last days, months, years, and even decades, the body periodically is alarmed by stressors and mounts an aggressive anti-stress response to reduce stress levels. (The stressors could be physical or psychological, or, typically, a combination of stressors that trigger the alarm reaction.) Common examples include events of daily life we often take for granted as normal, such as change of career, physical relocation, excessive exercise, and skipping meals on a regular basis. Some physicians refer to this as the "early fatigue" stage. In this state, brain norepinephrine output is increased, leading to a state of arousal and alertness. We use this alertness to keep us awake when it is time to go to sleep. We also see increased ACTH (a hormone produced by the anterior lobe of the pituitary gland), which stimulates the adrenal cortex into making more cortisol, DHEA, pregnenolone, and aldosterone, among others. These hormones' collective physiological actions result in a second wind to keep us going physically and emotionally when it is time to rest.

Individuals do not report symptoms at this stage, and their daily activities are unaffected, although they may note feeling tired. In order to maintain or boost their energy level, many rely on coffee or other caffeinated drinks to start their day. They may find they need increasing amounts of caffeine to feel revved up for the day. Unfortunately, the social acceptance of addiction to coffee gives us the excuse to carry a coffee cup around in the office. Some even consider this type of external stimulant normal. In fact, not to be part of the coffee culture can be considered unsociable.

Stage 1 is a common occurrence. Because the body's stress response is effective and no damage is perceived, no attention is paid to the fine detail of how the body is already drawing on its nutritional reserves at this stage. Almost all adults at one point or another have multiple such experiences. Many already have their first experience in their teenage years on retrospect. As long as the stress lessens and the normal rhythm of daily life returns, most people in this stage recover with extra rest. Most individuals pass in and out of Stage 1 without realizing they have experienced even a brief episode of adrenal fatigue. Routine blood laboratory tests are normal. Saliva cortisol testing is generally normal as well, but the morning cortisol usually starts trending up as Stage 1 progresses. In the absence of any outward symptoms other than occasional fatigue, this lack of energy is compensated by the socially acceptable use of stimuli to boost energy. Unfortunately, based on the premise that stimulating energy with coffee and sweets is harmless, for the most part, our society has inadvertently condoned this approach. In reality, suppressing symptoms only worsens the progression of those with Stage 1 AFS over time.

Stage 2: Resistance Response

Greater exposure to life stress, or psychological vulnerability to stress, increases cortisol demand. The neuroendocrine response is to put the HPA axis on overdrive to increase output of cortisol and other anti-stress hormones. Socioeconomic and psychosocial handicaps are probably central inducers of hyperactivity of the HPA axis. Alcohol, smoking, and traits of psychiatric disease may also be involved. The HPA axis starts to be overtaxed but at this stage is not yet dysfunctional.

Cortisol is the primary anti-stress hormone systemically. Its release from the adrenal glands helps to provide for and regulate our fuel requirement during stress. At the same time, it helps reduce inflammation and calm the nerves during highly stressful events. It serves as both an acceleration and braking mechanism at the same time via different pathways, ensuring our ability to successfully deal with stress and yet have normal physiological functioning. This is a temporary fix, however. One cannot drive a car successfully without damage over time if one foot is applied on the gas pedal, and the other one is applied on the brakes at the same time, though in varying degrees.

Cortisol and Metabolic Dysregulation

A consistently high cortisol level in the body has many unintended consequences. Studies have shown that rising cortisol is associated with overeating, a common finding in those with Stage 2 AFS. Cortisol stimulates the appetite and provokes cravings for sugar. It may explain why some people tend to eat more when they feel stress, especially craving sweets such as chocolate, which can lead to weight gain. Cortisol directly influences food intake by binding to receptors in the brain, thus regulating other chemicals released during stress.

Studies have shown that premenopausal women who secrete more cortisol during stress also choose to consume more foods high in sugar and fat. The craving for donuts and other sugary food and drinks in times of stress could be an indication of a body in Stage 2 AFS. Let us be clear that not all people under stress overeat, and some people experience loss of appetite instead. We still don't fully understand the precise mechanism of this, and many factors are likely involved.

Chronically high cortisol (but not high enough to warrant a diagnosis of Cushing's disease) has negative consequences. While cortisol has been shown to promote overeating, it also blunts the normal rise in the metabolic rate that occurs after a meal. When accompanied with excessive caloric intake, stress induced obesity is a risk. This kind of obesity is particularly harmful because the fat tends to accumulate centrally around the abdomen. Some call this "sick fat" or "toxic fat." This is also called adiposopathy and results in pathophysiologic endocrine and immune responses that promote metabolic disease. This process affects men and women differently. Studies have shown that lean women who are vulnerable to the effects of stress are more likely to have abdominal fat as well as a higher level of cortisol in their body. Lean women with abdominal fat tend to have exaggerated responses to cortisol, more negative moods, and higher levels of life stress. In other words, in lean women central fat may indicate an underlying sensitivity to stress and greater vulnerability to AFS.

Central Obesity

When you eat more than you need, calories not burned must be diverted. Adipose (fat) tissue is specialized tissue that functions as the major storage site for fats. When you consume more daily calories than you burn off, especially a diet high in carbohydrates, you usually end up with excess triglycerides, free fatty acid, and body fat. An abnormally high triglyceride level in a healthy person may sometimes be considered an early warning sign and an indirect surrogate marker of high cortisol in a setting of stress and AFS.

When deposited in the liver, fat can lead to fatty liver and cysts. This may take years to develop. It comes as no surprise that high cortisol promotes fatty liver. Those afflicted with Cushing's syndrome, a condition where the cortisol output is constantly raised, usually have high blood sugar and frequently develop fatty liver. Fatty liver increases the risk of metabolic diseases.

In addition, cortisol regulates the overall energy of the body by selecting and delivering the right type and amount of fuel needed to meet physiological demands during times of stress. This is accomplished by tapping into the body's fat stores and moving fat from one location to another, or when needed, delivering it to hungry tissues such as working muscle.

In the peripheral tissue, cortisol concentrations are controlled by a specific enzyme called 11-beta-steroid dehydrogenase, located in the adipose tissues, which converts cortisol to inactive cortisone. Cortisol has much greater glucocorticoid activity than cortisone; thus, cortisone can be considered an inactive metabolite of cortisol. However, this enzyme can catalyze the reverse reaction as well. Therefore, cortisone is also the inactive precursor molecule of the active hormone cortisol. Human visceral fat cells, such as those surrounding the abdomen, have more of these enzymes as compared to subcutaneous (under the skin) fat cells. In addition, deep abdominal fat has greater blood flow and four times more cortisol receptors compared to subcutaneous fat. This may also increase cortisol's fat accumulating and fat cell size enlarging effect. Together, they may increase the risk of central obesity. Along with a host of other factors including insulin resistance, they contribute to the "muffin top" look that many carry around with them in their abdominal area. These individuals generally have a high waist-to-hip ratio, which identifies visceral obesity.

Central obesity is the hallmark of, and a required finding for, diagnosis of metabolic syndrome. This syndrome is an epidemic afflicting many adults in developed countries. Metabolic syndrome is a powerful predictor for disease. The combination of fatty liver, obesity, diabetes, and hypertension is the forerunning and primary cause of life threatening vascular events such as myocardial infarction and stroke. It is clear that disturbances in cortisol and HPA axis function are involved in central or abdominal obesity. Cushing's syndrome and subclinical Cushing's disease (both of which are characterized by elevated cortisol output) are associated with increased waist/hip ratio, risk of insulin resistance, high amounts of fats in the blood (hyperlipidemia), and cardiovascular disease risk.

Cholesterol is a fat and a key raw material that your adrenal glands need to make steroidal hormones such as cortisol. Cholesterol levels that are too high, however, can increase your chance of getting heart disease, stroke, and other problems. A rising cortisol associated with this stage can produce similar signs of dysregulated lipid profile in the blood (dyslipidemia), though they are often quite marginal and thus passed over as non-AFS related.

Cortisol and Dyslipidemia

Using salivary cortisol measurements throughout the day, studies have shown that stress-related elevated cortisol secretion is often associated with dyslipidemia, as demonstrated by an abnormal blood lipid panel on a routine screening test.

Dyslipidemia is a risk factor for cardiovascular disease. Historically, this usually happens to those in their midlife years. However, we are seeing an alarming rise in the rate of secondary (acquired and not familial) dyslipidemia starting with many in their mid-twenties. Much of the blame of this abnormal lipid picture is placed on improper diet, alcohol, and lack of exercise, but stress as a root cause is often missed. Even if fatigue is absent, those with clinical signs of secondary dyslipidemia should be on alert for AFS, especially if there is a history of stress.

What is confusing is that for reasons we don't yet know, not everyone with Stage 2 AFS has abnormal fat levels in the blood. In addition, not everyone with dyslipidemia has AFS. Clearly there is a complex neuroendocrine background to metabolic syndrome, where the mechanisms regulating the HPA axis play a central role. While clinical symptoms of gross HPA axis dysfunction will only surface later in Stage 3, early onset of an abnormal laboratory lipid profile may serve as an advance marker of internal metabolic dysregulation. Typically, the total cholesterol is normal or high, with normal or high LDL (bad cholesterol), normal or low normal HDL (good cholesterol), and high normal or high triglyceride level. Such a dyslipidemia, especially if accompanied by high or rising triglycerides over time in an otherwise normal and healthy person, may be a warning sign that one may already be in early AFS and not know it. Many are placed on lipid lowering medications rather routinely and often prematurely. Others are placed on vigorous exercise and low-fat diets. Stress as a possible root cause is often under-investigated and not taken seriously.

Blood Pressure and Exercise in Stage 2

Blood pressure tends to be normal or borderline high at this stage. As this stage advances, aldosterone and central norepinephrine output rises. Aldosterone increases lead to sodium retention and thus increased fluid volume. The more fluid in the body, the higher the blood pressure if all else is equal. Separately, a systemic norepinephrine increase raises the blood pressure and heart rate. The bias is toward a higher than normal blood pressure. Because most are still in good health and relatively young at this stage, their vascular wall-support structure tends to be quite pliable. The automatic vascular relaxation response triggered by baroreceptors that are activated when blood volume and pressure rises, results in a compensatory reduction and, thus, normalization of blood pressure. Those who are older or unable to compensate may suffer from high blood pressure as a result. We will have much more to say about this in Chapter 7, *Stage 3A—Early System Dysfunction.*

While mild fatigue may be experienced from time to time under prolonged stress in this stage, a normal and active life continues. Exercise capacity is unrestricted. In fact, many report a sense of alertness and well-being after moderate aerobic exercise. During aerobic exercise, the body is manually put on alert as far as the neuroendocrine system is concerned. Norepinephrine and epinephrine output increase to help increase blood circulation and enhance oxygen delivery to the muscles and brain for optimum performance. Some are misled into thinking that such an approach is correct, and thus the more the better. They embark on an excessive exercise program almost as an addiction to combat fatigue brought on by stress.

Moderate exercise accompanied by proper rest and nutritional support is conducive to the overall healing process and recovery from Stage 2 AFS. Excessive aerobic exercise not accompanied by proper rest slowly drains the body of internal reserves, and can accelerate the decompensation over time.

> **Excessive exercise can be destructive, and many experience their first major adrenal crash after what appears to be a normal workout at the gym.**

If the crash was severe, then even after rest and recovery they do not feel quite the same as before. Some fail to fully recover from that point on and quickly slide into advanced stages of AFS. Others are able to recover slowly, but unless exercise is reduced quickly and proper nutritional healing and rest instituted consistently, the likelihood of repeat crashing is high. We see that high-performance athletes are particularly vulnerable. They often crash and succumb after a heavy training session, as well as after a competitive event.

Cellular Damage

As you can see from the diagram below, cortisol output reaches its peak in this stage. After that, cortisol output starts to decline back to a normal level as Stage 2 progresses. ACTH remains high throughout. This process can play out over years if not decades. When measured through saliva testing, the morning, noon, or afternoon cortisol levels may be high, early on, in this stage, and tend to return to normal or low normal after peaking as this stage advances. Nighttime cortisol level is usually normal throughout, though for reasons not well understood, we do see high nighttime cortisol in some individuals. Figure 4. below shows how highly variable cortisol and DHEA production is as a function of Stage.

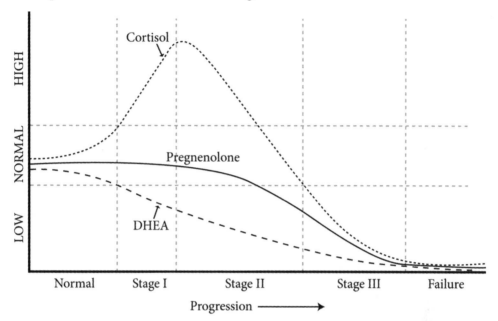

Figure 4. Production of Cortisol and DHEA at Each Stage is Highly Variable (Note: Figure 4 is also seen on page 25)

What makes this stage so dangerous is that much of the damage is subclinical and usually goes totally unnoticed. On the outside, one looks perfectly fine, but internal cellular damage is well under way.

Stage 2 often starts in the twenties or thirties and usually lasts for years into decades. Since, like Stage 1, it often goes undetected, it most often is evident only in retrospect. Intermittent fatigue, borderline or abnormal lipid panels, normal to borderline high blood pressure symptoms, and weight gain suggestive of reduced metabolism are treated as separate isolated problems, often with medications. The AFS picture is usually missed, especially early on. Most in this stage continue with their normal and active life on this track, thinking that all is well. Without considering AFS, they may be continually and unknowingly driving themselves into a path of slow destruction as cellular damage advances.

The Slow Death

Many in lifelong Stage 2 are unaware of the internal dysfunction caused by stress, but as aging sets in, borderline signs and symptoms may become more prevalent. By midlife, many are physically showing gross signs of central obesity with a "muffin top" belly or "spare tire" in the abdominal area, accompanied by lack of vitality and tolerance for exercise, hyperlipidemia (high cholesterol), dysglycemia (abnormal glucose level), mild but worsening food sensitivities, mild insomnia, and inability to lose weight despite strenuous exercise.

It is not uncommon to be taking a basket of prescription medications including those for persistent high blood pressure, the majority of which are classified as essential, another term for "unknown cause" in the medical world. Lipid lowering medications also are usually part of the regimen in order to normalize their dyslipidemia (generally high total cholesterol, with high LDL and low HDL), along with some type of sleep medication and possible sugar regulating medications.

Mislead by the normalization of blood pressure, blood sugar, and lipid profiles brought on by medications and confirmed by laboratory tests, many continue to live in the fast lane with its unrelenting stress. Ignoring Mother Nature's warnings, they are content to have been rescued by modern medicine with what appear to be harmless prescription drugs. After all, their blood pressure and blood sugar are normal, and their cholesterol numbers are now under control. Little do they know that, over time, such a symptom-patching approach often leaves the body vulnerable to other potentially more serious dysfunctions.

Remember that dyslipidemia, high blood pressure, and sugar imbalances are all symptoms of internal dysregulation, though they are now labeled as diseases and treated as such. Many factors combine to lead to these symptoms. Stress is one often overlooked factor. The wakeup call often comes only after a massive heart attack or a paralyzing stroke, both of which can be permanently disabling or even fatal. Unfortunately, it is often too late to completely reverse AFS and recover after such physically catastrophic events.

It is important to remember that the absence of fatigue as the predominant symptom in Stage 2 does not mean that the body is not under stress. The body's well equipped neuroendocrine compensatory response is simply working extra hard and has successfully overcome stressors. This results in a relatively normal state of energy flow. Therefore, most at this stage are mislead into thinking that all is well.

Having a healthy adrenal system is critical for overall well-being at any age. Whether it is to prevent onset of AFS, help the body fight infections, support recovery from surgery, or reduce fatigue, those who are on alert for signs of early stages of AFS and take appropriate remedial action are practicing good preventive medicine.

Sadly, most people are ignorant of this stage. They, along with those who are constitutionally weak or low in nutritional reserve, have an increased chance of progressing to the advanced stages, which we shall cover beginning in the next chapter.

Key Points to Remember

- There are four stages of Adrenal Fatigue Syndrome, from mild to serious.

- Stage 1 is called the Alarm Reaction. Fatigue is very mild and transient. The body has ample adrenal reserve. Physiologically, cortisol output increases. Full recovery comes with a good night's rest. Few are alert enough to know when this stage occurs and it becomes evident only in retrospect.

- Stage 2 is called Resistance Response. Fatigue becomes more bothersome and requires more rest than one night. A few days of vacation is often needed. Sugar fixes and an increased dependency on caffeinated drinks increases in order to overcome fatigue. Cortisol output peaks as demand continues from unrelenting stress. Clinical signs are few. We should always consider stress as a silent contributing factor to hypertension, dyslipidemia, and central obesity. Many stay in Stage 2 AFS throughout their adult life, unaware of internal damage.

Chapter 6

Advanced Adrenal Fatigue Syndrome: An Overview

Stages 3 and 4 are considered advanced stages of AFS, and for good reason. This is the major turning point where things can go bad quickly because the adrenal glands are exhausted. Those who have been only experiencing intermittent fatigue when stressed, characteristics of earlier stages, now start to face the uphill challenge of keeping up with their daily energy demand. Progressive increases in fatigue now mark their life. No longer are their daily activities unrestricted. For those who were healthy before, clinical symptoms start to surface and likely will get worse with time.

> **If not reversed, the ultimate fate awaits—adrenal failure.**

Stage 3: Adrenal Exhaustion

Recall in Stage 2 that unrelenting stress increases cortisol output from the adrenal glands. After peaking, the cortisol level starts to drop. Despite rising ACTH production from the pituitary gland and ongoing HPA axis stimulation, the adrenals are no longer able to keep up with the body's increased demand for cortisol production. Moderate to severe persistent fatigue is the norm as the body enters Stage 3, Adrenal Exhaustion. This stage is also called Neuroendocrine Exhaustion as the neuroendocrine system is now on full throttle, with eventual breakdown as this stage progresses. This stage may develop over a period of years as well, which is why lifestyle issues are so important in analyzing and discussing AFS.

As this stage progresses, total cortisol output drops below normal, and DHEA falls far below average. A twenty-four hour saliva cortisol test is likely to show a cortisol curve that has a tendency to flatten as AFS advances. In addition to the morning cortisol level being low, the nighttime cortisol level is usually reduced as well. The body's nervous and endocrine systems progressively become more dysregulated as this stage advances. The HPA axis becomes dysfunctional and eventually burns out. The emergency compensatory stress response system, mediated by the autonomic nervous system (ANS), starts to be put on overdrive. Most symptoms of advanced AFS, such as hypoglycemia, low blood pressure, and anxiety, start showing up here. Eventually, even the ANS system becomes dysfunctional, leading to Stage 4.

Stage 4: Adrenal Failure

Eventually, the adrenals and the neuroendocrine system become totally worn out and are defeated in their attempt to overcome stress. They surrender. This stage is also called Neuroendocrine Failure. When Adrenal Fatigue Syndrome has advanced to this stage, the line between AFS and subclinical and clinical Addison's disease, also called adrenal insufficiency, can be blurry. We may see the emergence of typical symptoms of Addison's disease: extreme fatigue, weight loss, muscle weakness, loss of appetite, nausea, vomiting, hypoglycemia, headache, sweating, irregular menstrual cycles, depression, orthostatic hypotension, dehydration, and electrolyte imbalances. The body appears to have lost its normal homeostasis and is breaking down. Intensive conventional multi-disciplinary medical attention is needed to achieve stabilization well beyond what can be done naturally. Hospitalization may be required. This stage will not be our concern in Adrenal Fatigue Syndrome.

For purposes of prevention and overall health trends, the information about Stages 1 and 2 is useful and important. However, most have slipped into Stage 3 by the time they see their doctors. Therefore, recovery concerns are foremost at this stage and, as you will see, other organ systems become involved.

A Closer Look at Stage 3 and the Speed of Functional Decline

So far, we've described the stages of AFS in general terms. However, in terms of recovery, we will keep our focus on Stage 3, Adrenal Exhaustion, and its phases. We do so because those in Stages 1 and 2 usually recover on their own and seldom seek professional help.

Stage 3 is important because most people begin to realize that something is wrong, and that they aren't snapping back to their normal energy levels. In addition, other symptoms, seemingly unrelated, might surface and persist.

As a general overview, we can understand how AFS progresses by reviewing the stages and phases, and match them with the following chart, *The Speed of Functional Decline.* As you can see, the vertical line shows fatigue levels, the horizontal line marks Stages 1 to 4, and in the case of Stage 3, Phases 3A to 3D. You will also see a horizontal line, the Adrenal Symptoms Threshold (AST). Symptoms of AFS start to be clinically visible when this threshold is penetrated on the downside. The curved line, then, traces the progress of symptoms and stages downward from asymptomatic to below the AST. The lowest line represents the level at which the adrenals are no longer able to produce sufficient hormones for basic normal function, though there is enough for survival.

This diagram shows the way in which Adrenal Fatigue Syndrome usually progresses through the stages over time, based on our experience. We caution, though, that the diagram is not meant to help you self-diagnose AFS, which is not a disease. However, it helps to paint a broad picture of the clinical presentation based on a typical history. We see tremendous variation in each person's progression.

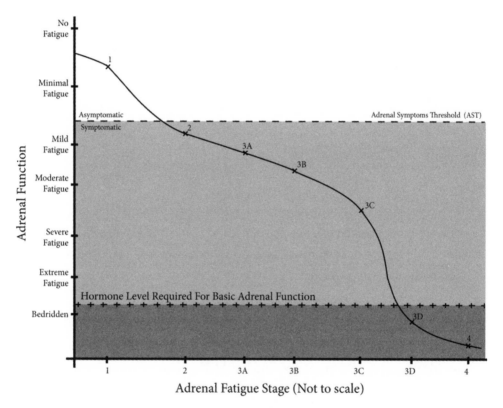

Figure 5. Adrenal Functional Decline as a Function of Stage

You can see from the chart that by Stage 3A, early exhaustion, the sufferer has noticeable mild to moderate fatigue that is nearly constant and stays below the AST. This may occur because of prolonged stress or the individual has ignored the warning signs of Stage 2.

Unresolved stressors are the main triggers from Stage 2 into 3A. By the time Stage 3A hits, rest helps, but the fatigue doesn't go away totally, even after rest. Generally, without effective intervention, things get worse over time and eventually get to Stage 3B where fatigue is constant. You can see from the graph that the curve is like a ski slope from 3B to 3C, which means we see increased velocity of the symptoms. At this stage, AFS is progressing quickly.

The journey from 3C to 3D is steeper and more like a cliff than a gentle ski slope. It takes the individual below the line at which the hormone level drops below what is needed for basic normal adrenal function. This is the point, between 3C and 3D, at which AFS is severe enough to render sufferers bedridden most of the time.

> **To be clear, falling below this adrenal threshold doesn't mean that the person can't sustain life, but it does mean that the other hormones are not easily primed. The body can still survive, but is in slowdown mode to conserve energy. That's why 3D is called near failure.**

The General Anatomy of Stage 3

Using fatigue as an indicator within Stage 3:

- In Stage 3A, mild fatigue is constant, and the person could have low thyroid, or a woman could experience premenstrual syndrome (PMS). Rest usually doesn't bring about total recovery, but individuals in this stage function at about 75-100 percent of normal capacity.

- In Stage 3B, mild to moderate fatigue is constant and these individuals do not get 100 percent recovery with rest. In terms of daily activities, they function at about 50-75 percent capacity. Symptoms of thyroid problems, estrogen dominance, and low libido often occur concurrently. Exercise becomes problematic.

- In 3C, the capacity to carry out normal activities is severely curtailed, down to 25-50 percent. These individuals might have to work part time, or often they are unable to work, or they try to work from home.

- In 3D, most are unable to work and are incapacitated.

Our clinical experience shows that in the early stages of AFS, those with mild to moderate fatigue often feel recovered after a nap of thirty minutes or so, but by Stage 3A it takes an hour-long nap to feel fine again. By 3B they need a nap of thirty minutes to two hours, but by 3C they need one to four hours to be fine. By the time sufferers reach late 3C or 3D, they need six to twelve hours of rest or more. Clearly, considerably more rest is needed between Stages 3C and 3D. It should be noted that these nap times are *above and beyond regular sleep time*. This is particularly important for those in advanced stages of AFS because their sleep cycle is usually disrupted and sleep quality goes down.

At 3D many sufferers are essentially bedridden. Those with symptoms of Stage 3D are in an extremely sensitive state, often feeling worse if they take supplements, for example. In addition, they often are in a catabolic state, which means the body's protein is breaking down and these individuals are losing weight. Digestion is usually breaking down, too, and these people may become constipated or unable to tolerate regular food well.

The Contrast and the Progress of Stage 3

As you can see, Stage 3D starkly contrasts with Stage 1. For sure, many people mask fatigue with coffee and sugar, but they don't see a problem doing so and consider treating fatigue this way as normal. When people notice themselves using stimulants like caffeine and sugar more and more, they may begin to sense that something is wrong. For example, their symptoms may slip below the AST and into Stage 2. Perhaps they see what is happening as a lifestyle issue, which then prompts them to take supplements, exercise, and make dietary changes they assume are beneficial (that may or may not be). In essence, Stage 2 is a little more symptomatic than Stage 1.

The steep decline that occurs in Stage 3 produces many symptoms that often confuse patients. As we've said, in 3A, sufferers experience fatigue and perhaps PMS or low thyroid function, but they don't feel too bad, all in all. They may miss identifying this stage totally if they are not alert.

Early in Stage 3A, symptoms characteristic of Stages 1 and 2, although mild and inconsistent, now become noticeable, and, in fact, chronic. Most see their doctor for the first time during this phase. This phase signals the onset of internal systems malfunction.

If the condition worsens, multiple endocrine axis imbalances tend to occur, which signals 3B. In women, we commonly see 3B manifested as *ovarian-adrenal-thyroid (OAT) axis imbalance*; in men, it manifests as adrenal-thyroid axis (AT) imbalance (see Chapter 8, *Stage 3B—Hormonal Axis Imbalances*). OAT axis disturbance can signal symptoms consistent with estrogen dominance, such as irregular menses, fibrocystic breast, low libido, possible uterine fibroids, and endometriosis. Those already taking thyroid replacement medications may need increased dosages to achieve the same result. Both men and women report low libido and increased fatigue.

As AFS progresses through these phases in Stage 3, other changes occur. For example, slightly elevated blood pressure, common in Stage 2, might change and become low throughout the day as Stage 3 progresses; mild musculoskeletal pain could turn into chronic myalgia of unknown origin; frequent recurrent infections are the norm (as compared to intermittent infections); feeling blue becomes mild depression, and disrupted sleep patterns become chronic insomnia; and fatigue that occurs at the end of a *stressful* day becomes an everyday event. Individuals may note a subtle, moderate change in their ability to carry out normal daily activities.

Not all organs are dysfunctional to the same degree and at the same time. The organ system that is constitutionally weakest is the first one to decompensate, while other organ systems appear to be intact.

For example, a person may complain of severe insomnia, but is otherwise feeling okay, relatively speaking. Usually, these sufferers continue activities and follow self-guided programs or regimens under the care of health professionals.

As Stages 3A and 3B gather steam, the body continues its downward path to greater impaired function, gradually becoming severely compromised in its attempt to maintain the fine controls of homeostasis. Normal equilibrium is lost, and the body enters a state of *disequilibrium* (Stage 3C). Mild to moderate fatigue characterizes the early phases; moderate to severe fatigue becomes the norm in Stage 3C and beyond. The body has lost its internal balance. Emergency systems are being activated as the alarm bell sounds.

Your body will try its hardest to maintain equilibrium with the activation of the *autonomic nervous system* (ANS) as a reactive compensatory mechanism. The ANS is an adaptive system, largely working outside the range of consciousness, to adapt to changing internal and external conditions.

By late Stage 3C, the ANS may itself be dysfunction due to overwork. Along with previous hormonal axes imbalances and receptor site dysregulation, the body is left with impaired metabolic, clearance, and detoxification pathways. This damage often gives rise to paradoxical, unpredictable, and exaggerated reactions and outcomes. For example, a person might have reactive blood sugar imbalances, that is, a quick rise in blood sugar after a meal, followed by a precipitous drop. Blood pressure might become fragile and unstable. It might drop suddenly when going from a supine to a sitting position (postural hypotension) along with a rapid increase in the heart rate, a phenomenon resembling subclinical POTS (postural orthostatic tachycardia syndrome).

Symptoms indicative of advanced Adrenal Exhaustion include heart palpitations, dizziness, sudden onset of anxiety, a feeling of being wired-and-tired, internal dysbiosis (imbalance in intestinal flora), acid-based imbalances, and adrenaline rushes. We may also see fluid and electrolyte imbalance, such as insufficient sodium (salt) in fluids outside the cells (hyponatremia).

> **The boundaries of each phase are decidedly *indistinct* and do not represent an absolute sequential gradation process. Most of those suffering from Adrenal Exhaustion usually report concurrent signs and symptoms in varying degrees of each of the earlier phases. That is the norm. The more advanced the exhaustion, however, the more we see late phase manifestations.**

If left unattended and as AFS advances, the body's key hormones, such as cortisol and aldosterone, might fall close or below the minimum required reserve for normal function and output. When this occurs, the body may down-regulate the amount of hormones needed in order to preserve what is on hand for only the most essential body functions. Extreme fatigue is common. We characterize this near failure state as Stage 3D. The body goes into full surrender as it gives up trying and simply does what it can to reduce energy-out to stay alive. In other words, the body is now in survival mode.

Dealing with Stage 4

When it comes to Stage 4, without aggressive conventional medical management, the body can continue to deteriorate and may ultimately collapse; we are talking about a situation in which the adrenals have become totally exhausted. The body's neuroendocrine response mechanism gives up and surrenders. The symptoms are extreme. Addison's disease now becomes part of the differential diagnosis. Patients suffer severe symptoms, including, of course, extreme fatigue. The body is in a catabolic state and most at this stage lose weight. Many are unable to eat regularly and become weaker. Medical attention is mandatory, and, unless there is intervention, the body can continue to deteriorate, leading to collapse.

The Big Picture

Taking a step back and looking at the big picture, we hope you can see that Adrenal Fatigue Syndrome is nature's systematic and logical neuroendocrine response in an orchestrated collapse when the body's complexity handling ability has been overwhelmed. AFS progression tends to be confusing for most because many organ systems are involved concurrently. The body, in its infinite wisdom, is in full control of the level of neuroendocrine stress response it sees fit to activate. Symptoms appear to defy conventional medical logic, not because they are illogical, but because we fail to look at them from a neuroendocrine perspective where the stress response is primarily regulated.

> **We need to look at the body as a whole unit. The more one focuses on each symptom, the easier it is to miss the big picture.**

It is important to take a step back. The big picture will emerge and will clearly point to a breakdown in bodily functions as the body struggles for survival.

We can see the progress of Adrenal Fatigue Syndrome most clearly when we look at the phases that appear in Stage 3, which we discuss in the chapters that follow.

Key Points to Remember

- Stage 3 is called Adrenal Exhaustion. The adrenals are no longer able to keep up with the body's demand for cortisol and start to fall below normal.

- Stage 3 is further divided into 4 phases, A through D.

- Stage 3A is called Early System Dysfunction. Fatigue characteristic of Stages 1 and 2 worsens. One sees early onset of a variety of medical conditions such as mild forms of insomnia, back pain, low blood pressure, hypoglycemia, anxiety, depression, and recurrent infection.

- Stage 3B is called Hormonal Axis Imbalances. The ovarian-adrenal-thyroid (OAT) axis in women and adrenal-thyroid (AT) axis in men are involved.

- Stage 3C is called Disequilibrium. The entire body is on full alert, and the autonomic nervous system is on full throttle as emergency measures are activated as the body tries to compensate on its own. Crude reserve systems are activated and a strong mind-body connection is evident. Symptoms such as depression, panic attacks, and dizziness may occur. The deepest decline in function and the greatest fatigue occurs from Stages 3C to 3D.

- Stage 3D is called Near Failure. The adrenal reserves are near depletion. Basic normal adrenal function is in jeopardy as the amount of hormones needed to prime other hormones becomes dangerously low. The body starts surrendering.

Stage 4 is called Adrenal Failure. The adrenals are totally exhausted and the body enters an emergency mode of operation for survival. Medical intervention is needed.

Chapter 7

Stage 3A—Early System Dysfunction

As you have seen from the overview of Adrenal Fatigue Syndrome, many experience symptoms that seem unrelated, confusing, and even mysterious. For this reason, it is easy even for health professionals to miss the big picture, which is why many patients sense that their physicians don't view the symptoms as seriously as merited. These issues begin to magnify in Stage 3, which is why we're taking a closer look at this stage and its phases.

In this stage, one or more of the body systems has weakened to such a point that a pathological subclinical or clinical state of the affected system surfaces. The organ system that is constitutionally the weakest or most sensitive usually is the first to exhibit the most prominent weakness. Some of the more common symptoms include hypoglycemia, low blood pressure, brain fog, and recurrent infections. These symptoms represent the onset of underlying system dysfunction or dysregulation, in particular the hypothalamic-pituitary-adrenal (HPA) axis we discussed in Chapter 2, *Stress, Hormone Basics and the "Forgotten" Adrenals*.

Some of the commonly affected systems are worth examining in detail.

Metabolic System Dysfunction

Metabolic system dysfunction is considered a pre-diabetic state and shows itself as glucose intolerance, insulin resistance, hypoglycemia, central obesity, low HDL (the good cholesterol), and high triglycerides. Any or all of these signs and symptoms may already be present in the earlier stages of AFS. In fact, many individuals have already been taking prescription drugs for lipid abnormalities (such as high LDL and low HDL) for some time by the time they reach this phase. These signs and symptoms also may meet the criteria of metabolic syndrome discussed in Chapter 1, *The Adrenal Fatigue Syndrome*. If not present before, they start to become more prominent in Stage 3A as the adrenal cortisol level starts to drop below normal and other hormonal imbalances become more obvious.

If left unattended, these warning signs of metabolic syndrome can lead to diabetes and accelerated arthrosclerosis. The most important and common clinical and early warning sign of this impending danger in the presence of Adrenal Fatigue Syndrome is subclinical hypoglycemia, where there are signs of low blood sugar but the laboratory fasting sugar level is normal.

In a healthy body, blood sugar is maintained within a narrow range to ensure smooth functioning. We experience this as even energy throughout the day. This maintenance occurs quietly in the background without our knowledge. When Adrenal Fatigue Syndrome is present, this automatic mechanism can be dysfunctional. In other words, the body's effort to return to normal blood sugar is not well regulated. It can be overly reactive, slowed, delayed, or crude in its response. All these are possible. The clinical picture can be confusing and at times quite vague.

The onset of hypoglycemia can be acute or chronic. It can be precipitated by what appears to be something harmless. Consider the following history from Betty, a thirty-three year old corporate executive under constant stress:

I was very healthy and ran almost every day up until six months ago. I skipped breakfast for three straight days with late lunches because I was too busy and was sometimes without food sixteen hours at a stretch. By the third day, I felt weak, with dizziness, nausea, and diarrhea. I did not faint, but it was close.

Despite returning immediately to a regular eating schedule, my symptoms did not go away. In fact, they got worse. I have never been the same since.

I have seen six specialists, all without helping me. All my medical workups are normal. I now have to eat every few hours to avoid hypoglycemia. I have also started to develop sensitivity to many foods, including rice, pasta, chicken, beef, and certain types of fruits. Now my diet is severely restricted. I even have to bring my own food to restaurants.

Let's look at the physiology behind Betty's problem.

Hypoglycemia and Adrenal Fatigue Syndrome

In Adrenal Fatigue Syndrome, the body's need for a continuous supply of energy throughout the day is much greater than normal. This demand is usually met with food consumption, which we then convert to sugar. If this demand is not met adequately, as often happens with Adrenal Fatigue Syndrome, the body turns to existing resources of protein and fat in the body to use in order to keep up with the energy demand. This internal energy synthesis pathway is put on overdrive.

Key hormones regulating blood sugar in the body include insulin, cortisol, and growth hormone. The role of cortisol is particularly important. Its level must be adequate to facilitate the conversion of glycogen, fats, and proteins to new glucose supplies, thereby elevating blood sugar levels. If cortisol is inadequate then it is difficult or even impossible to meet this increased demand and hypoglycemia can result. In the absence of other medical reasons for episodes of hypoglycemia, we must consider Adrenal Fatigue Syndrome as a possible cause.

When a person suffers from Adrenal Fatigue Syndrome, hypoglycemia is often associated with a combination of low cortisol and high insulin levels. This perfect storm commonly occurs when the body is under stress, either acutely or chronically. As AFS progresses into advanced stages of exhaustion, the output of cortisol lowers, and glucose release is slowed as well. This occurs along with insulin dysregulation, because the pancreas is put on overdrive as part of the ongoing stress response during earlier stages of Adrenal Fatigue Syndrome. Those who have a family history of or predisposition toward diabetes are particularly vulnerable. The body can be put in a position where it needs more glucose, but at the same time glucose regulation is not functioning properly. This combination of dysfunctions can lead to hypoglycemia and its common symptoms, among them are dizziness and fainting.

Clinical Definition of Hypoglycemia

Within a twenty-four hour cycle, healthy people generally maintain blood glucose levels between 4.4 to 6.1 mmol/L (82 to 110 mg/dL); or 3.3 or 3.9 mmol/L (60 to 70 mg/dL) are commonly cited as the lower limits of normal glucose.

> **Note: Millimoles per liter, expressed as mmol/L is the world standard unit for measuring glucose in the blood. The U.S. and a few other countries use mg/dL.**

Although the medical community agrees on what constitutes the normal blood sugar range, debate continues about what degree of hypoglycemia warrants medical evaluation and treatment, or that can potentially cause harm. The reasons are simple. Many healthy people can occasionally have glucose levels in the hypoglycemic range without any problem or signs of hypoglycemia. This adds to the difficulty of establishing hypoglycemia as a clinical state in the first place. They do well and are asymptomatic, but they routinely have a blood sugar level of under 90mg/dL. The situation is even more complex in those with Adrenal Fatigue Syndrome, because manifestations of hypoglycemia are more often than not subclinical. The individual has signs of hypoglycemia even though the blood plasma level is above 60-70 mg/dL. Fasting serum blood sugar and glucose tolerance tests are usually normal.

The diagram below shows how AFS can clinically affect hypoglycemia. After a meal, those in this phase tend to have a faster dip in blood sugar to below the hypoglycemic symptoms threshold (HST) level, which triggers symptoms of hypoglycemia such as irritability and fatigue. The more advanced the Adrenal Fatigue Syndrome, the more the blood sugar curve shifts toward the left. As a result, the time between finishing a meal to the onset of hypoglycemic symptoms shortens.

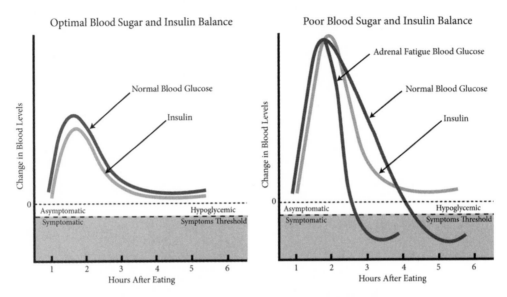

Figure 6. Optimal & Poor Blood Sugar and
Insulin Analysis vs. Hours after Eating

In AFS, hypoglycemic symptoms usually begin while the blood sugar is still within normal range. Therefore, we tend to believe that the underlying trigger of these symptoms is tied to the blood sugar drop itself more than the absolute level of blood sugar. In other words, it's the sensitivity to and perhaps the velocity of the drop that triggers hypoglycemic symptoms. That may be why the majority of sufferers of advanced AFS report some degree of such reactive hypoglycemia, even though their blood glucose is normal in laboratory testing.

The more advanced the AFS, the more intense the hypoglycemia in terms of symptoms and frequency. For this reason, those in Stage 3 AFS and beyond may need to eat every 2-3 hours, even if only a small snack, to prevent hypoglycemia during the day. As sufferers recover, then the time between meals and snacks can lengthen. In contrast, those in Stage 2 AFS can go 4-6 hours without food and not experience either hunger or symptoms of hypoglycemia. Many in Stage 1 can skip a meal and have no symptoms at all. Signs and symptoms of such reactive hypoglycemia usually improve as adrenal health is optimized.

Symptoms of Hypoglycemia

The symptoms of hypoglycemia are wide and varied. When they are subclinical, as they most often are at this phase, symptoms can be vague and therefore often miss detection. They include:

- hunger
- nausea
- headaches
- elevated heart rate
- a tendency to daydream
- confusion
- memory loss/amnesia
- dizziness
- irritability
- anxiety/jittery feelings
- rage
- in severe cases, fainting, coma, and seizures

During Stage 3A, hypoglycemic symptoms tend to be very mild. Because of this, they are more often than not under investigated and become evident only in retrospect, unless the hypoglycemia is severe.

We can temporarily reverse *acute* hypoglycemia by taking 10-20 grams of carbohydrate, the equivalent of 3-4 ounces of orange, apple, or grape juice. Unfortunately, too many people turn to one of the common sugar fixes that are so much a part of our society. They reach for a sugary drink or coffee or a sugary snack, but this is only a short-acting emergency remedy. It relieves symptoms immediately, but they return in an hour or two.

To reactivate and restore normal cell function, the body requires amounts of energy beyond what is normally required to maintain normal energy burn. In addition, with each hypoglycemic episode, more cells are damaged. Thus, the body reaches a new low. If this occurs at the same time the demand for glucose increases, the stage becomes set for an adrenal crisis. With each plunge of blood sugar, AFS increases and the hypoglycemia worsens. By the end of the day, a person might feel nearly exhausted but without having done anything. Episodes of low blood sugar are most likely to occur at around 10:00 AM and 2:00 PM, and/or between 3-4:00 PM.

Hypoglycemia Prevention Tips

You need a systematic and comprehensive approach to prevent and reverse the chronic subclinical hypoglycemia associated with Adrenal Fatigue Syndrome. We recommend following the guidelines in Chapter 23, *A Healing Diet for Adrenal Fatigue Syndrome*, which help those with blood sugar fluctuations and Adrenal Fatigue Syndrome. Below are key strategies you can implement now:

- Consume protein (such as nuts, meats, fish, poultry, beans, cottage cheese, whole milk yogurt) and fat (nuts, extra virgin olive oil, coconut, avocado) with each meal or snack. This leads to a slower release of sugar in the body and thus extends the time before you become hypoglycemic between meals.

- Plan frequent meals and snacks, i.e., 3 meals a day—breakfast, lunch, and dinner—plus midmorning, mid-afternoon, and bedtime snacks. Include protein and fat with each meal or snacks.

- Avoid the so-called sugar and flour foods—dessert foods and snack foods.

- Make sure you consume at least 1200 calories per day, even if you are trying to lose weight.

- Listen to your body. Sometimes you may need to eat something every two hours, especially if your work requires intense mental concentration or is very physical.

- Don't leave the house without taking along portable snacks, such as nuts, and keep them with you wherever you go.

- Follow the glycemic index (GI) described in Appendix B.

Snacks to Help Avoid Blood Sugar Dips

- whole milk yogurt and berries
- apple with almond butter
- nuts and fruit
- celery stick with cream cheese or nut butter
- refried beans
- cream cheese and salmon or tuna on a whole grain cracker.

Sample Breakfasts to Help Avoid Blood Sugar Dips

A good breakfast is important to replenish lost energy from a night's sleep. Consider the following:

- muesli (non-sweetened granola) with whole milk yogurt, nuts, and whole fruits
- nuts and green apples
- poached egg on sprouted wheat bread
- smoothie made with avocado, coconut, whole milk yogurt, nuts, and raw egg
- vegetable omelet
- cream cheese and salmon on whole grain bagel
- cooked oatmeal with nuts and fruits

Electrolyte Dysregulation Resulting in Low Blood Pressure (Hypotension)

Blood pressure is an important indicator of adrenal health and function. Stages 1 and 2 of Adrenal Fatigue Syndrome usually are accompanied by normal to high blood pressure as cortisol and aldosterone output peaks. As AFS advances, low blood pressure, at rest or related to posture, becomes more prevalent. Weak adrenals can drastically alter the blood pressure landscape in the body, leading to a wide variety of symptoms such as dizziness, lightheadedness, orthostatic (related to position of the body) hypotension (low blood pressure), and heart palpitations. Many of these symptoms show themselves for the first time during this phase.

Blood Pressure Basics

> Blood pressure is the force exerted by circulating blood on the walls of blood vessels. It constitutes one of the key vital signs of life, along with heartbeat, rate of breathing, and temperature. Blood pressure is generated by the heart pumping blood into the arteries and is regulated by the response of the arteries to the flow of blood.

Blood pressure is expressed as *systolic/diastolic*, for example, 120/80 is 120 systolic over 80 diastolic. The systolic blood pressure (the top number) represents the pressure in the arteries as the muscle of the heart contracts and pumps blood into them. The diastolic blood pressure (the bottom number) represents the pressure in the arteries as the muscle of the heart relaxes after it contracts. Blood pressure is always higher when the heart is pumping (squeezing) than when it is relaxing.

Systolic blood pressure for most healthy adults falls between 90 and 120 millimeters of mercury (mm Hg). Diastolic blood pressure falls between 60 and 80 mm Hg. The commonly accepted guidelines define normal blood pressure as lower than 120/80. Unlike high blood pressure (hypertension), low blood pressure is defined primarily by signs and symptoms of low blood flow and not by a specific blood pressure number, meaning blood pressure readings that fall below a certain threshold. Vegetarians generally have low blood pressure readings, and at the same time, they can be healthy and asymptomatic. Individuals with a blood pressure of 90/50 might have no symptoms of low blood pressure. Therefore, they do not have clinical low blood pressure. However, those who normally have high blood pressure may develop symptoms of low blood pressure if the reading drops to 100/60.

> The body's organs may be damaged if the blood pressure is not high enough to deliver adequate blood flow to the organs of the body. Signs of insufficient blood flow to the brain/brain cells include lightheadedness, dizziness, or fainting. If the blood pressure is already low, standing up can make it drop further, potentially causing severe dizziness and even fainting episodes (*orthostatic hypotension*).

When a normal person stands after lying down, gravitational forces cause blood pressure to drop, which immediately triggers the autonomic nervous system (ANS), which regulates the blood pressure to return to normal. The rise in pressure on standing usually ranges from 10-20 mm Hg. This overshoot normalizes in a short time and the overall blood pressure returns to normal. Under normal circumstances, a healthy person doesn't feel this behind-the-scenes automatic adjustment. However, when dysfunction exists in the ANS, which we often see in advanced Adrenal Fatigue Syndrome, the blood pressure fails to normalize which may result in orthostatic hypotension (also called postural hypotension). Other causes of orthostatic hypotension include dehydration, dysautonomia, medication side effects, and heart disease. If you experience postural hypotension, then investigate the issue with your physician to see if the symptoms are clinically significant.

When at rest, it is not considered abnormal to have low blood pressure. Many individuals have resting blood pressure under 90/60 and function very well. We evaluate the clinical significance or insignificance of low blood pressure by whether it is accompanied by symptoms, and whether or not it is related to postural position.

Aldosterone and Blood Pressure

Aldosterone is a salt-retaining hormone. It is responsible for maintaining the concentration of sodium and potassium inside and outside the cells, which in turn has a direct effect on the amount of fluid in the body. Therefore, aldosterone plays a significant role in regulating blood pressure.

As you may recall, aldosterone is a hormone manufactured in the adrenal cortex under the direction of ACTH (adrenocorticotropic hormone), produced by the anterior pituitary gland. ACTH stimulates the adrenal cortex via the HPA axis to secrete a wide variety of hormones including aldosterone and cortisol. Like cortisol, aldosterone follows a daily secretion pattern peaking at 8:00 AM. Its lowest point is between 12:00 AM to 4:00 AM.

A sequence of events can change fluid balance and blood pressure. Remember that sodium and water go hand in hand—where sodium goes, water follows. In addition, sodium and potassium oppose each other. As the concentration of aldosterone in the body rises, the concentration of sodium and water rises and more fluid is retained in the body, and then blood pressure rises. Conversely, when the level of aldosterone lowers, the amount of sodium and water in the body is reduced, and blood pressure goes down. Excessive aldosterone leads to high blood pressure, high sodium, and low potassium. Deficiencies of aldosterone in the dysregulation of the HPA axis can lead to low blood pressure, a compensatory high pulse rate, dizziness especially on standing, salt cravings, and palpitations. Severe cases may lead to high potassium and low sodium in the blood.

Unlike cortisol, aldosterone does not have its own negative feedback loop. If the aldosterone level is too high, aldosterone receptor sites will be down-regulated and their sensitivity to aldosterone reduced. Because stress stimulates ACTH production, in the early stages of Adrenal Fatigue Syndrome the amount of cortisol and aldosterone increases. As a result, the body retains sodium and water, which causes a bloated feeling. As blood pressure starts to rise due to increased blood volume, the baroreceptors (receptors that are sensitive to pressure) of the blood vessels are triggered. This automatically sends muscles within the blood vessels into relaxation mode. Blood pressure comes down and is normalized.

This auto-regulation helps to maintain stable blood pressure at a time when the total fluid volume increases because stress has triggered high levels of aldosterone.

With stress, the adrenal glands also secrete *norepinephrine* and *epinephrine*, hormones that constrict the blood vessels and increases blood pressure. This ensures that our brains have adequate blood flow and oxygen to help us deal with impending danger. The adrenals also release cortisol in response to stress. Cortisol also contracts mid-size blood vessels, though with less potency than epinephrine. In early stages of AFS, it is not unusual for our blood pressure to be high if not normal.

As AFS progresses to Stage 3A, output of cortisol and aldosterone generally start falling because of the reasons explained above. We start to see subclinical deficiency of cortisol, aldosterone, or both. Despite compensatory efforts to increase blood pressure by the body, the overall net blood pressure tends to fall.

AFS and Low Blood Pressure

Ultimately, several factors determine blood pressure readings at any point in time, including the actions of aldosterone, renin (an enzyme released by the kidneys), cortisol, epinephrine, norepinephrine, blood volume, HPA axis integrity, and the autonomic relaxation response. As you can see, it's a complicated process. When the body is under stress, it releases chemicals that raise blood pressure, and this sets off a series of compensatory responses that lowers blood pressure if the body is otherwise intact and functioning normally. If the body is unable to overcome the high aldosterone and epinephrine response, then *elevated* blood pressure results. Therefore, as most of us have heard, stress often causes increased blood pressure.

If the adrenals are exhausted because of stress, the picture changes drastically, because the adrenals are unable to mount a compensatory response. We start to see reduced aldosterone production, and sodium and water retention is compromised. Fluid volume is reduced, and the blood pressure becomes *low*. As a result of this process, cells become easily dehydrated and deficient in sodium.

To complicate matters further, most people with *advanced* AFS invariably also have some degree of autonomic nervous system dysfunction. ANS is one of three modulators of a hormone called renin. Renin activates the renin-angiotensin hormonal axis system (RAS), which ultimately leads to an increase in blood pressure. Many with severe adrenal weakness might also have symptoms consistent with subclinically low levels of renin and aldosterone. When this occurs, we can see low blood pressure along with salt cravings. This can exacerbate preexisting fatigue because oxygen delivery to the brain is reduced. Other symptoms, though less common, can include reduced hearing function, vertigo, visual disturbances of unknown origin, tingling, anxiety, and headaches.

In order to compensate for this fluid imbalance, the body leaks potassium out of the cells so that the sodium to potassium ratio remains constant. The loss of potassium is less than that of sodium, and as a result, the potassium to sodium ratio is increased. Therefore, most with advanced AFS have higher potassium relative to sodium load, although laboratory tests of both continued to be within or slightly outside the normal range. Sufferers may also experience a drop in blood pressure and an increase in pulse rate upon standing. Symptoms closely resembling POTS (postural orthostatic tachycardia syndrome) at a subclinical level may arise.

Other Common Causes of Low Blood Pressure

Prior to considering Adrenal Fatigue Syndrome as the culprit, we recommend investigating these other causes of low blood pressure:

Heart disease: Heart disease has many manifestations, such as weakened heart muscle, pericarditis (inflammation of the pericardium, the sac that envelopes the heart), bradycardia (slower than normal heart action), arrhythmias (irregular heart beat), and heart block (defective coordination of heart rhythms). Tachycardia (rapid heartbeat) can also lead to low blood pressure, as the heart is unable to maintain the stroke volume (volume of blood pumped in one beat) to supply adequate blood flow to the body.

Arrhythmia is more prevalent in those with ANS (autonomic nervous system) dysfunction. Persistent overtone of the SNS (sympathetic nervous system) increases the release of norepinephrine; chronic increases of norepinephrine can lower the heart's threshold for cardiac arrhythmia, including atrial fibrillation. We see this situation in advanced Adrenal Exhaustion.

Medications: Medications such as calcium channel blockers, beta-blockers, and digoxin (Lanoxin®) can slow the rate at which the heart contracts. Elderly people are especially susceptible, because these days, they typically take medications to treat high blood pressure. However, these medications can lower blood pressure too much, thereby producing symptomatic low blood pressure as well. Water pills (diuretics) often taken with other medications for hypertension, such as furosemide (Lasix®) can decrease blood volume by causing excessive urination.

Other drugs that can cause low blood pressure include: Medications used to treat Parkinson's disease, such as levodopa-carbidopa (Sinemet®); medications used for treating depression, such as amitriptyline (Elavil®); drugs used to treat erectile dysfunction (impotence), such as sidenafil (Viagra®), vardenafil (Levitra®), and tadafil (Cialis®) (when used in combination with nitroglycerine).

Less common causes of low blood pressure include septicemia (blood infections), alcoholism, diabetes, shock, kidney disease, vasovagal (involves both blood vessels and the vagus nerve) reaction, micturition syncope (cessation or interruption of urinary function), anaphylaxis (hypersensitivity to certain agents), and certain rare neurological syndromes such as Shy-Drager syndrome, which damage the ANS, and Addison's disease.

Dehydration and Fluid Imbalance

Aside from low blood pressure, sodium and potassium imbalance often lead to fluid depletion. In a person with advanced AFS, dehydration is quite common, but often overlooked as a relevant symptom associated with AFS. Such sensitivity to fluid depletion can be extreme. For example, those with advanced AFS may find a few minutes of exposure to strong sunlight a draining experience. This is particularly challenging for men and women who live in a hot and humid environment, especially when they're outdoors. These are signs of low marginal fluid reserve within the body.

When the fluid balance within the body is off, temperature control becomes a problem; many report temperature intolerance as well. The more fluid and electrolytes are dysregulated, the higher the chances that dehydration will trigger adrenal crashes. This is why we recommend that AFS sufferers carry a water bottle with them at all times, with a bit of salt or lemon added. These individuals should consume fluids with adequate electrolytes many times a day in intermittent dosages, while avoiding coffee, alcohol, and tea (with the exception of herbal tea).

Lost fluids should be replaced carefully and slowly. When lost fluid is replaced too quickly, without adequate sodium, the amount of sodium in the body may be diluted, resulting in an even lower sodium level, a state called *dilutional hyponatremia*. Low sodium can produce non-specific symptoms of confusion, lethargy, nausea, headache, seizure, weakness, and restlessness. This in turn worsens AFS.

In Stage 3A of AFS, fluid and electrolyte imbalances are usually in a mild sub-clinical state, whereas laboratory tests are normal. Because of its mildness, most are passed over as insignificant.

As AFS progresses, however, the clinical picture can change drastically. Dehydration, along with low sodium, leads to a convoluted picture that often defies conventional medical logic. We see many sufferers who have gone to the local emergency room because of these disturbing symptoms, only to have an extensive workup and then be told that all is normal. For example, in those who are severely decompensated and in a highly sensitive state consistent with advanced weakness, the electrolytes may fall within the normal range, even while symptoms persist. In severe cases, hospital admissions may be required and diuretics taken to reduce fluid load, while sodium is being replaced.

Commercially available electrolyte replacement drinks (i.e., Gatorade®) are designed for people who have normal adrenal function, but experience excessive loss of electrolytes during exercise. This is why these drinks are high in sodium, low in potassium, but quite high in sugar. If AFS is very mild, it's okay to consume these drinks as a fluid replacement, but those with advanced Adrenal Fatigue Syndrome usually have sugar imbalances and low sodium level. This is why we recommend drinking filtered water with a bit of salt added, especially in the morning upon awakening, for those who are stable. If blood pressure increases, or signs of edema (water retention) occur and nausea develops, stop the salt and tell a qualified health practitioner about what has occurred.

Only a small number of people in advanced stages of Adrenal Fatigue Syndrome have concurrent high blood pressure, and those falling into this category should check their blood pressure carefully during fluid replacement.

Suboptimal Detoxification Leads to Low Clearance

As the body adapts to an environment of lower energy supply, by necessity, the function of all major systems starts to slow down to prevent the body from entering a net negative energy state. Processing and excreting waste byproducts after nutrients have been assimilated by the cells is an important function. In the presence of advanced AFS, this function is invariably compromised, along with the body's digestive and absorptive mechanisms.

The liver is the major detoxification center, acting as a filter to remove foreign substances and wastes from the blood. For example, the liver clears toxins such as alcohol, solvents, formaldehyde, pesticides, herbicides, and food additives. The liver functions to convert toxins into compounds that the body can safely handle and remove through the kidneys (as urine), skin (as sweat), lungs (as expelled air) and bowels (as feces). The liver is also responsible for breaking down nutrients, medications, vitamins, and hormones into small, inert metabolites.

Unwanted waste byproducts and metabolites are normally excreted out of the body on a timely basis. With suboptimal or slowed clearance, the body might slowly accumulate undesirable waste byproducts or metabolites. They remain in circulation. The more advanced the fatigue, the more serious this problem becomes. Unwanted metabolites accumulate and can turn toxic inside the body. This leads to a variety of undesirable symptoms tied to inflammatory responses.

When excessive circulating metabolites find a home in the extracellular spaces of joints, joint pain of unknown origin may result. Some are deposited into the muscles, contributing to myalgia. Excessive circulating metabolites tend to be very damaging to our central nervous system as well. Many of these metabolites are fat soluble and cross the blood-brain barrier into the brain, resulting in the often cited brain fog, anxiety, and insomnia. Other complaints can include psychological and neurological symptoms such as depression, headache, abnormal nerve reflexes, and tingling in the hands.

If the internal pH is affected, the incidence of yeast infection (candidiasis) and interstitial cystitis can go up as well. Again, liver function laboratory tests are usually normal at this time. Unfortunately, we have no test sensitive enough to accurately measure clearance, other than a detailed and accurate patient history.

> Bear in mind that many healthy adults start to develop food and chemical sensitivities as they grow older, even without developing Adrenal Fatigue Syndrome. Intolerance to wheat, corn, and dairy products is common and can be early warning signs of suboptimal liver function. Unfortunately, this newly occurring symptom is often dismissed as a normal sign of aging.

Brain Fog—a Common Symptom of Impaired Clearance

Many individuals report brain fog at this phase. It is an important clue that something is wrong with the liver and other detoxification centers of the body, even when medical workups are negative. Brain fog is a descriptive phrase, and implies a mental state where memory is clouded and unclear, rather than a loss of immediate or past memory. Instead, individuals tell us that in brain fog their memory is "so close and yet so far" in terms of the recollection ability. They have trouble remembering where they put their keys or what they did yesterday, or they may not be able to concentrate or memorize simple things like phone numbers. However, long term memory remains intact. The ability to concentrate is usually compromised. They might double and triple check their work, yet still be wrong. When severe, this cognitive toll can impair those who work in intellectually intensive careers and jobs; eventually they might be unable to perform their normal duty.

Most brain fog usually is transient, lasting anywhere from hours to days. Assuming no other pathology is present, the duration of brain fog is often related to the degree of liver overload. The more the liver is overtaxed, the longer the brain fog lasts.

Time, proper nutritional support, and increased water intake gently enhance the detoxification process and helps lift the fog.

Brain fog usually spontaneously resolves as the body's detoxification system improves, which usually happens automatically as adrenal function improves.

> If the adrenal system is not performing optimally, brain fog may stay for a long time. Sometimes self initiated detoxification helps, but if not done properly, brain fog can worsen because of a retoxification reaction.

Focusing on adrenal recovery as a way to reduce brain fog is a much better way to go.

The Catabolic State and Loss of Muscle Mass

When responding to stress, the adrenal glands produce steroidal hormones, primarily cortisol. As previously stated, cortisol output is usually high in Stages 1 and 2 of Adrenal Fatigue Syndrome, but as AFS progresses, cortisol output is often pushed to its limit. Over time, high cortisol results in excessive breakdown of collagen and protein without sufficient replenishment (catabolic state). Along with reduced liver function, as discussed above, metabolites of the catabolic state increase, leading to chronic pain syndromes, joint pain, chronic fatigue, and fibromyalgia. If not reversed, protein breakdown starts to accelerate in this stage, leading to a gradual loss of muscle mass. The catabolic state results from a chronically high cortisol output. A high cortisol to DHEA-S ratio seen in blood tests can offer clues of this.

The cycle of catabolism is normally followed by a process of rebuilding or anabolism. The rebuilding process is normally carried out by androgens, such as testosterone. Unfortunately, testosterone output also starts to fall as the body slows the nonessential reproductive function. Therefore, the rebuilding process will be slow and sluggish.

This catabolic state usually begins slowly undetected, starting at Stage 3A. In addition to metabolite buildup discussed above, collagen break-down as part of normal living is not adequately replenished. As this happens, wrinkles begin to develop and premature aging sets in. Strenuous exercise or heavy lifting only further weakens the already fragile collagen support structure further. Outwardly, the loss of large chest muscle mass is not evident yet. However, certain fitness exercises, such as push-ups, can become more difficult.

With advancing AFS, the intercostal muscles (muscles connecting the ribs to each other) start losing mass, and taking a deep breath becomes a chore. Handshakes become weak as small muscles of the hand are also involved and lose muscle mass. If we pay careful attention, we see that no body part is spared. Of course, a person may look normal from afar but is physically frail on close examination. In severe cases, usually in advanced Stage 3C or 3D, some complain that it takes energy just to take a breath. Clearly, under normal circumstances this should be an automatic function.

As the collagen structures of internal organs break down, their functions are compromised. For example, gastrointestinal track motility (movement) and contraction forces are reduced. Adrenal Fatigue Syndrome is therefore often associated with poor ability to breakdown proteins, and common symptoms include indigestion, bloating, gas, and constipation. The body's acid production might be insufficient to help break down digested foods, resulting in further digestive problems.

It's no surprise, then, that secondary fibromyalgia and chronic fatigue syndrome are commonly associated with later stages of AFS. Clinically, we often see Adrenal Fatigue Syndrome symptoms consistent with fibromyalgia and chronic fatigue. Indeed, we could eventually find that these syndromes, which generally do not have agreed upon origins, are part of the cluster of symptoms of adrenal dysfunction.

Neurological System Dysfunction

While the rest of the body is adapting to a lower energy environment in the phase, the brain does not have this luxury. To function properly, energy to the brain cannot be compromised, or a cognitive toll begins. Brain function is the top priority of the body. Mechanisms involved in regulating blood sugar are designed to ensure that the brain always gets an adequate supply of glucose. Symptoms of reduced brain support can trigger a host of neurochemical imbalances leading to symptoms of sluggishness, anxiety, tremors, irritability, and mild depression.

Brain norepinephrine is the primary dysregulated neurotransmitter responsible for many of these symptoms. Depression has been further linked to low levels of cortisol, DHEA, and testosterone, which are linked to reduced adrenal function. So it's not surprising that Adrenal Exhaustion is strongly associated with increased fears, anxiety, depression, brain fog, and difficulties in concentrating. In addition, those in Adrenal Exhaustion often find themselves intolerant and easily frustrated.

The brain is also relatively isolated from the rest of the body because of the blood-brain barrier. It is lipophilic, meaning that it attracts fat-soluble molecules, such as steroidal hormones. It is easily affected by the lipophilic toxic metabolite buildup mentioned earlier. Hence, brain fog and sleep disturbances naturally follow.

Sleep problems are generally secondary responses to AFS, but they add a significant burden on the body, because sleep deprivation compromises the body's ability to self-repair. Sleep problems further contribute to AFS, thus setting off a vicious downward spiral of cascading dysfunction, including decreased immunity, impaired glucose tolerance, decreased morning cortisol levels, and decreased alertness and concentration. Again, we must not forget that at this phase, these symptoms are generally mild and escape detection.

Hormonal System Dysfunction

The various glands of the endocrine system have special significance when considering Stages 3A and 3B—early Adrenal Exhaustion. In order to regulate the complexity of the body's functions, hormonal systems are grouped into networks or axes. These axes are direct conduits and represent another advanced self-regulatory system which is built in to ensure that the body runs smoothly. Chapter 2, *Stress, Hormone Basics and the "Forgotten" Adrenals*, explained the hypothalamic-pituitary-adrenal (HPA) axis, which controls adrenal gland function. Key hormones such as cortisol, aldosterone, estrogen, and progesterone are regulated through this axis.

Problems with hormonal dysregulation start becoming evident in this stage, though signs are usually mild and symptoms generally subclinical. Dysfunction of sugar metabolism leads to hypoglycemia, and salt craving is a common symptom of aldosterone deficiency. Both hypoglycemia and aldosterone deficiency are symptoms of HPA axis dysregulation. The more advanced the AFS, the more hormones become dysregulated.

Remember that hormones are regulatory compounds vital to well-being. For example, testosterone deficiency leads to a loss of muscle mass and low libido. Too much estrogen can lead to fluid retention, fibrocystic changes in the breast, PMS, and endometriosis. Low thyroid leads to dry skin, fatigue, and weight gain. In order to feel good, the amount of each hormone must be maintained. A comprehensive hormonal evaluation requires that we look at them from the following perspectives:

- The absolute excess or deficiency of a specific hormone. This can be measured by laboratory tests. For example, too much cortisol or too little DHEA.

- The relative excess or deficiency of a specific hormone. This is not easily measured by routine laboratory tests. Specialized tests can help but are not diagnostic, and the best assessment tool is a careful history. Estrogen dominance is one example of relative excess or deficiency.

- The imbalance of hormones due to hormonal axis dysregulation, which can only be assessed by careful history. HPA axis dysregulation (discussed in this chapter) and OAT axis imbalance (discussed in the next chapter) are good examples.

In Stage 3A, we see subclinical or clinical evidence of all three categories of dysfunction, which results in early onset of symptoms of hormonal dysregulation.

How One Hormone Dysregulation Affects Another

We learned in Chapter 2, *Stress, Hormone Basics, and the "Forgotten" Adrenals*, that imbalances of estrogen and progesterone can lead to estrogen dominance and a continuum of associated conditions, including premenstrual syndrome (PMS), endometriosis, polycystic ovary syndrome (PCOS), cystic breast disease, fibroids, and irregular menstrual periods. Just as estrogen dominance can be attributed to adrenal weakness, the reverse is also true, and AFS can exacerbate estrogen dominance. Remember that cortisol is made from progesterone in the adrenal cortex. Weakened adrenals tend to favor cortisol production, which may lead to lower progesterone levels and promote estrogen dominance. This becomes a vicious cycle.

Thyroid hormone imbalances are common in AFS. In Adrenal Exhaustion, we often see reduced thyroid function which is the body's way of conserving energy. Low adrenal function, therefore, can worsen thyroid function. Many are told they have hypothyroidism, but in actuality, their adrenals are weak. Those who are already on thyroid replacement medication may in fact need a higher dose in the presence of AFS. In addition, the thyroid is intricately related to the ovarian system. Thyroid hormones stimulate progesterone production in the ovaries. As thyroid hormone output is reduced as AFS progresses, progesterone production is compromised. Without adequate progesterone to offset estrogen, we commonly see menstrual cycle irregularity, putting fertilization at risk. Miscarriages are common especially in the first trimester when progesterone demand is not met. Those who have recurrent first trimester miscarriages should always consider AFS as a possible cause. Fortunately, it is not unusual for women to overcome infertility problems when AFS resolves.

The adrenal cortex secretes both male and female sex hormones, but the quantities are small and their effects are usually masked by the same hormones produced in the testes and ovaries. In Adrenal Exhaustion, androgen secretion dysregulation may lead to masculinization, which means that women with estrogen dominance or other hormonal imbalances can develop secondary sex characteristics, such as excessive facial or body hair (hirsutism) and hair loss. Other consequences can include conditions such as PCOS, seborrhea (a skin inflammation with no known cause), and acne.

> **Most perimenopausal or postmenopausal women who experience hair loss invariably have some level of adrenal dysfunction.**

In males, low libido is an important sign of Adrenal Exhaustion, because the body is gearing up to survive, and reproductive hormones are less important. Sex drive is reduced in both men and women.

We will have much more to say about hormonal system imbalances later. Clearly, in this phase, many of the hormonal systems are way off normal function, including the critical HPA axis, but symptoms are subclinical and relatively mild. More often than not, conventional medical workups remain negative, that is, produce findings in the normal range.

Dysfunction in Immune Mediated Conditions

When the adrenals are overtaxed, the immune system is unable to function optimally. As a result, we often see exaggerated autoimmune or what are known as immune mediated responses such as:

- rheumatoid arthritis (RA)
- Hashimoto's thyroiditis
- allergic rhinitis (nasal inflammation not associated with the common cold)
- skin sensitivities, including psoriasis (a chronic condition marked by scaly, red patches)
- hypoactive (lowered) immune function
- frequent infections
- internal dysbiosis (imbalance in intestinal flora)
- candidiasis (fungal infections)
- recurrent herpes infections

While their onset may begin in Stage 3A and are mild and subclinical in nature, these can become full blown medical conditions by the time AFS reaches Stage 3C or 3D.

Allergies: Allergic reactions usually have strong adrenal components. Most allergies involve the release of histamine and other pro-inflammatory substances. To counteract this, the body releases cortisol, a strong anti-inflammatory hormone. The level of circulating cortisol correlates directly to the degree of inflammation in the body and the resulting symptoms of allergies. The weaker the adrenals, the stronger the effects of allergies because more histamine is released. It then takes more cortisol to control the inflammatory response and the adrenals need to work even harder to produce cortisol.

When the adrenals are exhausted, cortisol output is compromised, allowing unopposed histamine to further inflame the tissues. This vicious cycle can lead to progressively deepening adrenal exhaustion and more severe allergic reactions. People with food and environmental allergies often have weak adrenal function. (We explore this in great detail in Chapter 25, *Food and Chemical Sensitivities*). Suffice it to say that Stage 3A is where many of these symptoms start surfacing.

Autoimmune Disease: Autoimmune diseases, such as Hashimoto's disease or rheumatoid arthritis, represent a spectrum of diseases in which the white blood cells of the immune system become overactive. Chemical messengers called *cytokines* form an integral part of the immune system, and as messengers, cytokines inform and trigger other immune cells to activate, grow, or possibly die. Excessive pro-inflammatory cytokines are elevated in fibromyalgia and chronic fatigue, leading to aggravated inflammation and flu-like symptoms. Chronic inflammation can reflect an improperly functioning immune system.

Anti-inflammatory effects of cortisol restrain various physiological mechanisms in order to prevent them from causing havoc inside the body, which is what occurs when an autoimmune disease is present and over-reactive white blood cells secrete toxins and exacerbate the condition. In this way, cortisol protects the body from autoimmune processes and uncontrolled inflammation. We see insufficient levels of cortisol in people with advanced Adrenal Fatigue Syndrome, resulting in compromised and overactive white blood cells that lead to unrestrained damage to the body.

Infections: Chronic infections of all kinds are often the root cause of Adrenal Fatigue Syndrome and tend to predispose individuals to developing respiratory problems. Symptoms of Lyme disease and H. Pylori infection, in particular, can mimic AFS. Recurrent respiratory infections and delayed healing also add to the difficulty of recovering from Adrenal Fatigue Syndrome. Even a single infection can trigger AFS. Both chronic infections and acute infections, such as pneumonia, are triggers of AFS. Be especially careful about dental procedures that are incomplete or poorly performed which can serve as a source of toxins in the body.

Commonly overlooked chronic infections include viruses that lurk in the body and do not produce symptoms. Parasites and fungi also do their damage silently, but over time, the stress they cause chronically overloads the adrenals and weakens the body's immune system. This cascade of processes that weakens immunity makes it harder to fight off the infection. Therefore, it follows that Adrenal Exhaustion is commonly associated with frequent and repeated infections with slower than normal healing times. We must consider adrenal dysfunction if we see a longer than normal recovery period after an illness or flu, with decreased stamina and pronounced morning fatigue.

Unfortunately, the temptation to treat symptoms is great in order to provide immediate relief. This often leads to excessive prescription of antibiotics and medications rather than allowing the body to heal itself.

As Adrenal Fatigue Syndrome progresses, more and more of the body's systems become involved. Confusion is normal. Sufferers end up being treated for a variety of symptoms that are mistakenly taken as disease.

How You Know You Are in Stage 3A

As you can see, most symptoms of Stage 3A tend to be mild. Whether it is occasional brain fog, mild food sensitivities, intermittent hypoglycemia, salt cravings, or dizziness on arising, they are invariably overlooked until well past this phase and only become obvious in retrospect. That is why this phase can be so destructive to our overall health. Our central control has already been infiltrated by enemy forces. But alarm bells have been rung if one only listens carefully.

Stage 3A usually goes on for many years unnoticed. Extensive medical workups are invariably normal. Those who pay attention to their body know something is wrong, but they remain entwined in cognitive dissonance as they are told all is well. Most people in this circumstance tend to be confused.

If Stage 3A is not reversed, continued deterioration is the natural progression of AFS. Hormonal axes are the main conduits of maintaining internal well-being within the command center of our body. These axes begin losing their integrity—stability and predictability—as we enter Phase B of Stage 3. We examine that in the next chapter.

Key Points to Remember

- As AFS progresses, early clinical signs of organ system dysfunction are evident. This is usually when patients go see their physician for the first time.

- Symptoms of Stage 3A are associated closely to HPA axis dysregulation.

- Metabolic system dysfunction and imbalance leads to the onset of mild hypoglycemia. Low blood pressure and salt cravings reflect aldosterone deficiency. Both are signs of HPA axis dysregulation. Dysfunction in detoxification pathways, primarily in the liver, leads to a low clearance state, causing numerous symptoms from brain fog to hypoglycemia.

- Musculoskeletal system dysfunction leads to onset of joint and muscular pain of unknown origin as the body enters a catabolic state.

- Neurological system dysfunction leads to worsening insomnia, tremor, anxiety, and depression.

- Hormonal system dysfunction and imbalances lead to the onset of subclinical hypothyroidism, PMS, PCOS, and endometriosis.

- Immune system dysfunction leads to recurrent infection and yeast overgrowth, with exaggerated autoimmune response at times.

- The body is losing its ability to perform normally, but the symptoms are so mild they are invariably overlooked.

Chapter 8

Stage 3B—Hormonal Axes Imbalances

In the previous chapter, it was revealed that many Stage 3A symptoms, such as hypoglycemia and low blood pressure, are consistent with dysregulation of the HPA hormonal axis. This upstream axis is particularly important because it bridges the brain to the adrenal gland. Dysfunction of this axis serves as a warning sign that the worst is yet to come if AFS is allowed to progress. As AFS worsens to Stage 3B, downstream hormonal axes become dysregulated. Imbalances of such axes are the hallmarks of stage 3B Adrenal Fatigue Syndrome.

> In women, the axis involved is called the ovarian-adrenal-axis (OAT); in men, it's called the adrenal-thyroid (AT) axis.

Although we generally focus on the OAT axis, both women and men will find that this chapter is the foundation that supports your overall understanding of Adrenal Exhaustion.

The OAT Axis

In Chapter 2, *Stress, Hormone Basics, and the "Forgotten" Adrenals*, we discussed the HPA axis and HPG axis, which are important regulators of stress and menses respectively. In Adrenal Exhaustion, another axis dysregulates. This axis ties together the ovaries, adrenals, and the thyroid gland, hence the term *ovarian-adrenal-thyroid* (OAT) axis The diagram below shows how the HPG, HPA and OAT axes are interconnected.

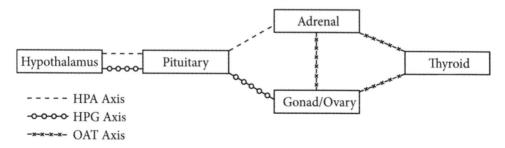

Figure 7. Relation between HPG, HPA and OAT Hormonal Axes

What happens to one organ of the three affects the other organs physiologically, clinically or subclinically. This makes these three organs hormonally interdependent. For example, if adrenals are weak, we often see concurrent thyroid malfunction and menstrual cycle irregularity. An underactive thyroid often aggravates adrenal weakness. Likewise, ovarian hormonal imbalances, such as estrogen dominance, often exacerbate any preexisting subclinical or clinical hypothyroidism.

We can liken the OAT axis to a three-legged stool; it isn't safe to sit unless all three legs are in perfect balance. So, for women to feel their best, all three organs in the OAT axis must be in harmony. Imbalances within the OAT axis lead to a variety of conditions. When mild, the conditions are bothersome and perhaps annoying, but when severe, they are incapacitating.

Symptoms of OAT axis imbalance often suggest concurrent estrogen dominance (ovarian), fatigue (adrenal), and hypothyroidism (thyroid). Because the symptoms overlap within the three organ systems, groups or clusters of symptoms can be very misleading. Consider this array of symptoms: insomnia, fatigue, myalgia, weight gain, joint pain, exercise intolerance, brain fog, sugar intolerance, diabetes, dry skin, feeling cold, slow metabolism, inability to lose weight, PMS, endometriosis, irregular menstrual cycle, fibrocystic breast disease, anxiety, depression, and accumulation of fat at the waist line. Hormonally, many are low in cortisol, progesterone, and thyroid. They appear clinically convoluted because the onset is simultaneous.

As you can see, these symptoms are linked to a variety of diseases. Many individuals are treated for thyroid problems alone. Some are evaluated for both ovarian and thyroid problems. However, few healthcare practitioners pay attention to the entire triad of ovarian, adrenal, and thyroid dysfunction.

Note: Women whose ovaries have been removed can still have OAT axis imbalances; imbalances in estrogen are involved and the ovaries are not the only place where estrogen is produced. The adrenal glands, as well as fat cells (adipose tissue), also produce estrogen. Therefore, those who are constantly stressed as well as overweight are particularly at risk.

OAT axis imbalance is not well researched, but we know it involves a clinical convolution of multiple hormonal axes imbalances. Unfortunately, no definitive test can isolate and identify this imbalanced state with pinpoint accuracy. At this point, what we do understand comes primarily from clinical experiences and case studies.

We view OAT axis imbalances as a clinical state, not as a disease state. The clinical state unifies common imbalances of the ovarian, adrenal, and thyroid systems into a triad. To better understand the OAT axis, we first look at key hormonal actions of the ovaries, adrenals, and thyroid glands individually, and we explain the way they affect each other.

Ovarian Hormones: Estrogen and Progesterone

You likely know that the ovaries regulate two sex hormones: estrogen and its opposing hormone *progesterone*, with the following features:

- Estrogen is produced by the ovaries, egg follicles, the adrenal glands, and in fat cells.

- Progesterone is produced almost entirely by the corpus luteum, which is the small mass of fat cells left over from the follicle after the egg leaves it at ovulation.

Progesterone acts as the *antagonist* to estrogen, meaning it balances and opposes the actions of estrogen. For example, estrogen stimulates the formation and growth of breast cysts, but progesterone is on the job to protect against breast cysts. Estrogen enhances salt and water retention, but progesterone acts as a natural diuretic. Estrogen has been associated with breast and endometrial cancers, while, generally speaking, progesterone has a cancer protective effect. (The endometrium is the mucous membrane that lines the uterus.) Women need both hormones to achieve optimum function. For example, progesterone does not do its job effectively without some estrogen in the body to "prime the pump."

The table below clarifies the balancing functions of each hormone:

Estrogen Effect	Progesterone Effect
Causes endometrium to proliferate	Maintains secretory endometrium
Causes breast stimulation that can lead to breast cancer	Protects against fibrocystic breast prevents breast cancer
Increases body fat	Helps use fat for energy
Increases endometrial cancer risk	Prevents endometrial cancer
Reduces vascular tone	Restores vascular tone
Increases blood clot risk	Normalizes blood clotting

As you can see from the table above, estrogen and progesterone act as checks and balances in order to achieve hormonal harmony. The relative dominance of estrogen and relative deficiency of progesterone leading to a state of estrogen dominance is the main culprit in the ovarian portion of the OAT axis imbalance.

Estrogen Dominance (Progesterone Deficiency)

Sex hormones, such as estrogen and progesterone, gradually decline with age, but we see a drastic change in the rate of decline during the perimenopausal and menopausal years. For example, from ages thirty-five to fifty, women experience a 75 percent reduction in progesterone production; in the same period, estrogen declines by about 35 percent. By menopause, women's bodies produce very little progesterone, but estrogen is present at about half its premenopausal level. Hence, we see a state called estrogen dominance. In other words, the body is bathed in a sea of estrogen because there is insufficient progesterone to offset it. This has serious pathological effects. The estrogen load is also exacerbated by stress and environmental factors, so the state of estrogen dominance adversely affects millions of healthy women from about the mid-thirties and up. Those who are exposed to excessive weight gain and stress may be afflicted much earlier, starting from late young adulthood. Men are also affected due to excessive environmental estrogen, though at a reduced intensity.

This phenomenon is illustrated in the graph below:

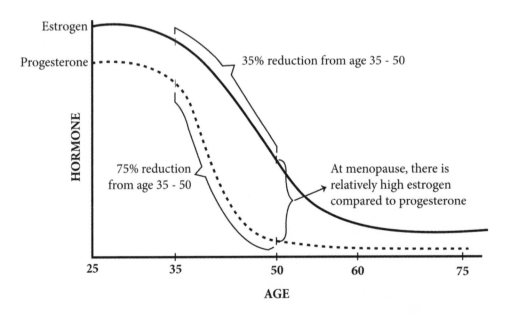

Figure 8. Estrogen and Progesterone Production as a Function of Age

Other factors contributing to estrogen dominance include excessive environmental estrogen, obesity, stress, poor diet, lack of exercise, and unopposed estrogen given as part of natural or synthetic hormone replacement therapy (HRT). In addition, an underactive thyroid can worsen the symptoms of estrogen dominance. AFS is also a commonly overlooked reason. Recall that pregnenolone is the precursor to progesterone. As AFS progresses, progesterone output can be reduced, which can then worsen estrogen dominance.

Symptoms of Estrogen Dominance

Women suffering from estrogen dominance typically experience some or even all of the following:

- swollen breasts and ring fingers
- impatience and irritability
- cramps before the menstrual cycle
- irregular periods
- fluid retention
- foggy thinking
- depression
- fatigue

These symptoms form the underlying common denominator for a variety of illnesses and syndromes previously regarded as unrelated entities. However, they represent different expressions of the same illness affecting different organs and body systems. If we put a lifetime of excessive estrogen on a continuum, then we might see the following manifestations at different times, starting with:

- **Premenstrual syndrome (PMS).** With numerous physical and psychological symptoms, such as abdominal pain, water retention, headaches, food cravings, irritability, and so forth.

- **Endometriosis.** A condition in which cells from the endometrium (the lining of the uterus) travel outside the uterus and attach to other pelvic organs. In addition to being a painful condition, endometriosis is a leading cause of infertility.

- **PCOS (polycystic ovary syndrome).** A hormonal imbalance that leads to irregular menstrual periods or lack of menstruation, along with other symptoms such as weight gain, diabetes, metabolic syndrome, and infertility.

- **Fibrocystic breast disease.** Fluid filled cysts developing in the breasts.

- **Fibroids.** Benign tumors that grow on the uterine wall and, if large, cause heavy menstrual bleeding and menstrual pain.

- **Breast cancer.** Malignant growths in the breast tissue.

Estrogen Dominance and Adrenal Fatigue Syndrome

Most women in Stage 3B AFS (or higher) suffer from estrogen dominance to varying degrees. Because treatments commonly focus on rebalancing estrogen, the root cause of adrenal weakness is easily missed. Because estrogen deficiency and estrogen dominance can have similar symptoms, such as hot flashes and PMS, some are prescribed estrogen replacement, which, in effect, increases the already high estrogen load in the body. While the initial clinical response may be positive for the lucky few, this approach invariably fails over time as Adrenal Fatigue Syndrome worsens.

The key is to focus on the adrenals first whenever clinically possible, as symptoms of estrogen dominance tend to subside when optimum adrenal health returns. If this is not possible, as sometimes happens when ovarian symptoms are overwhelming and demand immediate attention, proper balancing between ovarian and adrenal restoration is necessary. Long term, focusing only on rebalancing the ovarian hormones without concurrent adrenal support, increases the risk of recovery failure.

Remember that estrogen dominance is simply another way of saying progesterone deficiency on a relative basis. Low progesterone levels also occur in anovulatory cycles (menstrual cycles in which ovulation does not take place). In the presence of Adrenal Fatigue Syndrome, the body's emergency repair system is activated, however, and the body's priority is stabilizing basic bodily functions, such as blood pressure and blood sugar. In times of scarcity or stress, reproductive functions are considered low priority and ovulation might temporarily shut down. Women living under high stress conditions often experience irregular menstrual cycles or even the absence of their cycles (amenorrhea). In the absence of ovulation, the body doesn't produce additional progesterone for the cycle. Again, here, lower progesterone levels mean estrogen is higher and the hormonal orchestra is out of harmony.

Estrogen dominance can also be caused by excessive stimulation of estrogen through other sources. As adrenal weakness progresses, most individuals gain weight as the metabolism slows to conserve energy and food intake increases due to the cortisol effect in the brain (discussed in Chapter 5, *Early Adrenal Fatigue Syndrome: Stages 1 and 2*). When this happens, excessive fat cells accumulate, leading to an increased output of estrogen, thereby worsening any preexisting estrogen dominance. However, this is not the case by Stage 3D, a point at which most individuals lose weight.

Almost everyone is exposed to environmental estrogen-like compounds known as xenoestrogen, or you may hear the term *exogenous estrogen*. This is a relatively new phenomenon, starting primarily after World War II when the plastic and chemical revolution began and environmental effects soon appeared. These external estrogens are found in products containing chemicals that mimic estrogen. For example, many plastic products contain chemicals that enter the food chain when microwaving food in plastic dishes or using plastic wraps and containers. These xenoestrogens may also leach from cheaply produced soft plastic used in bottled water. Estrogen-like compounds can also come from certain foods, like cruciferous vegetables and unfermented soy products such as tofu. Chronic build up can worsen estrogen dominance, which in turn worsens Adrenal Fatigue Syndrome.

Clearly, excessive estrogen is to be avoided at all cost under normal conditions. This is even more critical in Adrenal Fatigue Syndrome.

Estrogen Dominance and the OAT Axis

In addition to the conditions above, estrogen dominance shows itself in ways that are not obvious, particularly because it influences the other organs in the axis. Consider the following:

- **Estrogen dominance may increase thyroid binding proteins in the bloodstream.** Thyroid hormones are trapped in protein and less available to the cells where it is needed. This means that total thyroid blood testing may show normal, but the tissues may be insufficient in free thyroid hormone, resulting in subclinical or clinical hypothyroidism.

- **When estrogen levels are high, the adrenal cortex fails to respond to signals from the brain.** In other words, the brain might send a signal to produce more cortisol, but the adrenal response is blunted. As a result, cortisol output is suboptimal relative to the demand signal. Estrogen also impairs adrenal function by interfering with the release of cortisol from the adrenal cortex. High levels of estrogen can lead to a corresponding increase in the level of cortisol-binding globulin (proteins), which, in turn, interferes with hormonal functions and circulates in the bloodstream, binding to cortisol, and rendering it inactive.

A woman with estrogen dominance may have adequate levels of total cortisol in her bloodstream, so testing the cortisol level in the blood may render results well within the normal range. However, her free (available) cortisol level may be low. Since only free cortisol can activate receptors inside the cells, the effectiveness of cortisol is blunted at the cellular level.

Pat (age 55) in her own words:

Looking back, I experienced so many symptoms that I know identify as part of Adrenal Fatigue Syndrome. Even as a young woman, I suffered severe menstrual cramps. In my thirties, PMS symptoms became difficult to cope with. I'm a nurse, and even with medical training I didn't understand what was causing these problems. I ended up using over-the-counter PMS products, including vitamin supplements, but the bloating, sugar cravings, and breast tenderness continued to get worse.

Then, in my late thirties, I was diagnosed with large uterine fibroids along with thickened endometrial lining. When my doctor recommended a hysterectomy, I agreed to have the surgery. I experienced such heavy bleeding and irregular periods which had become another issue to cope with. Today, looking back, I regret not having more information, because if I'd known more I wouldn't have had the surgery, although I do still have my ovaries.

After the surgery I went through years of hot flashes, and I gained weight in my abdomen. Then my hair began thinning, too, and I had heart palpitations. I also lost my sex drive and had vaginal dryness. All this and a sense of apathy left me with a poor quality of life.

In my early fifties, I went through menopause, which meant I had post-menopausal levels of estrogen and progesterone, measured with several saliva tests. I used hormone creams off and on for quite a long time, but they didn't make much difference in how I felt—which was pretty awful most of the time.

Through these years I began to feel more and more tired and, ironically, I didn't sleep well either. It was no wonder I was depressed. For a time, I wondered if I could manage to keep working. A friend told me about Adrenal Fatigue Syndrome, and I did my own research. It was disturbing to learn how little information exists within the conventional medical world. I believe my doctors, and I saw a few, were well intentioned, but they offered treatments within their range of knowledge. This was too narrow, and I believe my symptoms were treated as "women's" problems, when I now understand they were related to estrogen dominance and imbalance in the OAT axis. I didn't learn that in nursing school. I made those connections when I worked with Dr. Lam and started a personalized nutritional recovery program. Today, I can trace my symptoms and AFS back to my twenties, but I also feel as if I've discovered a healthy way to live over the next phase of my life.

A Two-way Street

Just as estrogen dominance can contribute to Adrenal Fatigue Syndrome, the reverse is also true. Cortisol is made in the adrenal cortex from progesterone, and when the adrenals are weak, we see a tendency in favor of cortisol production. If the progesterone level falls, a state of relative estrogen dominance develops. This situation creates an adverse feedback loop and in everyday terms, a vicious cycle. Excessive estrogen adversely affects both thyroid and adrenal function, and, in turn, thyroid dysfunction and Adrenal Fatigue Syndrome make estrogen dominance worse.

Progesterone Deficiency and Pregnancy

Pregnancy is impossible unless sufficient progesterone is present to provide a supportive environment for the egg in the uterus throughout the gestation period. Those in Stage 3B are particularly at risk, especially if estrogen dominance exists. Even if pregnancy is achieved, frequent miscarriages occur during the first trimester. This is the time when the need for progesterone increases.

Women with severe OAT axis imbalance are invariably unable to meet this need on a sustained basis. Resulting miscarriages usually occur in the late first trimester. Those who experience serial miscarriages should therefore be on the alert for AFS and progesterone deficiency. Fortunately, this is reversible in most cases. As adrenal function is optimized, many find themselves able to regain normal pregnancy. A frequent clinical oversight is the failure to consider AFS as a possible cause of serial miscarriages among those who have a history of high stress.

Adrenals and the OAT Axis Imbalance

The adrenal glands are usually the first of the endocrine functions to break down when stress has overwhelmed the body's normal compensatory response. Unfortunately, this is seldom recognized early on as a pathological state. Individuals use socially acceptable actions to compensate for feeling tired or otherwise off. For example, increasing coffee intake often masks the underlying problem as the adrenals are put in overdrive to cover up the early signs and symptoms of Adrenal Fatigue Syndrome—and this can go on for years.

The next endocrine gland to be affected is the insulin producing portion of the pancreas. Then, blood sugar becomes imbalanced and this dysfunction is temporarily fixed by drinking sodas or various energy boosting concoctions or by eating pastries and other sweets.

The thyroid follows the pancreas. Sluggishness, feeling cold most of the time, and weight gain are the predominant symptoms that bring patients to their physicians. This is often when hypothyroidism is first diagnosed. Physicians then routinely prescribe thyroid replacement medication. However, over time, many patients taking thyroid medications remain symptomatic. Along with hypothyroidism, we see symptoms of estrogen dominance. Symptoms include PMS, endometriosis, lumpy breasts (fibrocystic changes), and irregular menstrual cycles. Hormone replacement medication may work short term, but unless the adrenals are first attended to, the patient's response is often blunted and ultimately fails.

Finally, as the body advances toward Stage 3D, the parathyroid glands, the pineal gland, the autonomic nervous system (ANS) and the hypothalamus become affected. By this time, the OAT axis is severely imbalanced.

In Stage 3B, the many symptoms of adrenal dysregulation such as hypoglycemia and low blood pressure characteristic of Stage 3A progressively worsen. Much of this is due to the continued dysregulation of the HPA axis and cortisol dysregulation. As the adrenal function is compromised, estrogen dominance increases, and thyroid function worsens.

The Picture of Hypothyroidism

The thyroid gland, which sits at the front of the neck just below the larynx (voice box), acts as the body's metabolic barometer and helps cells convert oxygen and calories into energy. It is responsible for regulating heart rate, blood pressure, body temperature, metabolism, and growth.

Thyroid 101

To explain thyroid function simply, just remember that control starts at the pituitary gland with the release of thyroid stimulating hormone (TSH). TSH signals the thyroid gland to secrete a hormone called T4 (thyroxine). T4 in turn becomes T3 (triodothyronine) or Reverse T3 (RT3). T3 then causes the cells to generate energy in the form of ATP (adenosine triphosphate, a compound that supplies large amounts of energy to the cells).

T3 is responsible for most of the biological activity of thyroid hormones. It has a higher affinity for thyroid receptors and is much more potent than T4. RT3 acts as a braking system to T3. Not only is RT3 inactive, it binds to T3 receptors and blocks the action of T3. T4 should be considered a precursor to T3 and RT3.

> **A properly functioning thyroid gland requires a perfect balance of T4, T3, and RT3. The normal production ratio of T4 to T3 is 3.3:1.**

Causes and Symptoms of Hypothyroidism

A variety of factors can contribute to the development of thyroid problems. These include:

- exposure to external environmental radiation
- radioactive iodine used for treatment of hyperthyroidism (overactive thyroid)
- special X-ray dyes
- drugs such as lithium that have anti-thyroid effects
- overconsumption of uncooked goitrogenic foods, such as broccoli, turnips, radishes, cauliflower, unfermented soy such as tofu and soy milk, and Brussels sprouts
- mercury toxicity (dental amalgams are 50 percent mercury)
- autoimmune diseases
- infection
- brain tumors

Low thyroid function generates a global or whole body response. Symptoms include:

- Fatigue and low energy with a need for daytime naps, which is caused by a defect in cellular energy conversion and difficulty in converting from T4 to T3.

- Skin that becomes dry, scaly, rough, and cold because of increased demands on metabolism, such as cold weather, with little thyroid reserve.

- Excessive unexplained hair loss due to slowing down of cell turnover and tissue/hair production.

- Sensitivity to cold in a room when others are warm, which is caused by sluggish conversion of nutrients and oxygen to heat.

- Memory impairment and/or depression due to inadequate levels of thyroid in the brain.

- Constipation that is resistant to magnesium supplementation.

- Unexplained weight gain due to reduced metabolism, which enlarges fat cells that sequester T4, causing depletion and further sluggishness.

- High cholesterol which is resistant to cholesterol lowering drugs.

- Low libido, PMS, miscarriage, and infertility, which are linked to the disruption of testosterone, estrogen, and progesterone.

- Abdominal cramping and irritable bowel syndrome (IBS) caused by reduced muscular activity of the bowel wall due to thyroid depletion.

As you can see, thyroid gland dysfunction can be linked to many of the most common health complaints, but that link—the underlying cause of many symptoms—is often missed. This is not an uncommon situation.

Thyroid Laboratory Tests

- The most important tests of thyroid function are TSH, free T4, and free T3. Free T4 and free T3 measures the biologically active (free) forms of T4 and T3 respectively. As compared to total T4 and total T3, free T4 and free T3 measure the quantity of T4 and T3 that is not bound to the blood proteins and are thus most biologically available. Normal laboratory range is 0.8-1.8 ng/L for free T4, 2.3-4.2 pg/ml for free T3, and 90-350 pg/ml for RT3.

- TSH testing reflects the blood level of TSH. The *standard reference range* for adults is between 0.5 to 5.0 µIU/mL (equivalent to mIU/L) historically. A high number means the thyroid is hard at work, thus a sign of low thyroid function. Conversely, a low number means that the thyroid is working hard, or hyperthyroid. The typical reference was changed to 0.3 to 3.0 µIU/mL in recent years to reflect a growing consensus among endocrinologists that many suffer from mild hypothyroid disorder. It was unrecognized due to an upper limit of TSH, based on epidemiological data, that was too liberal. *The therapeutic target range* TSH level for patients on treatment ranges between 0.3 to 3.0 µIU/mL. The interpretation depends also on what the blood levels of thyroid hormones (T3 and T4) are.

Primary vs. Secondary Hypothyroidism

Hypothyroidism, or low functioning thyroid, can be *primary*, which means first in order of development, or *secondary*, which develops as a result of changing conditions in other parts of the body.

Primary hypothyroidism means that the thyroid cannot make the hormones T3 and T4 because of a problem with the gland itself. In the U.S., the most common cause is destruction of the thyroid gland by the immune system. This condition is called Hashimoto's thyroiditis. Treatment usually involves thyroid replacement therapy. Primary hypothyroidism can also be caused by surgical removal of the thyroid gland, which is then followed by inadequate thyroid replacement therapy. In primary hypothyroidism, TSH is usually high. However, if hypothyroid symptoms, such as low body temperature, fatigue, dry skin, and weight gain persist, despite thyroid replacement therapy and regardless of laboratory test results, we must look elsewhere for the cause of low thyroid function.

Secondary hypothyroidism is commonly thought to be linked with issues involving the pituitary gland, hypothalamus, and/or medications such as dopamine and lithium. In recent decades, we also include what is known as non-thyroid illness syndrome (NTIS). In this situation, patients have physical signs of hypothyroidism but do not have structural problems with the thyroid gland, and the TSH is normal. For example, in those suffering from *anorexia nervosa* (an eating disorder), the thyroid dysfunction has metabolic causes that do not fit the criteria for classic hypothyroidism as defined by endocrinologists. Treatment is usually directed toward the underlying cause, and steroid replacement is usually employed in addition to surgery as needed.

Adrenal Fatigue Syndrome perhaps is a common but frequently overlooked and unrecognized condition, closely associated with and possibly a cause of secondary clinical and subclinical hypothyroidism. Thyroid test results in advanced AFS usually show normal or low free T4 and free T3. TSH can be normal or high, but body temperature is generally low consistently. Fortunately, such secondary hypothyroidism can be reversed if indeed AFS is the cause. We see many with Adrenal Fatigue Syndrome who are on thyroid medication reduce their thyroid medicine as their adrenal health improves.

Hashimoto's Thyroiditis and AFS

Hashimoto's thyroiditis is a common autoimmune condition in which individuals develop an allergy toward their thyroid gland. Thyroid gland destruction and spillage of T4 early on in the disease can lead to symptoms and the state of *hyper*thyroidism, which stresses the adrenal glands, contributing to AFS. As a compensatory reaction, the pituitary releases less TSH in order to slow down thyroid hormone production. When enough destruction has occurred, thyroid production ultimately goes down, and the person then enters the *hypo*thyroid phase. At this time, both adrenal and thyroid function becomes compromised. Anti-thyroglobulin antibodies (ATA), autoimmune antibodies, and thyroid peroxidase antibodies (TPO) are invariably present in blood tests. In early stages, we see low TSH, high free T3 and free T4. In late stages, we see normal or high TSH, low free T3, and low free T4.

Grave's disease is an autoimmune disease in which an antibody is produced that mimics the action of TSH. As a result, the thyroid gland is put on overdrive to make T4. As the T4 level rises, the pituitary compensates and tries to reduce the T4 level by reducing TSH output. Typically, we find elevation of thyroid stimulating immunoglobulin or TSI, high free T3 and free T4. Needless to say, the adrenals are extremely stressed with this type of rollercoaster ride.

As you can see, Adrenal Fatigue Syndrome only worsens if you have Hashimoto's thyroiditis or Grave's disease.

How the Thyroid Affects Other Hormones

Thyroid hormone imbalance is perhaps the single most confusing and difficult to manage of all endocrine disorders. In addition to the already complex clinical picture, treatment errors are common if the intricate OAT axis involvement is not clearly understood.

Because the thyroid regulates metabolism, it also influences the reproductive glands. For example, the thyroid influences the menstrual cycle and fertility because of its role in producing SHBG (sex hormone binding globulin), prolactin (a pituitary hormone), and GnRH (gonadotropin releasing hormone, produced in the hypothalamus). All these hormones influence the menstrual cycle and fertility. Thyroid hormones also stimulate progesterone production in the ovaries. For example, women in childbearing years who suffer from PCOS and infertility problems usually have chronically low progesterone. Untreated thyroid problems could be behind the inadequate progesterone production, and, therefore, a contributing factor in a woman's infertility. When hypothyroidism is resolved, women often spontaneously overcome infertility problems.

Likewise, thyroid abnormalities influence PMS and symptoms of menopause. It is clear that thyroid function and estrogen dominance are closely linked. Iodine, a key supportive compound for the thyroid, is one of the best natural cures for fibrocystic breast diseases, a symptom of estrogen dominance.

In addition, thyroid hormones have similarities with certain metabolites of estrogen and progesterone. Estrogen and progesterone can block or facilitate receptor sites for thyroid hormones. In practical terms, this means that imbalances of thyroid hormones T3 and T4, combined with imbalances of estrogen and progesterone, can mimic symptoms of menopause. For example, women may notice sleep disturbances, mood issues, fluid retention, body temperature issues, and reduced energy. Then, based on books or articles they've read or TV health segments they've watched, they likely believe they are approaching menopause. Testing might show normal TSH values, but these women could be in a state of subclinical hypothyroidism and not know it.

Are You Hypothyroid?

Classic symptoms of thyroid dysfunction for both women and men include fatigue, dry skin, weight gain, low body temperature, and insomnia. Given these symptoms, physicians generally order lab tests to measure thyroid function. We recommend tests measuring TSH, free T4, and free T3 tests.

Results typically show:

- normal or high TSH (thyroid stimulating hormone);
- normal or low T3 and free T3 (triodothyronine); and
- normal or low T4 and free T4 (thyroxine).

Because the range of results can be wide, laboratory tests are typically inconclusive. Clinicians lean toward a bias of diagnosing hypothyroidism if clinical symptoms are consistent with low metabolism and reduced energy output. Typically, thyroid replacement medications are then prescribed, which should bring about improvement if indeed the thyroid gland is malfunctioning.

When Thyroid Replacement is Ill Advised

We often see TSH, T4, and T3 testing in the normal range, but at the same time, the person has classic symptoms of hypothyroidism such as weight gain and fatigue. Alternatively, test results of free T4 and free T3 may be low while TSH is normal or high. Many are started on thyroid replacement medication based on symptoms alone. This is a common conventional medicine practice.

In both scenarios, thyroid replacement with T4 and T3 without first considering adrenal involvement is a common pitfall and often aggravates the OAT axis imbalance. The reason is simple: Thyroid replacement tends to increase metabolic function, which is akin to putting all systems of the body into overdrive at a time when the body is trying to rest through the down regulation mechanisms. The body wants to slow down, but the medications are designed to speed it up.

In the case of *advanced* Adrenal Fatigue Syndrome, taking thyroid medication without concurrent attention to adrenal recovery often is analogous to pouring oil onto a fire. An already weak adrenal system may not be able to carry the burden of extra energy output. This confusing situation is made worse because thyroid medication may lead to a *temporary* boost of energy and improvement of other symptoms.

Fatigue usually returns over time, because the thyroid medication further undermines the preexisting adrenal weakness and often precipitates adrenal crisis. Moreover, the fatigue increases well beyond what the thyroid medication is trying to combat. Rather than stepping back and considering that other hormonal issues may be involved, specifically, adrenal hormones, it is tempting to increase the medication dosage or switch to more powerful thyroid medication. Again, this boosts energy and relieves symptoms temporarily, but does not address the underlying problem.

Meanwhile, once patients take thyroid medications, lab tests of T4, T3, and TSH might show improvement, but the individuals don't feel better and many actually feel worse. As stated earlier, many on thyroid replacement medications continue to complain of unresolved symptoms. Sufferers and clinicians alike are easily misled by what look like improving lab test results, and they may assume that the therapy is on the right track.

When symptoms fail to improve, we see a tendency to switch from one medication to another. Physicians may start with synthetic T4, to T4/T3 blends, and ultimately, to potent T3. It's all a matter of trial and error, but meanwhile, the patient often continues to get worse. Sometimes, adverse side effects of the medications, such as heart palpitations and tremors, surface as dosages increase and the patient continues to feel fatigued and sluggish. We call this state being "wired and tired," the worst of both worlds. Being "wired and tired" occurs too frequently and just as often goes unnoted.

Then, as physicians run out of options to control symptoms, they often prescribe antidepressants. These drugs seldom work in the long run in this situation. Rather, they often make the OAT imbalance worse. These solutions do not address the reality that adrenal function plays a key role in this imbalance.

Focus on the Adrenals when Thyroid Replacement Fails

Clinicians should be on the alert that if symptoms of hypothyroidism fail to resolve, or if an ever increasing dose of thyroid medicine is necessary, AFS should be considered. When the adrenals are weak, nearly all other hormone regulated organs are affected, including the ovaries, the thyroid, and the pancreas. Put another way, in the presence of Adrenal Fatigue Syndrome, few hormones are allowed to work at their optimal levels, and that includes thyroid, insulin (produced by the pancreas), cortisol, progesterone, estrogen, and testosterone. When the adrenals are weak, the normal negative feedback loop is compromised and carrier hormones in the blood can be disrupted, which compromises the ability of each hormone to regulate and fine tune its target organ to achieve homeostasis. That might sound abstract, but this multiple hormone disruption can lead to noticeable, distressing symptoms.

The more complaints the sufferers make, the more they end up being treated for symptoms of Stage 3A, or for the weak thyroid and ovarian systems' dysfunction of Stage 3B, while the most important component, adrenal dysfunction, is ignored. This is the case with most healthy individuals seeing their doctor for fatigue and lethargy.

Those who are concurrently chronically ill fare even worse. Their adrenal functions are invariably already compromised due to preexisting conditions, such as diabetes and heart disease, just to name a few. Concurrent low adrenal and thyroid function is the clinical norm. Generally speaking, problems with adrenal function are not considered or investigated, and the focus appears to be on low thyroid function, either by symptoms alone or a combination of symptoms and abnormal laboratory test results.

> **The recovery process is best served by supporting the adrenal glands before raising the thyroid hormone.**

Again, increased circulation of the thyroid hormone often further strains the already weak adrenal glands, leading to adrenal crashes and further decompensation.

Therefore, this thyroid-only treatment does not consider the axis imbalance and so not only fails, but might make the condition worse. Conversely, an approach focusing on adrenals first often leads to spectacular results, with the ovarian and thyroid hormones rebalancing themselves as the adrenal glands recover.

> If the situation described here sounds similar to what you or someone you know is experiencing, then it goes without saying that you should investigate Adrenal Fatigue Syndrome as a possible cause of your thyroid problem. The good news is that as adrenal function normalizes, those erroneously placed on thyroid replacement invariably find they need less medication. Some may not need thyroid replacement at all as their AFS improves. Those who continue to take thyroid medicine as the adrenal recovers need to be careful to avoid being overmedicated and thus run the risk of hyperthyroidism. The ability to reduce thyroid medication represents a good gauge of improvement in adrenal function, and the credit goes to the adrenal glands, not the thyroid gland. In improving adrenal health, the need for down-regulation subsides and thyroid function suppression is lifted, leading the way to normalizing thyroid function.

Caution: Do not abruptly discontinue thyroid medications (and other natural compounds that may have stimulatory effects such as herbs and glandulars) without professional guidance. You could experience unpleasant, even intolerable, withdrawal symptoms. In rare cases, adrenal crisis may be precipitated.

Sometimes patients improve, but their lab test results lag behind. For example, free T3 and T4 continue to be low. However, patients note that their body temperature is back to normal, their energy has increased, and weight management has improved. The lesson is simple—do not rely only on laboratory tests.

Weight loss plans usually fail when the OAT axis imbalance goes unaddressed. However, once the underlying cause of the myriad symptoms is dealt with, weight loss often naturally follows.

Adrenal Fatigue Syndrome vs. Hypothyroidism—Clearing Up Confusion

For many, experiencing both low adrenal and low thyroid function is the norm rather than the exception. This is especially prevalent in women with OAT axis imbalance. They may report a consistently low body temperature. This is one big difference between primary hypothyroidism and hypothyroidism associated with AFS. The table below clarifies the key signs, symptoms, and differences between Adrenal Fatigue Syndrome and hypothyroidism:

Characteristics	Adrenal Fatigue Syndrome	Hypothyroidism
Body Measurements		
Weight	Early: gain weight; severe - cannot gain weight	Generalized weight gain
Body Temp	Consistently 97.8 or lower	Low 90s to 98.6
Temp regulation	Fluctuating and exaggerated	Steady
Mental Function		
Mental Function	Brain fog	Slow thinking
Depression	Sometimes	Frequent
Physical Looks		
Eyebrows	Full	Sparse outer 1/3
Hair	Thin, sparse on extremities	Coarse and sparse
Hair loss	Sometimes	Common
Nails	Thin, brittle	Normal to thick
Peri-orbital Tissue	Sunken	Puffy
Skin	Thin	Normal
Internal Feeling		
Ligaments Flexibility	Good	Poor
Fluid retention	No	Yes
Pain	Headache, muscular, migraines	Joints, muscles
Reactivity	Heightened and hyper-reactive	Hypo-reactive

Characteristics	Adrenal Fatigue Syndrome	Hypothyroidism
Medical Condition		
History of Infections	Common	Occasional
Chronic Fatigue	Yes	Yes
Orthostatic Hypotension	Frequent	No
Blood Sugar	Tendency toward hypoglycemia	Normal to *hyper*glycemia
Heart Palpitation	Frequent	No
GI function	Irritable or hyperactive	Constipation and hypoactive
Malabsorption	Yes	No
Sensitive to Medications	Frequent	Normal
Personality Trait		
Personality Traits	Type A	Type A or B
Obsessive Compulsive	Frequent	Mixed
Habits		
Sleep Pattern	Waking up 2-4 AM	Sleepy
Temperature Tolerance	Intolerance to cold and heat	Intolerance to heat
Food Craving	Craving for sweet and salty	Craving for fat

Despite the presence of both conditions, resolving Adrenal Fatigue Syndrome should take precedence if possible because it is the key to a total healing process.

Axis Component Dominance

Within the OAT axis imbalance, we frequently see that one component dominates, meaning that the ovaries, adrenals, and thyroid do not contribute in equal measure to the problems. The system that clinically dominates usually reflects the organ system that is constitutionally the weakest and thus most damaged. For example, symptoms of subclinical hypothyroidism may be more severe than those associated with adrenal and ovarian dysfunction.

Those who are thyroid dominant usually report lack of energy, dry skin, the inability to lose weight, and so forth. Fatigue is their chief complaint. These women are too tired to worry about PMS or being depressed, although they have symptoms of depression. The adrenal dominant type usually describes fragile emotional states such as anxiety and irritability. Like the thyroid dominant type, these individuals are tired, but the fatigue is minor in comparison to the emotional roller coaster ride they experience due to easily triggered anger or rage. Finally, the ovarian dominant type usually describes significant brain fog and memory loss, along with PMS and other symptoms of estrogen dominance.

Recognizing which component dominates the OAT axis is important in designing a comprehensive recovery program, because the nutritional support, diet, and lifestyle modifications are different for each.

During the recovery process, the type of dominance can change as well. For example, one can be thyroid dominant and progress to adrenal dominant. This can occur when the thyroid function improves or if there is an acute adrenal crash that overwhelms the thyroid. If we know which component is dominant, then clinicians can prioritize the recovery plan and time the correct support measures during the recovery period.

Because so many with Adrenal Fatigue Syndrome or a combination of hormonal imbalances are left to try to find the best remedies on their own, they are usually unaware of the OAT axis and they may not consider the way hormones work together. These individuals often adopt what we call self-guided or scattershot approaches. Some of the literature about AFS might offer a standardized approach, but without careful consideration to the types of dominance and their on-going progression, this often leads to delayed or failed recovery.

Greater Implications

We have discussed the organ systems that produce the major symptoms of OAT axis imbalance so prevalent in early Adrenal Exhaustion, but other organ systems often become involved, particularly as the imbalance advances. For example, consider digestive functions, specifically, processing and assimilating nutrients. If the OAT axis imbalance is left unattended, individuals may experience reduced absorption of nutrients from the GI track and other digestive conditions such as: leaky gut; irritable bowel syndrome (a syndrome that includes many unpleasant digestive symptoms, such as alternating diarrhea and constipation); food sensitivities that were not present before; internal dysbiosis (an imbalance of intestinal flora, which over time is linked to a variety of conditions); and reduced liver function, despite normal lab test results.

When the OAT axis is not well balanced, no organ system is spared from dysfunction.

Treatment Confusion

As we've discussed, women with OAT axis imbalance often end up seeing various specialists who may not be mindful of the organ system triad at work. The focus tends to be on either the thyroid, ovarian, or both. As long as the adrenal component is ignored, the body's ability to recover is marginalized. Not only that, unintended consequences emerge. For example, if a woman begins taking thyroid medication, she may see menstrual irregularities begin. This may be followed by problems dealing with stress and worsening fatigue.

Over time, patients are invariably disappointed and discouraged and usually move on to another specialist. Sometimes, patients give up. If they have taken antidepressants, thyroid replacements, ovarian hormones such as synthetic estrogen and progestin (or even the natural form of these hormones), or other medications, they may be worse off. Unfortunately, if patients resort to self-navigated programs, they usually end up futilely jumping from one nutritional or glandular supplement after another, or in a scattershot manner seek this or that exercise or meditation program that promises health improvements. This approach usually leads to frequent adrenal crashes and worsening conditions.

Recovery can be complex, and it is critical to address the needs of the individual based on how advanced the OAT or AT axis imbalance is. The state of estrogen dominance is an issue unto itself, and we urge you to educate yourself about this common situation. (Our mini-book Estrogen Dominance focuses on this topic and is available at *www.DrLam.com*.)

The OAT axis and the combination of symptoms and progression to Stage 3C can seem a bit abstract, but every day we see the steady path of AFS to this stage in the lives of women. In men we see the same progression to AFS through the AT axis imbalance. Fatigue, lethargy, low libido, anxiety, brain fog, and weight gain are the key symptoms for men.

Clearly, reversing Stage 3B is critical if one is to avoid the natural progression of AFS into Stage 3C, which we turn to next.

Key Points to Remember

- The body's hormonal organs are closely tied together through various axes. Though lesser known than the HPA axis, the ovarian-adrenal-thyroid (OAT) hormonal axis is extremely important.

- When the OAT axis is disrupted, there is an imbalance of hormones that leads to symptoms of estrogen dominance, low energy, and hypothyroidism.

- Each portion of the OAT axis affects the others. Imbalance of one will worsen the other and vice versa.

- Estrogen dominance worsens adrenal function, which in turn aggravates estrogen dominance.

- Adrenal Fatigue Syndrome lowers thyroid function, which in turn worsens AFS.

- The OAT axis imbalance is often missed. Symptoms of AFS and hypothyroidism are similar. Sufferers are treated for hypothyroidism when the underlying problem is adrenal function.

- It is common to stimulate thyroid function in an attempt to reduce fatigue. This strategy often fails and over time AFS tends to worsen.

- Within the OAT axis, each of the components is not equally damaged. One of the components is usually more damaged than the others, presents itself as the dominant symptom, and thus masks the other components of the axis. Knowing which component is dominant is important in the overall assessment and recovery plan.

Chapter 9

Stage 3C—Disequilibrium

As we saw in Stage 3B of Adrenal Exhaustion, sufferers experience many symptoms resulting from the disruption of major adrenal related hormonal axes. However, despite the range of symptoms, including subclinical hypothyroidism, low energy, estrogen dominance, irregular periods, and low libido in men and women, critical body functions remain relatively intact. In other words, the body as a whole still functions relatively well. Most sufferers continue to work fulltime. However, as the adrenals decompensate and enter into Phase C of Adrenal Exhaustion, the body continues to weaken, which triggers its various reserve systems to spring into action as the body loses its homeostasis and equilibrium.

Although by this time, many individuals have already sought medical help for a confusing array of symptoms that manifest in Adrenal Fatigue Syndrome, reaching this stage might drive them to look for a different approach.

Homeostasis

Homeostasis, derived from Greek, means to *stand equally*. It developed from a theory of physiology first put forth by Claude Bernard. Briefly, the theory holds that in order for a closed system to maintain equilibrium with its surrounding environment, the system requires many minute changes and dynamic internal adjustments to maintain the status quo. The human body is comprised of more than 70 trillion cells, and to be in optimum health each cell must maintain its equilibrium or homeostasis with its surrounding environment. For homeostasis to occur, the cells need to excrete waste and take in new materials in equal measure. Regulatory systems, such as the negative feedback loop and the autonomic nervous system, are needed to maintain cellular equilibrium. Therefore, we define homeostasis as the stability of the physiological systems that maintain life.

Without this equilibrium, the body is unable to perform such mundane function as standing up, maintaining stable body temperature and heart rate, and so forth. Depending on the stress placed on the regulatory systems, the needs of cells change. Outside our conscious awareness, the regulatory systems are activated automatically in order to maintain internal harmony in the body.

These systems are jeopardized in 3C of Adrenal Exhaustion. The key regulatory systems for internal equilibrium are the nervous system and the endocrine system. While the functions of both of these systems may be compromised in earlier phases, they enter into a steep slope of declining function during this phase as seen in Figure 9 below:

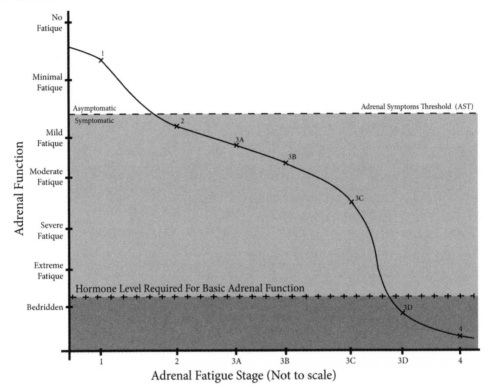

Figure 9. Adrenal Functional Decline vs. Adrenal Fatigue Stage

Put simply, the internal thermostat of the body is broken in this phase. In order to maintain normal function, the body activates compensatory systems, but unfortunately, these reserves and compensatory systems are crude at best and they lack the finely tuned capabilities of the regular systems. The key functions of the body are saved, but a variety of side effects surface. Side effects in themselves are the body's way of alerting us that it is in trouble.

In practical terms, in addition to the same symptoms seen in Stages 3A and 3B, those in 3C Adrenal Exhaustion often report the gradual or sudden onset of any of the following as this phase progresses:

- panic attacks
- onset of heart palpitations despite normal cardiac function
- onset of dizziness and lightheadedness at rest

- waking up in the middle of the night for no reason and inability to go back to sleep
- onset of fragile emotional states such as crying for no apparent reason
- fragile reactive fluid state with edema and sodium imbalance
- POTS-like symptoms (postural orthostatic tachycardia syndrome, which is rapid heart rate while arising from a supine position)

Dysfunction of the autonomic nervous system (ANS) is responsible for many of Stage 3C symptoms. In order to grasp how this occurs, it's important to take a quick and partial tour of the nervous system to see its myriad functions.

Ben (age 39) talks about his experience with Adrenal Fatigue Syndrome:

I struggled with fatigue on and off for more than ten years. I ignored it for a long time and pushed myself to overcome it. But, over a three to four year period, I reached a point where fatigue was interfering with my daily life. As a senior executive for a major corporation, I'm on the road 60-75 nights a year, and that travel drained my energy. In order to keep functioning, I needed to go to bed early, usually before 9:00 or 9:30 on a typical weeknight. Unfortunately, even after several hours sleep, I felt groggy and tired in the morning.

As my fatigue worsened, I had to give up playing golf on the weekend with my friends. I needed all my energy to keep up with my job. As time went on, I had difficulty working out, and gradually it seemed I could no longer build muscle. I experienced severe brain fog, and my blood pressure dropped and became too low. It was so frustrating to see new symptoms appear along the way, from insomnia to shakiness, if I didn't eat every two or three hours.

Of course, I saw my doctor who ordered a variety of tests, but they all came back normal, so he sent me to an endocrinologist, who ordered more tests. Then I went to an allergist and found I had some food allergies that could be causing fatigue. The change in diet didn't help, though, and neither did the herbs and vitamins my wife found for me. At one point, my family physician told me that my fatigue was in my head and antidepressants might help. Skeptical as I was, I gave the antidepressant a try but it had no effect on my exhaustion or anything else. I still felt weak and short of breath during exercise, and I didn't sleep any better, either. When the doctor said, "I guess you'll have to learn to live with this exhaustion," I knew I needed a new direction.

A Nervous System Primer

Without question, the nervous system is one of the most complex of the body's organ systems, but even a superficial understanding helps understand the manifestation of some symptoms associated with advancing Adrenal Exhaustion. Here are the basics:

The body is divided into the central nervous system (CNS, comprising the brain and spinal cord), and the peripheral nervous system.

The peripheral nervous system is in turn divided into two parts: the *somatic nervous system* that regulates skeletal muscle functions that help us deal with the outside world, and the *autonomic nervous system* (ANS) that regulates functions of the smooth muscles and glands.

The ANS is further divided into five branches:

- the parasympathetic nervous system (PNS)
- the sympathetic nervous system (SNS)
- the enteric nervous system (ENS), which regulates intestinal (enteric) functions
- the sympathetic cholinergic system (SCS) that regulates sweating
- the adrenomedullary hormonal system (AHS), also called the sympathetic adrenergic system

The nervous systems are illustrated in the following diagram:

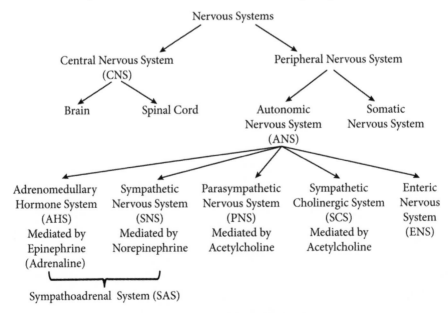

Figure 10. Nervous Systems

The PNS regulates the so-called vegetative processes such as urination and digestive functions. Dysfunction of the PNS leads to a wide variety of illnesses including abnormal gastric acid secretion, erectile dysfunction, and loss of urinary control and bowel movement irregularities.

The SNS regulates the unconscious housekeeping functions of the body at rest and during normal daily living, including blood pressure, body temperature, force of the heartbeat, and heart rate around the clock. It is absolutely necessary for handling simple stressors such as exercise, standing up, and adaptation to change in environmental temperature. Therefore, the SNS is working in the background around the clock without our knowledge. It is not only activated when we face severe stress, but in times of emergency.

The AHS regulates the emergency and distress functions such as those responsible for the body's fight-or-flight response and it has properties similar to the sympathetic nervous system (SNS), plus more. It is truly the body's responder of last resort when faced with extreme stress. Different from the SNS structurally, the nerve fibers of this system innervate the adrenal medulla directly from the spinal cord via the splanchnic nerve (paired nerves carrying fibers of the ANS) and is preganglionic (a ganglion is a biological tissue mass, most commonly a mass of nerve cell bodies). This direct highway of nerve transmission occurs at superfast speed, providing instant response by way of epinephrine (also called adrenaline) release from the adrenal medulla when the body is under stress. The AHS is activated in fainting, shock, extreme fear, hypoglycemia, and low body temperature.

The combination of SNS and the AHS constitutes the sympathoadrenal system (SAS). Maintaining a normal balance of the SAS within the autonomic nervous system is vital to optimal body function and homeostasis. This is of particular importance in the case of Adrenal Exhaustion. Dysregulation of the SAS is the hallmark of Stage 3C Adrenal Exhaustion symptoms.

Norepinephrine vs. Epinephrine

We provided information about norepinephrine in Chapter 2, *Stress, Hormone Basics, and the "Forgotten" Adrenals*, explaining that it has duo roles. It is the principle stress signaling neurotransmitter in the brain. Outside the brain, norepinephrine acts as the hormonal messenger of the sympathetic nervous system (SNS) and is responsible for making sure that our daily activities proceed smoothly.

We need to keep in mind the following:

• Norepinephrine is the chemical mother of epinephrine and they share many similar functions.

- Epinephrine is the chemical messenger of the AHS released from the adrenal medulla.

- Epinephrine is much more potent when compared to norepinephrine. Therefore, epinephrine is the ultimate emergency fight or flight hormone, with norepinephrine a helper.

- Epinephrine primarily deals with emergency functions of the body. It is also involved in the mundane functions of daily living, such as standing up and normal exercise, though in much smaller amounts.

- The exact pathophysiological mechanisms of how these two catecholamines play in many of the resulting symptoms are still not known. Many other factors are likely involved.

> Clinically, however, it appears the more advanced the adrenal weakness, the more dominant role epinephrine plays. This is likely due to an increased amount of epinephrine being released the more stress is experienced.

The Sympathoadrenal System (SAS)

Proper understanding of the SAS is a cornerstone in accurately deciphering the convoluted symptoms often present in Stage 3C. The SNS and the AHS (defined above) are two components of the SAS. Remember that norepinephrine in the brain acts as a neurotransmitter that stimulates arousal. Low levels of brain norepinephrine are associated with loss of mental alertness, poor memory, and depression. This is why medications for depression often target both dopamine and norepinephrine in an attempt to restore them to normal levels.

Mild elevations of the norepinephrine level produce heightened arousal, similar to what we experience with stimulants. This arousal is considered pleasurable and several so-called recreational/street drugs, such as cocaine and amphetamines, work by increasing the level of norepinephrine in the brain.

Moderately high levels of norepinephrine take arousal from pleasant to a level that makes us uncomfortable, such as anxiety, increased startle reflex, jumpiness, fear of crowds and tight places, impaired concentration, restless sleep, and physical changes. The physical symptoms may include rapid fatigue, muscle tension/cramps, irritability, and a sense of being on edge. Almost all anxiety disorders involve elevation in norepinephrine levels. Severe and sudden increases in norepinephrine levels are also associated with panic attacks.

Chemically, epinephrine is the son of norepinephrine, and in turn, norepinephrine is the chemical son of *dopamine*. These three chemicals, epinephrine, norepinephrine, and dopamine, fall within a family called *catecholamines* and they represent three different ways the body is regulated internally.

Transported by the blood stream once it is released from the adrenal glands, epinephrine has wide ranging effects throughout the body. Norepinephrine is also released from the adrenal medulla in smaller amounts relative to epinephrine. Released from the nerves of the SNS, norepinephrine primarily acts locally on nearby target cells such as the heart. For example, when released into the heart by the SNS, norepinephrine regulates the heart rate and it must be highly concentrated in the blood stream before it can exert its effects as a hormone.

Epinephrine is one of the most powerful vasopressor (causing a rise in blood pressure) drugs known. It increases the heart rate and the strength of heart muscle contractions. It constricts blood vessels and veins, and is also a powerful bronchodilator (relaxes the airways) and inhibits the release of histamines. Histamines are triggered by an allergic reaction. It triggers the inflammatory response. Finally, as previously mentioned, epinephrine (adrenaline) is primarily responsible for the body's emergency fight-or-flight response, not norepinephrine.

At rest, concentrations of epinephrine and norepinephrine in the blood are low, but they can rise under certain physiological (adaptation) or pathological conditions. For example, when one goes from the supine to the standing position, norepinephrine concentration increases two fold. In patients with pheochromocytoma plasma (a tumor in the adrenal gland where large amounts of catecholamines are released), symptoms consistent with excessive norepinephrine and epinephrine can surface, including: headaches, sweating, palpitations, elevated blood pressure, and anxiety.

The actions of epinephrine and norepinephrine are generally similar, but norepinephrine constricts most blood vessels, while epinephrine (adrenaline) causes constriction in many networks of minute blood vessels but dilates (opens or widens) the blood vessels in the skeletal muscles and liver. Both hormones increase the rate and force of contraction of the heart, thus increasing the output of blood from the heart and increasing the blood pressure under normal conditions.

Epinephrine and norepinephrine also have important metabolic actions. Epinephrine stimulates the breakdown of glycogen into glucose in the liver, which then causes blood sugar levels to rise. Both hormones increase the level of circulating free fatty acids. The body can then use the extra amounts of glucose and fatty acids as fuel in times of stress or danger, when increased alertness or exertion is required.

Because epinephrine is much more powerful than norepinephrine, its deployment is more tightly controlled and it is released in great amounts during times of extreme distress. It is sometimes called the emergency hormone because it is released during stress, and its stimulatory effects will fortify and prepare an animal for either fight or flight.

When the SAS is activated as a response to stress, both norepinephrine and epinephrine are released into the body.

Norepinephrine and Epinephrine (Adrenaline) Overload

Chronic or acute stress leading to Adrenal Exhaustion increases SNS as well as AHS activity as a compensatory response, which raises the absolute level of both norepinephrine and epinephrine in the body. Usually, the SNS is already in operation 24/7, helping us deal with the routine stressors of daily living. The AHS involvement is relatively minor when the body is calm. Because norepinephrine is a much weaker hormone compared to epinephrine, its systemic effects are not as prominent unless the overproduction is severe.

As Stage 3C progresses, we see clinical signs of norepinephrine overload first as the SNS is put on overdrive. The result is occasional mild heart palpitation, but it is not worrisome. Anxiety levels may increase, but not out of control. Epinephrine overload comes later as the body further weakens which puts the AHS on overdrive. Symptoms are similar to norepinephrine, only worse and more intense. Heart palpitations may be more severe requiring visits to the emergency room at times. Atrial fibrillation may be triggered. Full blown panic attacks may surface.

The following symptoms are associated with both norepinephrine and epinephrine overload. The key difference lies in intensity. The more epinephrine circulating in the body, relative to norepinephrine, the higher the intensity of symptoms. They include:

- increase in heart rate
- increase in blood sugar
- increase in respiration
- sense of impending doom
- relaxation of skeletal muscle blood vessels
- increase in energy that does not feel natural

- increase in emotional sweating

- constriction of skin blood vessels (pallor)

- trembling

Both epinephrine and norepinephrine overload worsen existing ANS imbalance, usually already present in a lesser degree in earlier phases of Adrenal Exhaustion. Because our hormones are interconnected, severe dysregulation of the SAS as seen in late Stage 3C (or borderline Stage 3D) can trigger other systems' dysfunction, including:

- severe orthostatic hypotension

- extreme fragile blood pressure

- inability to stand for more than a few minutes

- sudden onset of lightheadedness, "spaciness," and dizziness

- atrial fibrillation and premature ventricular contractions (PVCs)

- extreme temperature intolerance

- fragile body fluid and electrolyte state

- sudden onset of fainting

- sudden loss of bowel and urinary control

The Problem with the SAS

When healthy people are stressed, excess epinephrine released from the adrenal glands is quickly swept up by efficient epinephrine transporters that carry it away before it can wreak havoc inside the body. For example, standing requires blood vessels to contract to keep gravity from allowing all your blood to pool in your legs. The burden of this primarily falls on norepinephrine. Epinephrine is also released, though in a much smaller amount. The body releases just the right amount of this hormone throughout the day as we move around and change positions. Any excessive amounts of epinephrine are cleared out of the body quickly. The body's blood pressure is thus maintained in a normal state. Proper balance of epinephrine and norepinephrine within the SAS system is of paramount importance for us to feel good. Anyone who is healthy will not notice the continuous rebalancing process happening throughout the day.

On the other hand, in Stage 3C of Adrenal Exhaustion, over activation of the SAS can lead to the release of larger than normal amounts of both epinephrine and norepinephrine, especially if the AHS component is put on overdrive. This is more evident in late Stage 3C, where epinephrine seems to be the most prominent hormone flooding the body. Adrenaline rushes are common. Consistently high levels of epinephrine (and to a lesser degree, norepinephrine) may also lower the threshold of normal cardiac rhythm, triggering abnormal cardiac arrhythmias, such as atrial fibrillation and premature ventricular contraction (PVC).

As if this is not enough, those with a weak constitution may already have a reduced capacity to clear unwanted epinephrine and its metabolites from the body. This further contributes to excessive amounts circulating in the body. Increased production along with reduced clearance leads to toxic buildup of metabolites, which manifests symptoms such as panic attacks, a sense of impending doom, rage, brain fog, severe insomnia, and fatigue. Those on steroidal hormone replacement already are particularly vulnerable as their liver is invariably overtaxed much of the time serving as the major breakdown center of such medications.

While the SAS ensures the body's survival by bringing more blood supply to the brain, the fine control of the rest of the body is compromised, including the metabolic, endocrine, and central nervous systems. As a result, the body often experiences exaggerated and wild metabolic and hormonal rollercoaster rides, with accompanying fluctuations in blood sugar level, body temperature, blood pressure, heart rate, sleep, and emotional states. During an adrenal crash in this stage, AFS symptoms can become drastically exaggerated. Once the SAS is activated, it may take hours or even weeks before the body is able to return to baseline.

Those with weak adrenals constitutionally have higher tendencies to be more sensitive to excessive epinephrine/norepinephrine, and are more prone to suffer symptoms resembling a clinical condition known as dysautonomia, meaning a clinical dysfunction of the ANS. The weaker the adrenals, the stronger this association will be.

Reactive Sympathoadrenal Response (RSR) vs. Sympathetic Overtone (SO)

In the context of Adrenal Fatigue Syndrome, over-stimulation of the SAS with its resulting epinephrine and norepinephrine overload is usually a compensatory reaction of the ANS, triggered by excessive stress well beyond what the body can handle. This in turn causes the SAS to be activated and put into overdrive. The SNS and the AHS are activated, hence the name sympathoadrenal. The resulting cascade of compensatory responses is called *reactive sympathoadrenal response* (RSR), that is, reactive to another action. To put it simply, the body is bathed in a sea of both epinephrine and norepinephrine.

In contrast, norepinephrine overload as a function of an overtaxed SNS is called *sympathetic overtone* (SO). SO is generally less severe compared to RSR because norepinephrine is a less potent hormone compared to epinephrine. It tends to be more prominent in early Stage 3C while RSR more so in late Stage 3C and beyond. This has important clinical ramifications when it comes to assessing the level of adrenal weakness and planning for recovery.

HPA, SNS, and SAS

Those who are in Stage 3C Adrenal Exhaustion often concurrently experience the worsening symptoms experienced in Stages 3A and 3B, the point at which we see early system dysfunction and hormonal axis imbalance. However, keep in mind that we see tremendous overlapping of symptoms among the three phases because they are closely related. For example, in Stage 3C disruptions of the SAS affect the HPA axis that controls adrenal cortex function. We also see concurrent imbalances of the OAT or AT axis.

Because the SNS is part of the SAS, the SNS is therefore related to the HPA axis. Stimulating one system tends to inhibit the activity in the other. As the SNS outflow is increased, glucocorticoid released from the adrenal cortex is reduced. In other words, the reactive sympathoadrenal response (RSR) seen in Stage 3C, with increased secretion of epinephrine and norepinephrine, will blunt cortisol and aldosterone output. As a result, salt craving increases and low blood pressure becomes more pronounced, exacerbating Stage 3A and 3B symptoms. The body is in a no-win situation.

Sensitivity to Stressors

In Stage 3C of Adrenal Exhaustion, the body can become extraordinarily sensitive to stressors. Mundane activities may act as triggers in this phase, although these ordinary stressors do not normally behave as triggers in early stages of AFS. The threshold for stressors to act as triggers is lowered for reasons we don't fully under-stand. For example, these mundane but potential triggers include such things as:

- eating a big meal high in refined carbohydrates
- watching an action movie
- being exposed to fluorescent lighting
- taking a cold drink

- prolonged sitting in front of a computer monitor
- taking a long car drive
- being startled by the phone ringing in a quiet room
- performing a short but intense dance or exercise
- being exposed to cold or hot temperatures that the body is not used to (even though most people consider the temperature normal)
- taking an uphill or long walk
- being exposed to indirect sunlight
- drinking soda pop, tea, or coffee
- eating chocolate
- eating food that is hard to digest such as corn

Symptoms of Adrenal Fatigue Syndrome usually become drastically exaggerated during an adrenal crash in Stage 3C. Once the SAS is activated, it may take hours or even weeks before the body is able to return to baseline. This state of acute adrenal weakness, an adrenal crash, may send sufferers to the emergency room, but complete medical workups are invariably negative and don't reveal the true cause of the problem. In addition, the weaker the adrenal function, the longer it takes to recover.

Just as happens in Stages 3A and 3B, most sufferers sadly continue taking prescribed drugs for symptoms management. By this time, antidepressants or antianxiety medications may have been added in order to control symptoms that have a mental/emotional component. In the interim, conventional laboratory tests continue to be normal.

Wired and Tired

Those in Stage 3C are often concurrently burdened by worsening symptoms of Stages 3A and 3B, such as hypoglycemia, brain fog, anxiety, and so forth, plus the symptoms of hormonal axis imbalance. Because sleep is invariably disrupted, many live in a state of persistent tiredness or chronic fatigue. This is expected because the body is essentially in a slow down mode in order to conserve energy. As far as the body is concerned, the less activity the better.

At the same time, the body at this stage is usually on high alert, a state of hyper-arousal, mediated by the SAS peripherally and brain norepinephrine centrally. This is the body's ultimate way of dealing with stress: stay alert while laying low. As mentioned before, we call this wired-and-tired. As a result of being on full alert, those in this phase are typically unable to relax. Severe insomnia is the norm. Some individuals don't sleep much at night but only catch catnaps during the day. Others fall asleep only after a long wakeful period, as the tired factor finally outweighs the wired factor. However, the wired factor tends to return and periods of sleep are short. In other words, sleep patterns are severely disrupted.

As more epinephrine is released without the dampening effect of cortisol, blood pressure can suddenly rise and spike on a reactive basis, leading to an abrupt onset of intermittent higher than normal blood pressure, anxiety, and heart palpitations. When the rush is over, the body drops back down to a lower than normal level of function, resulting in lower than normal blood pressure and one becomes exhausted. Blood sugar levels can similarly be affected, with resulting subclinical *hyper*glycemia first leading to a *hypo*glycemic state characteristic of an unstable blood glucose curve, while blood sugar remains within normal limits by conventional medical standards. It comes as no surprise that the body is constantly drained of energy just having to deal with this never ending parade of disequilibrium. This downward cascade of decompensation is a true nightmare in the making.

Unexpected and Paradoxical Reactions

Starting in Stage 3C, we commonly see unexpected and paradoxical reactions to strategies that worked in early stages. These reactions can be exaggerated, unexpected, or opposite. For example, as Adrenal Exhaustion progresses through 3C and into 3D, one may not be able to tolerate vitamins, herbs, or medications that were once helpful; these substances may now produce an unexpected and unpleasant reaction. Not only do these measures fail to improve fatigue, they may make it worse. Some of these reactions include:

- When taking steroids, experiencing fatigue or malaise instead of a sense of calm.

- A sudden onset of anxiety attacks and impending doom at rest.

- Sudden onset of heart palpitations, despite normal cardiac function.

- Sudden onset of dizziness and lightheadedness at rest, after stressful situations, or after consuming certain types of food, especially carbohydrates.

- Sudden onset of fluctuating blood pressure.

- Staying in bed for an extended period of time with no energy to get up, even after a full night's rest.

- After vigorous exercise, experiencing a sense of being beaten up that lasts for days.

- Inability to think clearly and difficulty recalling even a recent problem.

- Waking up in the middle of the night for no reason and then being unable to go back to sleep.

- Being constipated instead of having loose stools when taking high doses of ascorbic acid or magnesium.

- A sense of being wired up and anxious after taking vitamins, adrenal glandular, or herbs.

- Becoming more toxic instead of feeling better when going through a detoxification program like juice fasting or cleanses.

- Sudden onset of fragile emotional states such as crying for no apparent reason.

- A sense of well-being after taking selected nutrients, only to be followed by a crash.

- Fluid retention/depletion in a setting that is highly sensitive to sodium load, which in turn is hard to maintain.

- Intolerance to certain treatments, such as acupressure, acupuncture, cranial-sacral therapy, chiropractic manipulation, and others; or, after a brief honeymoon following treatments, a crash occurs.

One can experience any combination of the above, and we don't fully know the exact cause of each of these symptoms, though it is clear that an overall dysfunctional ANS and compromised liver clearance system is responsible for many of the symptoms. We've observed that the more advanced the Adrenal Exhaustion, the more prevalent the paradoxical and unusual symptoms become as the neuroendocrine system becomes dysregulated. Collectively, they point to a body that has lost the ability to maintain the fine control necessary for a stable internal homeostasis environment.

Cognitive Toll

Physiologically, our body is in a state of cognitive hyperarousal—flooded in a sea of ever increasing brain norepinephrine while cortisol output from the adrenal gland is waning. These are automatic responses to the experience of threat.

The consequences of chronic relentless demand on the brain can also become toxic. For example, our prefrontal cortex begins to slow down. We become impulsively reactive rather than logically reflective. Our decision making process becomes blunted as our capacity to think clearly is compromised. This cognitive toll is especially serious for anyone whose work requires extensive mental function, such as executives, teachers, scientists, engineers, lawyers/judges, managers/supervisors, healthcare professionals of all kinds, and so forth. It should come as no surprise that at this stage, sufferers are invariably confused, anxious, and very frustrated.

Clearly, Stage 3C can be very debilitating. Fortunately, corrective actions are possible and the outcome generally positive. If not properly reversed, progression to Stage 3D could be likely.

Key Points to Remember

- Stage 3C is also called disequilibrium. The body's emergency systems are being activated and called to action in order to stabilize internal functions.

- Much of this alarm response is driven by the sympathetic nervous system (SNS) with its chemical messenger norepinephrine, and the adrenomedullary hormonal system (AHS) with its chemical messenger epinephrine.

- The SNS and AHS are collectively called the sympathoadrenal system (SAS).

- The hallmark of this phase is the dysregulation of the chemical messengers epinephrine and norepinephrine of the SAS.

- Symptoms common in Stage 3C include anxiety attacks, heart palpitations, electrolyte imbalances, dizziness, severe insomnia, and paradoxical reactions to medications and supplements.

- Crashes with longer than usual recovery phases are more frequent, as the body becomes more sensitive to triggers and the crash threshold is lowered.

- Routine laboratory tests continue to be negative.

Chapter 10

Stage 3D—Near Failure

The body's strategy in dealing with unrelenting stress involves reduction in energy expenditure by down-regulating nonessential functions such as metabolism, while concurrently redirecting limited internal energy resources to vital organs, such as the brain and heart. This process is well underway in previous phases of Adrenal Exhaustion, mediated largely by adrenal hormones as well as the autonomic nervous system. By the time Stage 3D is reached, the body is nearly exhausted in its effort. In this phase, the body, in its all out heroic effort to maximize chances of survival, continues to down regulate. Unfortunately, this down regulation further reduces vital hormonal output, exaggerating a downward vicious cascade. Cortisol output is low throughout the day, with both epinephrine and norepinephrine flooding the body. No system is spared from this negative impact. No wonder the clinical symptoms are convoluted and confusing to say the least.

> While survival is not in question yet, the body is severely decompensated and hormonally struggling just to make ends meet. Indeed, the adrenal system of hormonal control is near failure. What makes this clinical state perplexing is that for the most part, routine laboratory tests continue to be within or slightly outside the normal range, yet one can see the body literally falling apart internally. Sufferers will describe themselves as the living dead.

Without adequate levels of hormones to regulate various bodily organs, along with the autonomic nervous system dysregulation, the body is in disarray. We see rapid weight loss, reduced gastric assimilation, and severe loss of muscle tone as the body enters into a shutdown mode to further conserve energy. No organ is spared. Put simply, the body is on the brink of surrendering, no longer having the energy to try to work its way out of this severe weakness.

In Stage 3D therefore, the adrenals have lost most of their ability to serve as the body's stress control center and they become hypersensitive, and for reasons we don't fully understand, they react negatively to any attempts to jump start them. Much of what we know in this phase comes from clinical observation. Fortunately, only a very small percentage of those with AFS progress to this phase.

Traditional medications and nutritional supplementation that are successful in earlier stages usually backfire in Stage 3D. The body is inherently unstable. In terms of physical activity, one is often incapacitated and bedridden due to fatigue. Many people need help with daily activities such as driving, shopping, and cooking, and some may only be able to stay up and walk around for a few minutes before they become so tired they need bed rest.

We know this is the body's last resort way to conserve energy. As this takes place in one organ system, the rest of the body down regulates, too. Digestion and the removal of metabolites decreases, with a drop in the basal metabolic rate. The reproduction system is essentially shut down, evidenced by non-existent libido in men, and amenorrhea in women. No system can escape from this body wide energy conserving effort. This is a slow motion controlled collapse engineered by the body as the only way it knows to ensure survival. Understanding this helps us better interpret the many signs and symptoms of this phase.

Signs and Symptoms of Stage 3D

Consistent with an unstable body, adrenal crashes occur frequently, with much delayed recovery. In addition to previously mentioned characteristics of Stage 3C, more unpleasant symptoms may surface as follows:

- **Gastric bloating with jaw tightness after eating, and only small amounts of food or liquid can be tolerated at one time.**

For reasons not fully understood, the body seems to enter a state of clamp down, where the digestive apparatus appears to reject any attempt to ingest food. The body may resist even nourishing liquid such as chicken or beef broth. In severe cases, the individual may tolerate only a few teaspoons at a time. Rest is often needed before the next attempt.

- **Extreme sensitivity to minute doses of iodine, herbs, glandulars, and vitamins—an extreme paradoxical reaction.**

The more advanced the phase, the more this sensitivity increases. An amount as little as 10 mg of vitamin C may be too much. We can't describe the exact physiological mechanism, but poor clearance is likely an important factor. The culprit may not be the natural compound itself but the inability of the body to clear the byproducts promptly, leading to an internal build up and resulting toxic state. Forcing the body to take in more nutrients often worsens the condition over time.

- **Extreme intolerance to many vegetables, especially those high in potassium. Potassium supports your body by maintaining the balance of water and acid.**

Most in Adrenal Fatigue Syndrome are high in potassium relative to sodium, although when measured, both are within normal laboratory range. Moreover, potassium is important because it metabolizes carbohydrates and protein and helps build muscle. High potassium vegetables such as tomatoes and sweet potatoes are often problematic at this phase. Tomatoes are one of the highest potassium vegetables, with 400 mg per tomato and tomato juice can contain as much as 535 mg of potassium. A baked sweet potato with skin is also a high potassium vegetable, with 508 mg of potassium. Other high potassium vegetables with 200-300 mg of potassium include one cup of asparagus, or one half cup of cooked pumpkin. Commercially available vegetable juices as well as many popular sports drinks are also high in potassium. These are best avoided if the body cannot tolerate them. Symptoms can include nervousness, agitation, heart palpitations, gastric bloating, and gastric pain. Those who over indulge in food high in potassium are at risk of adrenal crashes.

- **Extreme nervousness and a sense of impending doom.**

The exact cause is not known, but chemical and neurotransmitter imbalances are likely involved in the central nervous system. In particular, brain norepinephrine overload is the likely culprit. Peripherally, epinephrine overload from an overactive AHS may be implicated. This can lead to a wide variety of sympathetically driven responses including sweating, anxiety, and the irregular blood pressure we commonly associate with nervousness.

- **Uncomfortable chest and head contractions when arising from a supine position.**

When occurring in the chest, these contractions are usually sharp and very different from angina pain, which is generally dull in nature. Cardiac workups are usually completely negative, with no abnormal findings. It is unclear if these contractions are due to an exaggerated musculoskeletal reflex response; a loss of blood volume on postural changes, which trigger hormonal releases that lead to muscle contraction; or overstimulation of muscles that are already in a catabolic state.

- **Extreme sensitivity to gluten, wheat, and dairy products.**

These sensitivities are quite common in Stage 3C, but tend to get worse in this phase. Just touching wheat products may initiate a reaction for those who are extremely sensitive. In other words, sensitivity increases and symptoms are more intense. Those who are constitutionally weak may have concurrent pH imbalances, which lead to imbalances of intestinal flora (dysbiosis). Common symptoms include bloating, itchiness, gastric pain, diarrhea, irritability, joint pain of unknown origin, runny nose, heart palpitations, recurrent Candida infection, and insomnia.

- **Extreme sensitivity to massage, acupuncture, sauna, detoxification, or stretching.**

Any excessive movements of the musculoskeletal system may trigger further protein breakdown, already in a catabolic state. Muscles are now fragile. Without proper collagen support, they tend to break down easily. Deep tissue massages could exacerbate this and should be avoided. Even gentle lymphatic massages may worsen the condition in this phase. This is likely due to the concurrent inability of the liver to clear toxic metabolites from the body on a timely basis from lymphatic drainage overload during the massage. Most detoxification methods, even when executed gently, carry great risk of worsening the condition.

- **Extreme fluid and electrolyte imbalances, such as dilutional hyponatremia and fragile blood pressure.**

The body appears to be in a state of disarray and confusion in fluid and electrolyte balance. One can go in and out of such imbalances rather frequently. Too much water relative to sodium balance can lead to dilutional hyponatremia (insufficient salt in body fluids). The reverse is also true. Too little fluid intake can lead to dehydration. Too much salt intake can lead to edema (too much fluid collected in body tissues). These can be triggered with the smallest amount of fluid imbalance which we usually see only in those with severe infection, trauma, shock, or kidney disease. Laboratory electrolyte studies are usually normal at first until the condition is well advanced.

- **Extreme reliance on prescription medications for sleep.**

Natural compounds with sleep supporting properties, such as tryptophan, GABA, and melatonin, seldom work at this stage. Strong prescription medications are usually required, and even then, periods of sleep don't last long. Rather, waking frequently becomes the norm. That means the body never is fully rested during the night. Even the strongest sleep medication may only produce a few good hours of sleep at a time. It's also common to wake up groggy.

- **Extreme temperature intolerance to heat, such as sunlight or a hot bath, and cold, such as an open refrigerator, a cool room, and cold water.**

The body's internal thermostat seems to malfunction. The body is unable to tolerate the normal range of external temperatures and easily tires. It may be problematic to simply leave the house and go outside, where the temperature difference is only a few degrees. The body's sweat response also appears to be dulled and is easily dehydrated, especially when outdoors. A five minute exposure to sunlight may trigger an adrenal crash. Frequent fluid replenishment is necessary.

- **Extreme high frequency of racing thoughts where the mind is unable to stop and the person feels continuously wired.**

This symptom likely occurs because the body is flooded in a sea of brain norepinephrine, but is unable to clear it in a timely basis. The more advanced the phase, the more prominent this dysfunctional clearance becomes. Unwelcome toxic metabolites build up in the brain. When it is time to sleep, the body cannot relax to allow normal sleep function to take place. Invariably, this is associated to a high degree with sleep onset insomnia, and to a lesser degree, with sleep maintenance insomnia.

- **Extreme sensitivity to televisions, computer monitors, telephones, cell phones, fluorescent lights, microwaves, cordless telephone, electric blankets, and Wi-Fi signals.**

Constant emission of electric signals and radio frequencies from wireless technology can disturb heart rate variability. This can lead to autonomic nervous system disruption, with increased sympathetic tone and reduced parasympathetic tone. Heat and vibration from such emission at the cellular level is not well tolerated. Symptoms including fatigue, headache, tingling sensation in the face, chest pain, vision difficulties, nausea, vertigo, insomnia, tremor, tachycardia, irritability and heart palpitations, can be triggered. Microwave radiation is particular harmful. Those with such sensitivity should stay at least twenty feet from any electrical appliance. Those affected, should restrict their computer, cordless phone and cell phone use.

- **Extreme overall weakness that impedes normal talking or eating.**

Stage 3D sufferers are normally locked in an advanced, overall catabolic state, and muscle mass decreases as weakness progresses. Weight loss becomes a major problem. This in turn triggers further loss of appetite as the body tries to slow down to conserve energy. This unstable positive feedback loop system is undesirable and a clear sign of a body in deep trouble. Talking becomes stressful. One feels drained after a simple phone call. Eating food is draining, because the mere action of chewing food may require energy that the body does not have. Those at this state are truly in a living hell.

- **Extreme and persistent constipation requiring enema to empty bowels.**

This is quite common in this phase. The body, in its best attempt to conserve energy, slows down all nonessential functions. As gastric motility slows, constipation becomes the norm. This forms a vicious cycle. In addition to being uncomfortable, bowels not emptied properly can lead to toxic build up which worsens this phase of AFS. Enemas may be required to help emptying, but this can worsen the already slow bowel movement over time, as the bowels get lazy with repeated and persistent enemas.

- **Extreme sensitivity to chemicals in common household items such as perfume, shampoo, and other oil-based products.**

This usually occurs when using products containing petroleum based carbon compounds with chemical structures similar to estrogen (also called xenoestrogen). We recommend using simple organic compounds instead. For example, use vinegars as disinfectants, and clean vegetables with ozonated water.

- **Fatigue worsens with small dosages of steroidal medications such as Cortef® or Florinef®.**

While using steroidal medication in severe cases of Adrenal Fatigue Syndrome may be considered, these medications are not universally well tolerated. For some, this type of medication is helpful, but it usually takes a prolonged adjustment period before the therapeutic dose is reached. In others, the medications may be rejected outright, and they might trigger an adrenal crash. Careful titration is absolutely needed, but only under the guidance of a skilled healthcare provider. We will have much more to say about this in Chapter 22, *Tools of Last Resort.*

- **Amenorrhea (absence of menstrual period).**

Amenorrhea is the norm for many women during this phase, because the body continues to selectively down regulate any nonessential functions for survival. Women who still have menses might experience irregular cycles and light menstrual flow. They commonly have PMS related symptoms from day 4 to day 14 of the menstrual cycle, as well as the days surrounding the onset of menses. The body seems to be struggling to maintain hormonal normalcy amidst a very challenging environment. Regular menstruation might return as the body recovers, and indeed, can be seen as a sign of adrenal recovery.

- **Extreme sensitivity to vibration.**

Those traveling in a car on a bumpy road may find this challenging. Only a few minutes might be tolerated, with frequent yawning and shortness of breath. We do not know the exact mechanism that triggers this.

• **Reversal of the twenty-four hour saliva cortisol curve pattern may occur.**

This phenomenon occurs from time to time, with unknown etiology. Here, the cortisol to DHEA ratio is generally high.

Positive Feedback Loop—The Final Cascade Down

During Stage 3D, positive feedback loops of the autonomic nervous system (ANS) that are inherently unstable are now in full force. They may have already been activated in earlier phases, but the clinical presentations tend to be milder when compared to this phase. These inherently unstable loops are the leading causes for the final breakdown of the body. For example, over stimulation of the AHS and SNS in Stage 3C can lead to rapid and irregular heart rate. Cardiac output may be compromised. The ability to deliver the proper amount of blood and oxygen to the body can be reduced. In severe cases, this can result in the onset of heart failure. In Stage 3D, such heart failure will in turn trigger more SNS and AHS stimulation, and thus propel the viscous cycle downward. If not resolved, the ultimate picture is one of clinical collapse.

Positive feedback loops that often play a part in worsening paradoxical reactions are already common as Stage 3 progresses. In Stage 3D, this can become amplified and exaggerated. Many try to aggressively detox or increase nutritional supplementation. Even if well-being improves in the short term, the results are often transient and usually fail over time. The body appears to reject every external effort to support the adrenal glands.

Without question, this period demonstrates the reality of the unpleasant and unpredictable paradoxical responses. Traditional dietary approaches also are seldom helpful, and the clinical outcome over time is often blunted and may fail if the body continues to decompensate. In such a case, restoring equilibrium should be the key focus. The best strategy of reversal, therefore, involves first breaking the positive feedback loop and allowing the system to stabilize.

The Living Dead

During Stage 3D, sufferers usually become very frustrated as they are left to self navigate. Incredibly, laboratory tests continue to be normal, but in this stage the body is literally falling apart internally. Sufferers at this stage are often incapacitated and frequently refer to themselves as the living dead, existing, but not really living normally.

Progression to 3D from earlier phases can be gradual or abrupt. It is not uncommon to see a stressful event (e.g. death of a loved one, excessive exercise, overwork, medication intolerance, excessive overload of steroids from medications, and infectious processes, such as insect bites or pneumonia) overwhelm the already decompensated and constitutionally weak adrenals. In these situations, the descent into 3D can be rapid, even occurring within days or weeks.

Self navigation is *not* for Stage 3D. Unless the vital signs are unstable, laboratory tests usually do not help but simply add to the confusion. Without timely reversal, the natural progression of Stage 3D conditions to cause further decompensation and, ultimately, collapse. It is possible to improve with a comprehensive nutritional recovery program, but this requires considerable patience, with no guarantee of success. It may take months just to stabilize such a damaged body before any reversal can begin.

If you think this profile fits you, then please refer to Appendix A for guidelines for finding a practitioner to help you. That is your biggest task.

Key Points to Remember

- The level of key adrenal hormones such as cortisol or aldosterone fall below the level needed for normal basic adrenal function, but this is yet to be classified as severely pathological by conventional medical standards.

- The body is in full survival mode. The focus is to maintain all essential functions, while turning off all nonessential functions.

- Symptoms of fatigue and dysregulation become extreme. One is usually bedridden most of the day, and ambulatory help is needed to carry out normal daily chores and self care functions.

- Extreme sensitivity to all medication and nutritional supplements is the norm.

- Almost all attempts to jump start the adrenals that were previously successful backfire, and the body enters a shutdown mode to conserve remaining energy.

- Symptoms include extreme fatigue, extreme constipation, extreme food sensitivity, and extreme paradoxical reactions to nutrients and medications.

- Clinicians give up and patients are released to self navigate.

Chapter 11

Diagnostic Tests—What You Need to Know

Developments in modern medicine allow us a wide array of laboratory tests designed to help diagnose certain disease states, along with measuring the severity of the disease and the burden on the body. We have literally thousands of tests available to us, but your doctors must choose the correct ones to evaluate whether you have Adrenal Fatigue Syndrome, and they must understand the limitations of these tests.

Routine Laboratory Tests for Fatigue

The most common AFS symptoms patients report to their doctors include: lack of energy, lethargy, dizziness, insomnia, hypoglycemia, low blood pressure, and anxiety. In an otherwise healthy person, conventional medicine workups to investigate these symptoms include:

- Hematology, a complete blood count (CBC) to detect or rule out anemia which measures red cells, white cells, and platelets.

- Biochemistry to rule out systemic organ damage such as liver and kidney disease.

- Inflammation in the blood through the ESR, *erythrocyte sedimentation rate,* and *C reactive protein,* both markers for inflammation.

- Cancer markers for early detection of cancer.

- Blood sugar levels to rule out diabetes mellitus and glucose intolerance.

- Urine testing to rule out infection or kidney damage.

- Fecal occult blood to rule out bleeding from the gut and to screen for cancer.

- Electrolyte panel to assess kidney function.

- Thyroid stimulating hormone, T4, and T3 levels to rule out thyroid malfunction.

These tests can detect *macroscopic* pathology such as major organ failure in the form of diabetes, heart disease, metabolic dysfunction, cancer, liver failure, kidney failure, and thyroid diseases. Unfortunately, these routine tests do not detect organ dysfunction at the subclinical level, such as those afflicted with subclinical hypothyroidism, Adrenal Fatigue Syndrome, mild liver dysfunction, subclinical imbalanced electrolyte function, minor hormonal imbalances, and suboptimal detoxification capacity. In addition, many conventional physicians pay little if any attention to laboratory values that lie close to or just outside of normal range, both at the low- or high-normal levels.

We also have a wide array of standardized testing protocols. These protocols are well intentioned in that they are meant to efficiently detect most common medical problems with both accuracy and speed. However if patients' results fall within the statistical norm, regardless of symptoms, the patient is often considered normal even though they suffer from unpleasant symptoms. Conventional medicine testing is limited in these cases. Saying that nothing is wrong often leads patients to embark on various kinds of programs on their own.

Complex conditions like Adrenal Fatigue Syndrome, subclinical hypothyroidism, chronic fatigue syndrome and tension myositis syndrome are difficult to evaluate precisely because routine laboratory values usually fall into the standard normal range. Even when laboratory tests indicate abnormalities, many doctors are unable to correlate these clinical findings if the patient's symptoms, often referred to as "presentation," are confusing or convoluted, as we often see with AFS. It's no wonder patients are frustrated when they feel tired and lethargic, among other symptoms, but they are deemed well.

Before we had super-sophisticated testing, physicians relied primarily on detailed histories and physical examinations. Laboratory values were used to confirm a diagnosis or clear up doubt.

> Sadly, thorough examinations and taking detailed histories are fast becoming lost arts. The results are alarming because ill people are sent home after being told the laboratory says they are well. This is why so many patients struggle alone, going from one specialist to another. Often feeling abandoned, they fall into despair.

When Normal is *Not* Normal

Considering the sophistication of modern medicine, most find it hard to believe that a person with symptoms of AFS could end up with normal laboratory test results. Consider the following:

- Most AFS sufferers have low immune function, so they have frequent infections. However, a blood test shows a normal white cell count. What is poorly understood or ignored is that normal or low normal white cell counts can be a sign of poor immune function. As well, nutritional deficiencies, such as low zinc, magnesium, B vitamins, and essential fatty acids can contribute to poor immune functions, so a normal white cell count does not rule out these problems at the subclinical level.

- Normal platelet count does not rule out stealth viruses or a residual bacterial infection, such as that seen in post-acute Epstein-Barr (EBV) virus infection. This is a member of the herpes virus family and one of the most common human viruses. Low or low normal platelet count can be a sign of toxic stress from viral causes or emotional forces.

- A normal fasting blood sugar in absolute terms, but with symptoms of clinical hypoglycemia present, is common in advanced stages of AFS.

- Normal electrolyte levels do not rule out the presence of debilitating subclinical dilutional hyponatremia as seen in advanced Adrenal Fatigue Syndrome.

- A normal TSH, free T3, and free T4 do not rule out secondary subclinical hypothyroidism associated with adrenal and neuroendocrine dysfunction. Similarly, a normal TSH can be present in those with clinical hypothyroidism. In other words, you can be suffering from primary hypothyroidism clinically but have normal TSH levels. *In fact, current conventional medicine protocol calls for starting a patient on thyroid medication based on significant symptoms alone even if TSH is normal.*

- We often see normal blood aldosterone and sodium levels accompanied by salt craving and low blood pressure in sufferers of advanced AFS.

- Normal potassium levels do not rule out the need to reduce the internal potassium load. In Adrenal Fatigue Syndrome, sodium depletion is common, leading to a relative (and not absolute) potassium overload that when tested is still within normal laboratory range.

- High normal liver enzymes usually suggest liver dysfunction, typically from chemicals such as medications or resulting from poor nutritional status. Normal liver enzymes are commonly associated with suboptimal clearance of metabolites in AFS as the body slows down to conserve energy.

- High normal or high total cholesterol could mean low levels of vitamin D and is commonly associated with hypothyroidism.

> **Many chronic illnesses, including AFS, progress over time slowly. Relying solely on routine blood serum laboratory tests for a definitive assessment is an extremely incomplete approach.**

Functional Laboratory Testing

Functional and specialized laboratory testing go beyond standard testing and offer a window of insight into the way our bodies are working. These tests generally focus on the endocrine, gastrointestinal, immunology, and metabolic systems, along with the nutritional function of the body.

Some of the most popular specialized tests, but not necessarily what is needed in most cases, include:

- *Organic acids urinary analysis* to assess the efficiency of cellular energy production and metabolic toxicity.

- *Neurotransmitter assessments* to determine serotonin, dopamine, GABA, and epinephrine/norepinephrine levels.

- *Digestive stool analysis* to gain information about intestinal absorption, intestinal metabolism, enzyme level markers, stool pH, detection of pathogenic microorganisms, levels of beneficial bacteria, fecal color and occult blood, and gut immune function via IgA levels.

- Small intestine bacterial overgrowth breath test *for assessment of bloating, gas, diarrhea, and irregular abdominal pain.*

- *Intestinal permeability analysis for assessing leaky gut, irritable bowl, and malabsorption syndromes.*

- *Liver detoxification tests*, including various challenge tests to evaluate the detoxification pathway and capacity.

- *Immunoglobulin testing* to evaluate the classical immediate reaction (IgE allergy) to pollen, or the delayed reaction (IgG allergy) results from poor digestion and leaky gut syndrome. Both are prevalent in AFS and environmental illnesses. These tests can also be helpful to assess toxic reactions from residual infections such as that caused by Epstein-Barr virus and Candida.

Other potentially helpful tests include:

- *Lyme disease testing*, because this can mimic AFS.

- ATP/cellular energy tests to assess mitochondrial function (the energy producing structures in the cells).

- Bone resorption assessment to identify early bone loss.

- Melatonin profile for assessment of circadian pattern and seasonal affective disorder (SAD).

- Amino acid analysis to assess chronic fatigue, depression, and immune problems.

- Essential and metabolic fatty acids analysis to assess inflammatory reactions.

- Urine iodine with pre- and post-loading tests to identify iodine/iodide sufficiency.

- Helicobacter pylori specific antigen (HpSA) stool tests to determine if the stomach and duodenum contain H. pylori, which is a major cause of peptic ulcers.

As you can see, the list is long, and one can become overwhelmed. However, as with other tests, each functional test offers a narrow peek into the inner workings of the body from a specific perspective, but is seldom definitively diagnostic. Normal values do not rule out pathology, and abnormal values require clinical correlation to make sense.

> With modern technology there is a tendency to over-test. If we perform enough tests, it is almost impossible not to find some small abnormality. However, that doesn't mean that each abnormality needs to be acted on. In fact, some abnormalities may not pose a health threat at all, but the unnecessary treatment can actually hurt you. Some of the most common overused tests include whole body scans, virtual colonoscopies, and high tech mammography.

Treating the Numbers

We often see a rush to treat patients based on abnormal lab values rather than through the whole person approach. We can call this "medicine by the numbers." It's a common clinical approach, but as with regular blood tests, reference ranges for functional testing are not perfect. In addition, tremendous statistical variation exists. What is applicable to a general population group may not be applicable to any given individual. Patients need astute, open minded clinicians to know what tests to order and how to correlate the laboratory findings with the clinical history in order to make sense of these test results.

Experienced clinicians know what to look for, along with the pros and cons of each test. However, *patients* must be aware of the pros and cons of clinical tests, too. As an example, the following tests are frequently ordered but are seldom necessary for assessment of Adrenal Fatigue Syndrome, for reasons outlined:

- *Serum (blood) magnesium:* This test doesn't tell us about the magnesium where it counts—inside the cell. To really look at magnesium closely, an intracellular magnesium level test should be ordered.

- *Total T4 and total T3 (for thyroid function):* This test doesn't tell us what counts. A *free* T3 and *free* T4 are required.

- *Serum (blood) essential fatty acids:* Deficiencies are nearly universal, so we don't need to measure them.

- *Serum (blood) vitamins A, C, and E:* Since deficiencies are widespread, we don't need a test to confirm them.

- *Vitamin B profile, including thiamin (B1), riboflavin (B2), niacin (B3), vitamin B6, folic acid, vitamin B12:* Deficiencies are pandemic, so we don't need to test.

- *Serum test for estrogen and progesterone:* Doesn't tell us the free levels present, which is what is important.

Laboratory Tests Specific to Adrenal Fatigue Syndrome

As we've said, AFS is difficult to evaluate with traditional blood tests. Those available are designed to detect the severe, absolute deficiencies of adrenal hormones that characterize Addison's disease. Blood testing is also useful to detect extreme, excessive levels of adrenal hormones associated with Cushing's disease. In other words, available blood tests measure adrenal hormones only at the extremes.

For a minute, picture a bell curve. The ACTH (adrenocorticotropic hormone) challenge test is the standard acceptable test for definitive diagnosis of Addison's disease. It reveals extreme underproduction of adrenal cortisol output, as shown by the bottom few percent of the bell curve. This means adrenal function must be extremely low in order to fit a recognized diagnosis. However, symptoms of non-Addison's adrenal weakness and low cortisol output can begin to appear after a moderate deviation from the mean on the bell curve. Therefore, the adrenal glands could be functioning well below the norm and not be detected by the ACTH test.

What this tells us is that a test result showing so-called *normal* levels of adrenal hormones does not mean that one is free from adrenal malfunction at the subclinical level. As long as one is not on alert for AFS, these blood tests lead to misguided interpretations. Many tested for adrenal function are told the results are well within the *normal* range, but in reality, their adrenal glands are performing sub-optimally; meanwhile, clear signs and symptoms continue as the body cries out for help and attention.

Serum (blood) and *urine* laboratory studies are commonly used. Unfortunately, they cannot be relied upon for accurate diagnosis. They can indicate AFS indirectly. For example, a morning serum cortisol level of under 15 mcg/dL (normal range 5-23 mcg/dL), or a mid-afternoon level of under 10 mg/dL (normal range 3-16 mg/dL) may serve as warning of sign of underlying AFS when accompanied with symptoms of fatigue. A 24 hour urine cortisol with results in the lower 1/3 of normal reference range also serves as alert of AFS. It should be remembered that most AFS sufferers have normal serum and urine cortisol levels.

Serum tests of two surrogate markers of adrenal function, cortisol and DHEA (measured in the blood by way of DHEA-S) and their ratio can tell us if the body is in an anabolic state (build up) or catabolic state (breakdown). However, these blood levels alone do not provide clear evidence of AFS.

Saliva testing: We can test adrenal health by measuring levels of key adrenal hormones such as cortisol, progesterone, estrogen, testosterone and DHEA in the saliva. A saliva test is more accurate than blood tests to measure free and circulating amounts of both cortisol and DHEA, as opposed to the total amount, which is what is measured in the blood.

> We can measure DHEA at any time during the day, but cortisol levels vary throughout the day. Generally they're at their highest in the morning and lowest in the evening before bedtime. For this reason, the recommended tests require four saliva samples taken at 8:00 AM, 12:00 PM, 5:00 PM, and before bedtime.

Multiple saliva samples give us the ability to map the daily curve of free cortisol in the body relative to DHEA levels, allowing us to have a much clearer picture of adrenal function. The following are general correlations on how saliva cortisol and DHEA levels relate to Adrenal Fatigue Syndrome:

- Normal cortisol, normal DHEA does not rule out AFS.

- Normal cortisol, high DHEA points to early stages of AFS or excessive DHEA intake.

- High cortisol, normal DHEA points to early AFS as the body puts out more cortisol relative to DHEA as part of the stress response.

- High cortisol, low DHEA usually points to early phases of Stage 3 AFS.

- Low cortisol, low DHEA usually is associated with late phases of Adrenal Exhaustion.

The above correlations are very general, and we see many exceptions to the rule. It gives you a general idea that proper interpretation is much more than simply looking at the absolute numbers on a laboratory report. In addition, paradoxical values are common, especially in those who have a sensitive body or are in advanced AFS. Delayed response needs to be factored in as well.

How to Properly Interpret Saliva Cortisol Test

Saliva cortisol test has many limitations. Results can be confusing and oftentimes defy conventional medical logic. To be useful, saliva cortisol levels must be viewed in the proper context. Keep in mind the following:

- Morning free cortisol level is indicative of peak cortisol output modulated by the HPA axis.

- Lunch cortisol level points more toward cortisol adaptability.

- Mid-afternoon cortisol is highly associated with metabolic issues such as blood sugar imbalances.

- Evening cortisol level refers to baseline adrenal cortisol function. As AFS advances, the daily cortisol diurnal curve changes, as shown in Figure 11.

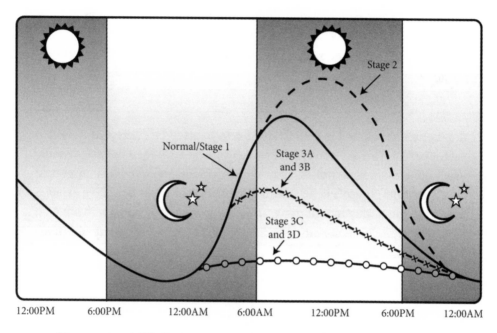

Figure 11. AFS Stages and Circadian Release Of Cortisol

Those in Stage 2 generally see a rise in total cortisol output, especially in the morning which can linger well into the afternoon as the adrenal cortex is put on overdrive. Those in early phases of Stage 3 will see morning cortisol declining from a high level back to normal, and then as Stage 3 progresses, the morning cortisol level becomes low. Most in Stage 3C or later experience flat cortisol output throughout the day. The 24 hour cortisol curve is flat, as shown above.

Many exceptions exist to the above generalizations, so we can't rely totally on a test result to make clinical decisions. For example, some who are in Stage 2 show high evening cortisol but low or normal morning cortisol. These individuals tend to have low energy in the morning but are alert as evening arrives. Then, despite high evening cortisol, they often sleep well and don't have sleep onset insomnia that commonly plagues those with elevated evening cortisol. Even after a night's rest, though, they tend to be sluggish in the morning. Others may show both high noon and nighttime cortisol levels, with normal morning and afternoon levels. This may be reflective of the body's erratic response to increase cortisol output during the day when faced with episodic stressor events.

For reasons not well understood, some clinically in Stage 3 may exhibit Stage 2 Adrenal Fatigue Syndrome cortisol curve pattern. A small number of people can have a totally normal cortisol curve while in late phases of Stage 3. This should alert us to further investigate whether other conditions are the ultimate root cause. It should be clear that proper clinical correlation is critical. Few test results are straightforward. Over reliance on cortisol values alone as a yardstick of adrenal function can therefore be misleading.

> Another pitfall is that it is easy to stay overly focused on cortisol as the main culprit of AFS. This is a common mistake. One doesn't need to have a statistically abnormal saliva cortisol curve to have AFS. In fact, some healthy people have abnormal cortisol curves, and not every abnormal cortisol curve exhibits itself as Adrenal Fatigue Syndrome. Those who are preoccupied with bringing the cortisol level back to normal as the main goal of recovery invariably fail.

Remember that AFS is a complex condition with many causes. In advance stages, the entire neuroendocrine system is dysregulated. Low cortisol is but one of many parameters to consider. As mentioned earlier, a small number of sufferers in advanced stages of AFS can present with totally normal twenty-four hour cortisol patterns, but yet they clinically present with all the classic symptoms. Saliva test as an absolute diagnostic tool for AFS leaves much to be desired and is far from perfect.

In addition, be wary of computerized laboratory interpretations, as they have limited value. In fact, it can be misleading if we fail to match the different cortisol values with the body's symptoms throughout the day along with the clinical state.

> Note: If you are taking oral hormones or applying topical supplemental hormone creams such as DHEA, steroid, insulin, or pregnenolone, the saliva or blood test results may be elevated. False elevation can also occur if the test is done within 90 minutes of exercise, in times of unusual stress, within 6 hours of caffeine intake, or within a few hours after a physical injury. It is best to avoid taking hormone supplements well before testing. Those who are on prescription medications are particularly vulnerable to inaccurate test results. Drugs such as oral contraceptives, thyroid medications, pain medications, SSRIs, benzodiazepines for anxiety, statins for lipid control, and

anti-epileptics can lead to a flattened 24 hour cortisol curve due to blunting of cortisol release.

Stress is another factor to consider at the time of testing. Cortisol levels tested after a quiet and relaxing morning may be different from those taken when you are under tremendous stress.

Warning: Cortisol and other hormonal levels vary widely among individuals; in addition, the body is in a constantly changing state. Because of these variables you should agree to undergo these laboratory tests only with professional guidance and the reassurance that these tests are both relevant and cost effective. Not to be forgotten is the fact that not all laboratories are of the same quality as well.

As you know by now, Adrenal Fatigue Syndrome symptoms can be numerous and severe while at the same time, laboratory results are normal. The reverse is also true. The test results could show abnormal levels of cortisol and DHEA, but one might not be experiencing symptoms. Furthermore, in advanced Adrenal Fatigue Syndrome, the twenty-four hour saliva cortisol curve invariably becomes flattened most of the time and can stay that way for an extended period, even during recovery. Sometimes we see a delayed response, which means the test results may be confusing and misleading and show no meaningful change while symptoms are improving.

Suffice it to say, overreliance on tests is a common adrenal recovery mistake.

Saliva testing is best used in serial studies performed only as needed for comparative purposes. Relying on a single hormonal snapshot to draw clinical conclusions is another common mistake in recovery. This is especially common among those who are not under professional guidance. For example, patients may rely on laboratory tests without understanding their limitations. They then embark on a self guided nutritional recovery program that eventually leads to improper use of nutrients, thus making the condition worse. Again, a thorough history taken by an astute and experienced clinician is superior to lab tests and is the most accurate way to assess AFS status. If you are not sure if you have AFS, need a baseline picture, or if you are not recovering from AFS, the saliva cortisol test can be very helpful, provided that it is always properly interpreted by an experienced and qualified health professional who knows your history.

Key Points to Remember

- Routine diagnostic tests as part of the workup for fatigue and a low energy state are normally negative.

- Normal test results may indicate underlying abnormal function, but this is often overlooked.

- Functional laboratory testing can be helpful, but most are not needed.

- Many are treated based on numbers and test results, especially those with abnormal laboratory thyroid function results. Some are given thyroid replacement medication based on symptoms alone.

- Laboratory tests specific for Adrenal Fatigue Syndrome also are not conclusive and, to be of value, require proper interpretation.

- Saliva cortisol tests, in particular, are often misinterpreted.

- Single saliva tests are often misleading as the results vary widely among individuals.

- Saliva testing is best used in serial studies and only as needed by a practitioner who knows what to look for.

- In determining AFS status, a thorough history taken by an astute and experienced clinician is far superior to laboratory tests.

Chapter 12

The Adrenal Crash and Recovery Cycle

Adrenal crashes are very common and almost every person with Adrenal Fatigue Syndrome has experienced them. We define adrenal crash as *a state of acute adrenal weakness*. The body's compensatory mechanism to stress has been overwhelmed. To ensure survival, the body initiates a series of actions designed to conserve energy. An adrenal crash represents such an effort by the body as it down regulates and returns us to the most basic form of survival—a vegetative state.

> **Crashes are usually characterized by severe fatigue, and, in extreme cases, incapacitation.**

Many individuals in Stages 1 and 2 of Adrenal Fatigue Syndrome have experienced adrenal crashes, but they often are not aware of it. They may be aware of incidents or periods of stress and fatigue, perhaps with loss of stamina and disturbed sleep. But these symptoms pass as the body recovers. These early stages of AFS can last for years and even decades before progressing to the later stages.

However, as AFS progresses, the crashes become more frequent and severe, ultimately, in many cases, moving into Stage 3 phases. As symptoms increase, many people report them to their doctors, at which point, they are often diagnosed as individual health problems, such as hypothyroidism, PMS, or depression. The adrenals are seldom identified as the potential source of the symptoms.

The First Alarm Bells Ring

Crashes are usually the first alarm bells to ring early on in Adrenal Fatigue Syndrome. However, more to the point, those who have never heard of AFS are also familiar with crashes. Given the general attitudes about cycles of fatigue, these crashes can appear completely harmless, even normal, which helps explain why Stage 1 and even Stage 2 can go on for years or decades.

For example, many people expect to have short periods of extreme fatigue or exhaustion, which spontaneously improve immediately after taking a nap or resorting to a sugar fix. In fact, in our society, a sugar fix has long been considered a normal response to a midmorning or mid-afternoon slump, which we can liken to a minor crash. Drinking a great deal of coffee can bring on a caffeine crash after the stimulating effect of caffeine has worn off. Overwork, excessive exercise, crowded schedules, and so forth can bring on fatigue, which is often viewed as a normal part of life. Many individuals often say aloud that all they need are "a few days off," or, "a good night's sleep," or "the emergency crisis at work to end."

With time, however, these crashes become more frequent and intense. As AFS becomes more severe, perhaps progressing into Stage 3, a crash can be triggered by something as simple as taking a longer than usual walk, and it can last for weeks and even months in extreme cases. Of course, these crashes can vary greatly in intensity, depending on the stage of Adrenal Fatigue Syndrome.

> With each crash, the body usually recovers on its own, or the individual perceives that things are back to normal. However, internally, the body gets weaker with each crash. A good recovery program is not measured only by the speed of recovery, but also by the absence of adrenal crashes along the way.

If not properly nurtured back to full function, these small crashes become more frequent and intense. Over time, as the body gets weaker, the recovery time also lengthens. This means that if no steps are taken to repair the damage, the body enters Stage 1 of Adrenal Fatigue Syndrome and slowly gets worse, advancing to Stages 2 and 3, and ultimately to adrenal failure. This is why everyone needs to be aware of AFS; understanding stress and the adrenals help us protect the body by living in such a way as to avoid the serious stages of AFS.

Minor crashes might be infrequent during the early stages of AFS (Stages 1 and 2), but can occur every few days in late stages (Stages 3 and 4). *Major* crashes usually occur only once every few years in early AFS, but can occur as frequently as every few weeks in Stage 3. In such cases, the body never has a chance to fully recover, but instead goes through one crash cycle after another. In the absence of corrective steps that nurture the adrenals back to health, the body becomes preoccupied with fighting the crashes, along with trying to recover and function normally.

Recurrent crashes mean that the body's emergency system is frequently reactivated in order to overcome the crash, and the body is in a constant state of alertness. This eventually drains the body of energy, finally leading to a state of chronic fatigue and physical exhaustion. In severe cases (Adrenal Exhaustion, Stage 3C or 3D or beyond), sufferers may be bedridden in a state of what we've heard described as the living dead. Further, on the outside, these individuals often appear normal, but internally they can barely function.

Adrenal Crash and Recovery Cycle Anatomy

The complete crash and recovery cycle is broken down into two phases:

- *Crash Phase*, where the body decompensates with worsening debilitation.

- *Recovery Phase*, where bodily functions are gradually restored to the pre-crash level of function.

The most prominent symptom during the crash phase is fatigue, which results from dysfunctional and dysregulated hormonal and metabolic pathways. Therefore, gauging the energy level during the crash phase gives us the most accurate indication of the severity of the crash over time. We lack laboratory tests to quantify this objectively, but we can say that the more symptoms experienced and the relative intensity of those symptoms indicates the depth and severity of the crash.

> **The recovery phase is marked by a gradual return to a pre-crash level of adrenal function and energy, with unpleasant symptoms resolving as recovery proceeds.**

Looking at the more advanced stages, Stage 3C specifically, the recovery phase is further broken down into a stabilization period followed by one or more mini-recovery cycles, each consisting of a *preparation* period, a *honeymoon* period, and a *plateau* period. Think of these three sequential periods as moving up a set of stairs, as the diagram below illustrates. Overall, successful recovery plans consist of multiple "S" curves in an upward sustained series without major downward crashes interfering.

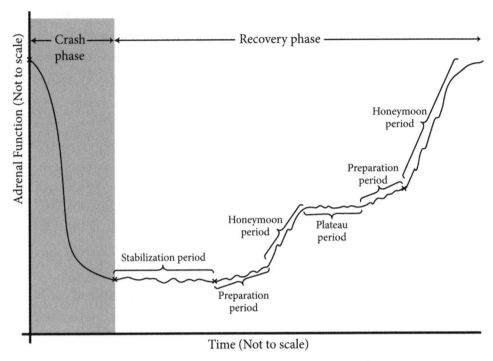

Figure 12. Adrenal Crash and Recovery Curve

The stair step graph above illustrates the following:

Stabilization Period: Immediately after an adrenal crash, and prior to the initial mini-recovery leg up, we usually see a stabilization period during which the body no longer decompensates, but instead, gradually settles into a steady state of lowered function. As we shall see, this stabilization period plays a significant role in the overall recovery phase. We understand that a person is relieved that the worst is over, but we also caution that the unpleasant symptoms can come back at any time.

Preparation Period: Depending on the stage of AFS, this period normally lasts from a few hours to a few weeks. When adrenal function is strong, as in early stages, the duration is short. During this time, sufferers may not feel any significant energy difference, even if they are taking new supplements or increased dosages of current supplements. However, they often feel a sense of improved control, along with a much lessened sense of impending doom. Although the fatigue continues, if individuals pay attention, they experience subtle improvement. In this phase, the body builds its lost reserve and becomes stronger internally. However, it's not uncommon to feel worse from time to time.

Honeymoon Period: Usually following the preparation period, this period can last a few days to weeks—if the preparation period is carried out properly. Here, too, the duration is highly dependent on the stage of AFS, and generally speaking, the earlier the stage the longer this period can last. The weaker the adrenal function, the more short-lived this period tends to be, unless patients are guided by experienced clinicians. During this time the body is better able to handle stress; we see reduced fatigue, heart palpitations and brain fog often dissipate, anxiety attacks diminish, blood pressure begins to stabilize, and functional sleep returns.

We might see mini-crashes and setbacks from time to time that last a few days. Many find these more tolerable than previous mini-crashes, and recovery is faster. Sufferers often report an overall sense of well being, as if a burden has been lifted from their shoulders, and they tend to generally be optimistic again.

Plateau Period: Here, the body has stabilized. The duration of the plateau varies, from a few weeks to a few months or more. In early stages of Adrenal Fatigue Syndrome, this generally asymptomatic phase can go on for years, but in later stages, we see a more dismal picture. For example, sufferers must slowly adapt to an overall lower energy level. If adrenal function is already at its maximum point, then individuals can be stuck, without upward progress, for a long time.

> We also see that many on self-guided programs are unable to rise to the next cycle, because they lack the knowledge needed for ample foresight and planning. Perhaps the most trying time in the recovery cycle, sufferers often grow impatient, usually because they interpret the lack of continued and sustained improvement as failure.

The temptation is to jump from one doctor to another in search of quick results. Especially among those with advanced weakness, most Adrenal Fatigue Syndrome sufferers go through multiple crash and recovery cycles over time. If we carefully analyze and compare triggers and accompanying symptoms of each cycle over time, we are often able to gauge overall adrenal function.

Looking for Causes of Adrenal Crashes

If we look deep enough, we can see that all adrenal crashes are precipitated by some kind of stressor event. Some might appear obvious, such as the death of a loved one or a major life change, such as loss of a job, a relationship, or a home. Or, the event is minor and frequently overlooked, such as taking an extra long walk, a sugar binge, or working a day or two of overtime.

Although small crashes often elude detection, it's extremely important that we investigate the cause of each crash, because history is likely to repeat itself and the same stressor will predictably trigger subsequent crashes. We must understand what triggered the current crash and take steps to prevent recurrence.

Throughout this book, we list various causes of AFS and the kinds of stressors that come into play. Just to emphasize the point that any kind of stress can trigger a crash, we've added another sample list of *everyday* situational stressors that can trigger adrenal crashes. They include: overwork; dehydration; long road trips; vacation; dental procedures; infection; overexposure to sun; lack of sleep; for males, sexual intercourse with ejaculation; drinking soda or coffee; medication withdrawals, especially steroids; thyroid medication sensitivity, especially T3; infection such as the flu or those caused by insect bites; overmedication, such as the use of steroids and anesthesia with epinephrine; and investigative procedures such as an ACTH stimulation test.

Still more stressor triggers include: overuse of stimulating supplements, heavy metal toxicity, excessive exercise, exposure to heat such as sauna or steam room, exposure to toxic fumes, prolonged standing, becoming overly anxious, relationship difficulties, long airplane trips, moving/relocating, overly aggressive detoxification such as enemas or high colonic treatments, certain kinds of massages or acupuncture, excessive improper breathing and use of stimulating breathing exercises, and stimulating entertainment, such as watching an action movie or riding a roller coaster.

> Note: The more advanced the Adrenal Fatigue Syndrome, the less intense the stressor needs to be in order to trigger an adrenal crash. In advanced AFS, the body's reserve is already low. It does not take much to trigger a crash.

In day-to-day life, it's fair to say that many of us are sometimes puzzled by our inability to handle certain kinds of events/stress like we used to. Sometimes people chalk the symptoms up to aging, but other times this essential change leads some to resolve to take better care of themselves or learn to handle stress better. This is a good instinct, but it might lead to self-guided programs or medical diagnoses that end up worsening the AFS.

Symptoms of an Adrenal Crash

Remember that not all adrenal crashes and recovery cycles are symptomatic. As we've said, it's likely that those experiencing Stage 1 and early Stage 2 AFS remain unaware of the crash, especially if sufficient adrenal reserves exist to compensate and ensure normal daily function. These stages can easily last for decades, or in situations of acute stress, the crashes may intensify, occur more frequently, and affect ever greater areas of one's life.

For those in Stages 3 and 4 of Adrenal Fatigue Syndrome, symptoms of varying severity are universally present in a crash. In these stages, symptoms of adrenal crash represent a sudden intensification or abrupt onset of many already existing pre-crash AFS symptoms. As you can see, these match the symptoms listed early in this book. Symptoms can include:

- Drastically reduced energy and increased fatigue.

- Drastic increases in brain fog and dizziness.

- Increased frequent hypoglycemic episodes, as sugar regulation becomes dysfunctional, with accompanying lightheadedness.

- Major change in mental and cognitive function, triggering severe depression, anxiety, irritability, and rage.

- Loss of the steroid hormone precursor DHEA, leading to low testosterone or imbalanced estrogen and progesterone levels. These hormonal changes are often seen in women as sudden increases in symptoms of estrogen dominance appear, i.e., water retention, hot flashes, insomnia, bloating, and emotional changes. In men, libido diminishes greatly.

- Poor digestion from the constant decrease of metabolism, with irregular bowel movements, constipation, and irritable bowel.

- Sudden onset of myalgia with joint pain as the body enters a catabolic (breakdown) state.

- Sudden worsening of symptoms of hypothyroidism, linked with the inhibition of thyroid hormone activation and also suppression of the controlled release of hormones from the thyroid. Dry skin and weight gain are common.

- The sensation of being wired-and-tired is common, with the inability to fall asleep.

- Metabolic imbalance and sugar dysregulation, with bouts of awakening in the middle of the night with cold sweats, palpitations, and hunger pangs.

- Arthritis flare-ups from the poorly regulated inflammatory pathways.

- Acne and hair loss from imbalance in hormones and poor immune response.

An adrenal crash doesn't necessarily include all of these symptoms, and some individuals have only a few, but the symptoms can be severe. Again, generally speaking, the more intense the symptoms, the more severe the crash. One can experience any degree of adrenal crash at any stage of Adrenal Fatigue Syndrome. We also can classify crash intensity into five levels.

The Levels of Adrenal Crash Intensity

Clinically, Adrenal Fatigue Syndrome crashes are classified into 5 levels based on subjective evaluation. This means that clinicians assign certain percentages of function, but patients are not expected to think in those same clinical terms. Rather, patients may describe how they feel, which clinicians then fit into the levels discussed below. However, for both clinicians and patients, these levels are subjective and few individuals are able to put percentages to their adrenal function. We consider levels 1 and 2 minor crashes with good recovery potential; levels 3, 4, and 5 are considered major crashes and hence, the recovery phase is less certain.

Level 1: There is a loss of 10-19 percent of immediate pre-crash baseline level of adrenal function in terms of energy, metabolic imbalance such as hypoglycemia, and emotional dysfunction such as irritability. Typically, sufferers say they are more tired than usual, more irritable, and they experience hunger before meals earlier than normal. These individuals can perform normally at their jobs and complete their household chores, but they feel quite tired at the end of the day. A nap or extra rest helps restore their well-being.

Level 2: There is a loss of 20-29 percent of immediate pre-crash baseline level of function mentioned above. Here, too, we typically see a definite reduction in energy, but at this level taking a nap or resting for thirty minutes is helpful. Many individuals report they are less emotionally stable than normal, and they find themselves easily irritated. They often feel relief when mealtime comes around. By this time, the ability to perform on the job or complete chores is compromised, but when individuals force themselves they can meet their obligations. Even with extra rest during the day, these individuals feel tired and they sense that something is not quite the same. The body is under strain.

Level 3: We see a loss of 30-39 percent of immediate pre-crash baseline level of function as discussed above. Typically, at this point, the energy level is low throughout the day. Extra rest and a nap are not as helpful, and the body remains very tired. By this time, we see moderate reductions in the ability to perform outside activities and household chores. At this level, individuals feel like staying home all day—not only for a few hours to rest. Emotionally, it's common to be short tempered and feel anger and rage. At times, the body craves sugar for energy. Insomnia is worse, and in many cases accompanied by cold sweats, heart palpitations, and dizziness in the middle of the night for no apparent reason.

Level 4: We see a loss of 40-49 percent of immediate pre-crash baseline level of function as discussed above. Typically, fatigue is severe throughout the day, and individuals are unable to perform most household chores. The body feels totally drained, and on an emotional level, individuals often feel depressed—sometimes, they're too emotionally weak and drained to get angry.

At this level, foods or nutritional supplements that once generated energy can make things worse. It's also characteristic to be unable to work or accomplish regular chores. In some cases, those who work are unable to keep their jobs. Irritability is high, and even TV noise can be very bothersome. Once in bed, the temptation is to stay in bed most of the time as the least draining experience.

Level 5: We see a loss of greater than 50 percent of immediate pre-crash baseline level of function as discussed above. At this level, individuals are bedridden most of the time, getting up only to accomplish the basic personal hygiene chores. It is not unusual to require assistance to walk around the house or even to take a shower or change clothes.

Adrenal Recovery Phase

The recovery phase covers the time from the peak of the crash when the energy is lowest until the body returns to its immediate pre-crash level of adrenal function and energy level. The recovery phase is harder to detect; it can be fast or slow, with frequent setbacks. The more advanced the adrenal fatigue, the less chance we see for a 100 percent recovery.

Under ideal or professionally managed conditions, the recovery phase is marked by multiple mini-cycles each consisting of three components: preparation, honeymoon, and plateau. Each mini-cycle can range from a few days to a few weeks. The weaker the adrenals, the more such mini-cycles are needed and the longer each mini-cycle will last in order to return to pre-crash levels of function.

If not handled properly, such mini-cycles may also be a setup for follow up rolling crashes.

Even in successful recovery, post-recovery energy is generally still below the level of pre-crash levels, and a second or third dip or setbacks are common during the entire recovery process. For some, we see a prolonged period of stabilization before the first recovery mini-cycle begins, especially among those with Adrenal Fatigue Syndrome Stage 3 or beyond. At the extreme, some do not recover at all but instead progress to the next crash after a period of stabilization.

Over time however, we usually can detect a definite recovery phase following each major crash. The following figure shows the various possible recovery curves.

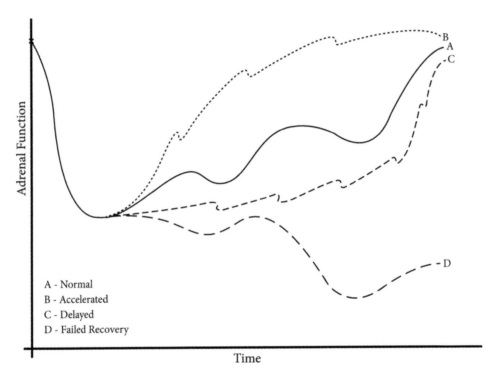

Figure 13. A Comparison of Adrenal Function Recovery Curves

Curve A represents a normal recovery with many mini-recovery cycles along with inevitable setbacks, but a gradual up trend in adrenal function.

Curve B represents an accelerated recovery usually occurring in those in Stages 1 and 2, or those with very strong constitution. We also associate this curve with those who are able to go from the crash phase to honeymoon period directly, usually under professional guidance. This is the most desirable curve.

Curve C represents a prolonged stabilization period and delayed recovery common in Stage 3.

Curve D represents a failed recovery after a moderate stabilization period. We see progression to a subsequent adrenal crash, which is common among those with weak constitutions. This is the least desirable.

All four types of recovery curve are possible in any stage of AFS, although the delayed (curve C) and failed (curve D) are more prominent in the more advanced stages of adrenal weakness as well as those with weak constitution. Unless stressors are removed and the adrenal glands are given the correct tools and nurtured back to health naturally, most recoveries are eventually followed by subsequent worsening crashes as part of the natural progression of this condition.

Common Signs of Adrenal Recovery

Signs of adrenal recovery include:

- Symptoms of the crash appear to be stabilizing, or at least not worsening.

- A sense of calm returns, along with a better ability to deal with stress.

- Reduced anxiety.

- Reduced sense of hypoglycemia.

- More energy for ordinary activities impossible during a crash (i.e., washing dishes or gardening).

- Less salt craving.

- Temporary *worsening* of estrogen dominance symptoms such as PMS and heavy menstrual bleeding.

- Temporary rejection of nutritional supplements that had been beneficial previously.

- Sudden positive and exaggerated response to nutrients, but followed by negative response.

- Return of dreaming during sleep.

- Return of menstrual period where there was amenorrhea (no menstrual cycle) before.

Individuals can have any number of minor or major crashes during any stage of Adrenal Fatigue Syndrome, but those in Stage 3 are the most confusing and difficult to understand. The question is how to manage these distressing situations and begin the process of recovery, which we address in a chapter later in Part II of this book.

Key Points to Remember

- Crashes are very common and inevitable for those in Stage 3 or higher Adrenal Fatigue Syndrome.

- Extreme fatigue is the hallmark of a crash. This is the body's way of forcing a return to a simpler state of survival, i.e. incapacitation. The body's ability to cope with complexity has been overwhelmed.

- A crash is usually followed by a recovery. The recovery phase is further divided into the stabilization, preparation, and honeymoon periods.

- Additional symptoms of an adrenal crash can include worsening hypoglycemia, depression, anxiety, fragile blood pressure, heart palpitations, poor digestion, feeling wired-and-tired, and pain of unknown origin.

- Crash intensity can be categorized into levels 1 to 5, with level 5 being the most serious where over 50 percent of immediate pre-crash function in terms of energy is lost.

- Recovery patterns can be normal, accelerated, delayed, or failed. The most ideal is the accelerated path which normally occurs under professional supervision.

- Common signs of recovery include reduced anxiety, increased energy, reduced salt craving, better sleep, and a sense of calm returning.

Chapter 13

Typical Adrenal Fatigue Syndrome and Crash Progression

By the time most women and men come to us for help, they are already in advanced stages of Adrenal Fatigue Syndrome. Many are surprised at the extent of damage done to their bodies, but few are surprised if we ask them to take a step back and do a detailed personal life history. Over the years, we've found that only a minority of sufferers developed Adrenal Fatigue Syndrome due to acute stressful events, such as accident, surgery, infection, and emotional traumas. Most have had signs and symptoms of AFS for many years and even decades, but have ignored them for far too long. Acute events merely serve as triggers of adrenal crashes more often than not.

A typical picture emerges, and you need to understand this. It's really quite simple: Your body behaves logically. Any history, while not 100 percent predictive of the future, often indicates what is likely to happen ahead. A thorough knowledge of AFS progression will help you anticipate and prepare for what may be coming ahead. Now that you understand the physiology behind AFS, especially the crashes, we think you will find this discussion vital.

We often reiterate that in Stages 1 and 2, most people experience symptoms, including fatigue, but recover quickly and never realize that Adrenal Fatigue Syndrome was a factor. In fact, except in the cases of extreme stress and rapid onset of Adrenal Exhaustion, most patients realize they have experienced many crashes and recoveries along the way to Stage 3 and its phases. A crash in Stage 1 is hardly noticeable, while a crash in Stage 3C will invariably land you in bed for days. Not all crashes are the same. Here, we examine more closely the nature of these crashes in each stage (previously described in this book).

The following diagram shows the typical general progression of Adrenal Fatigue Syndrome over time, with steady deterioration during the generally asymptomatic Stages 1 and 2. This is followed by a rapid and functional decline in Stage 3, which is especially severe in Stage 3C. If unattended, the natural progression is likely to end in adrenal failure. Note that the exact progression varies from person to person with wide variations in intensity and timing. Furthermore, multiple crashes usually occur along the way, and the entire progression typically lasts a decade or more.

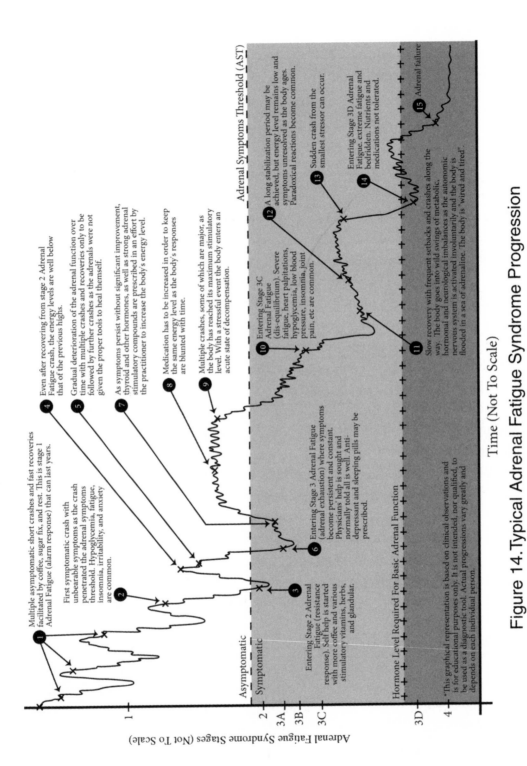

Figure 14. Typical Adrenal Fatigue Syndrome Progression

1. Multiple asymptomatic short crashes and fast recoveries facilitated by coffee, sugar fix, and rest. This is stage 1 Adrenal Fatigue (alarm response) that can last years.

2. First symptomatic crash with unbearable symptoms as the crash penetrated the adrenal symptoms threshold. Hypoglycemia, fatigue, insomnia, irritability, and anxiety are common.

3. Entering Stage 2 Adrenal Fatigue (resistance response). Self help is started with more coffee and various stimulatory vitamins, herbs, and glandular.

4. Even after recovering from stage 2 Adrenal Fatigue crash, the energy levels are well below that of the previous highs.

5. Gradual deterioration of the adrenal function over time with multiple crashes and recoveries only to be followed by further crashes as the adrenals were not given the proper tools to heal themself.

6. Entering Stage 3 Adrenal Fatigue (adrenal exhaustion) where symptoms become persistent and constant. Physicians' help is sought and normally told all is well. Anti-depressant and sleeping pills may be prescribed.

7. As symptoms persist without significant improvement, thyroid and other hormones, as well as strong adrenal stimulatory compounds are prescribed in an effort by the practitioner to increase the body's energy level.

8. Medication has to be increased in order to keep the same energy level as the body's responses are blunted with time.

9. Multiple crashes, some of which are major, as the body has reached its maximum stimulatory level. With a stressful event the body enters an acute state of decompensation.

10. Entering Stage 3C Adrenal Fatigue (dis-equilibrium). Severe fatigue, heart palpitations, hypoglycemia, low blood pressure, insomnia, joint pain, etc are common.

11. Slow recovery with frequent setbacks and crashes along the way. The body goes into wild swings of metabolic, hormonal and neurological imbalances as the autonomic nervous system is activated involuntarily and the body is flooded in a sea of adrenaline. The body is "wired and tired".

12. A long stabilization period may be achieved, but energy level remains low and symptoms unresolved as the body ages. Paradoxical reactions become common.

13. Sudden crash from the smallest stressor can occur.

14. Entering Stage 3D Adrenal Fatigue. extreme fatigue and bedridden. Nutrients and medications not tolerated.

15. Adrenal failure

Adrenal Symptoms Threshold (AST)

Asymptomatic

Symptomatic

Hormone Level Required For Basic Adrenal Function

"This graphical representation is based on clinical observations and is for educational purposes only. It is not intended, nor qualified, to be used as a diagnostic tool. Actual progressions vary greatly and depends on each individual person.

Time (Not To Scale)

Adrenal Fatigue Syndrome Stages (Not To Scale)

1
2
3A
3B
3C
3D
4

Stage 1 Adrenal Fatigue Syndrome
(Alarm Reaction, points 1-3 on the chart, previous page)

In this stage, the body is alarmed by stressors and mounts an aggressive anti-stress response to reduce stress levels. Brain norepinephrine is activated and the mind is put on alert. Unfortunately, this subclinical state is seldom recognized as a pathological condition. Blood sugar levels become imbalanced, resulting in low energy and usually remedied with quick fixes, such as soda drinks, energy potions, and high carbohydrate foods such as pastries and other sweets. Those who require coffee to start the day may already be in this stage but are unaware of it. If a major crash occurs, recovery usually takes a few days or weeks at most and full recovery is achieved. Crashes in this stage usually go unnoticed and are only evident in retrospect.

Stage 2 Adrenal Fatigue Syndrome (Resistance Response, points 3-5)

With chronic or severe stress, the adrenals eventually become unable to compensate. Those in this stage still carry out normal daily functions, but the sense of fatigue is pronounced at the end of each day as the body needs more rest than usual to recover. Despite a full night's rest, the person often doesn't feel refreshed in the morning. Anxiety and irritability begin to set in. Insomnia becomes more common, as it takes longer to fall asleep, and waking in the night several times is common. Infections become more recurrent. PMS and menstrual irregularities surface, and symptoms suggestive of hypothyroidism (such as a sensation of feeling cold and a sluggish metabolism) become prevalent. Those who require multiple cups of coffee to sustain them throughout the day may well be entrenched in this stage without knowing it.

Compared to Stage 1, the frequency of minor and major adrenal crashes is higher. The intensity is also increased. The Adrenal Symptoms Threshold (AST) has been penetrated on the downside. A mild degree of adrenal symptoms are usually present before the crash, but not always. During the adrenal crash, these symptoms worsen and may be exaggerated, but they're still manageable.

At this stage, many individuals recover fully with no symptoms after the crash as they rise above the AST, but not all are so fortunate. A significant number of people remain symptomatic below the AST after recovery. They might manifest symptoms that are slightly worse than the state they were in before the crash. These crashes are often what bring sufferers to their physicians for the first time. Medical workups are usually normal.

Crashes associated with Stage 2 Adrenal Fatigue Syndrome are characterized by a higher intensity of symptoms compared to crashes associated with Stage 1. To start, the pre-crash energy level is lower than Stage 1 Adrenal Fatigue Syndrome at the baseline. At the height of the crash, the adrenal function usually descends and penetrates the AST. Debilitating symptoms start to appear, including anxiety, insomnia, and low blood sugar. As with crashes associated with Stage 1 AFS, each crash and recovery cycle end at an adrenal function status that is slightly compromised. This is a gentle downward cascade of functions resembling a waterfall or a series of steps going down. The duration of the recovery phase is usually longer when compared to that experienced in Stage 1.

Stage 3A Adrenal Fatigue Syndrome
(Early System Dysfunction, points 6-9)

As the body enters Adrenal Exhaustion (Stage 3), the clinical picture drastically worsens. Mild symptoms characteristic of Stages 1 and 2 Adrenal Fatigue Syndrome continue to worsen and become clinically evident. Symptoms become persistent or chronic, including any of the following:

- The slightly elevated blood pressure now becomes low throughout the day.

- Mild musculoskeletal pain turns into chronic myalgia around the clock.

- Frequent recurrent infections are the norm in comparison to intermittent infections.

- Occasional mental feeling of blues becomes mild depression.

- Sleep patterns become more disrupted as insomnia becomes chronic.

- Fatigue that usually occurs during the end of occasional stressful days becomes an everyday event.

We see the ability to carry out normal daily activities moderately reduced. Most people are exhausted after a full day's work. However, not all organs are dysfunctional to the same degree at the same time. The organ system that is constitutionally weakest is the first one to decompensate, while another organ system appears to be intact. The HPA axis dysregulation is responsible for many of these symptoms.

Minor crashes become increasingly common, occurring once every few weeks. Major crashes usually occur farther apart. Symptoms are prevalent pre-crash, and because most are longstanding, most sufferers have adapted to them, although they live at a lower energy baseline level. During the adrenal crash, the symptoms worsen. Even after recovery, the body remains symptomatic, and below the AST most of the time.

Stage 3B Adrenal Fatigue Syndrome
(Hormonal Axis Imbalances, points 9-10)

The endocrine system in our body is linked hormonally in a series of axes for optimal function. Dysfunction in one system invariably affects the others, leading to a cascade of decompensation as the body weakens. In this phase, hormonal axes such as the ovarian-adrenal-thyroid (OAT) axis in women and adrenal-thyroid (AT) axis in men are particularly compromised.

When these axes become imbalanced, the adverse feedback loop creates a vicious cycle of cascading decompensation involving multiple organ systems at the same time. In women, this could typically involve symptoms associated with low thyroid, progesterone, and cortisol hormones. In the male, the adrenal-thyroid axis may be compromised. Sufferers' physical and emotional states continue to deteriorate and they enter into a state of confusion. By that we mean they are unable to logically dissect the myriad systemic manifestations of multiple hormonal axes imbalances.

Compared to those experiences in Stage 3A Adrenal Fatigue Syndrome, crashes are usually more intense and more frequent as the adrenal reserve is depleted. It is not uncommon to have minor crashes every few weeks, and major adrenal crashes every few months. The body never fully recovers to a point that the energy is consistently above the AST at any point in the crash and recovery cycle.

Stage 3C Adrenal Fatigue Syndrome
(Disequilibrium State, points 10-13)

The body gathers steam as it continues its downward path of impaired functions. Gradually, the body becomes severely compromised in trying to maintain the fine controls of homeostasis. Therefore, normal equilibrium is lost. The body will try its hardest to maintain equilibrium. The autonomic nervous system (ANS) is now put into overdrive as a way to overcome perceived danger and impending doom. The body is flooded in a sea of norepinephrine and epinephrine. However, the compensatory response systems can become dysregulated. Along with damaged receptor sites, impaired metabolic and detoxification pathways exist in what is now a low clearance state, leading to paradoxical and exaggerated responses.

Clinical manifestations include swings in blood sugar levels, with reactive hypoglycemia being the hallmark, along with fragile and low blood pressure, postural hypotension, and the inability to remain standing for a prolonged period of time. Reactive sympathoadrenal responses include heart palpitations, night sweats, and reactively driven anxiety followed by depression. Normal activities are usually very much restricted.

Crashes that occur in this phase are fast and furious. Minor adrenal crashes can occur every few days, and major ones are not far behind. There is a roller coaster ride of ever worsening symptoms. It is not unusual for one to go from a minor crash immediately into a major crash before the minor crash has even completed its recovery. A state of constant fatigue exists, with severe energy depletion. The highest rate of functional decline occurs at this phase. A major crash can be very scary and may require trips to the emergency room. The recovery phase for Stage 3C crashes can be many more times longer than that of Stage 1.

Stage 3D Adrenal Fatigue Syndrome (Near Failure, points 14-15)

As the body's various hormones, such as cortisol and aldosterone, fall below the minimum required reserve for basic normal function, the body continues to down regulate the amount needed in order to preserve what is on hand for only the most essential body functions. This down regulation further reduces cortisol output, exaggerating a vicious downward cycle. The body may not be able to tolerate steroids, or the response may be blunted. Even at low doses, normal nutrients are often systemically rejected by the body. Unstable hormonal positive feedback loops are activated which invariably worsen the condition.

Those who are in this stage often live in the hopeless state of constant crashes. The body is too drained to mount a productive response. Adrenal crash symptoms are usually extreme. Minor crashes can be intermingled with major crashes. Emergency room visits are common due to unstable blood pressure, irregular heart rate, and severe anxiety with a sense of impending doom. Sufferers are usually bedridden and require help to carry out daily self care and minimal chores.

In addition to a much longer recovery time compared to Stage 3C, sufferers remain symptomatic well below the AST throughout almost the entire crash and the recovery experience. Those in late Adrenal Exhaustion have a very low adrenal pre-crash reserve at baseline. Compared to earlier stages, stress triggers can be something that would not have triggered a crash in early stages. This may be a longer than usual walk or inadequate fluid intake. The body is much more sensitive to stressors as adrenal weakness progresses.

Fortunately, most adrenal crashes, even in advanced states, can be managed with the right tools and approach (discussed later in Part II). In the next chapter, we get a glimpse of what happened in the life of one woman when Adrenal Fatigue Syndrome advanced into Adrenal Exhaustion and remained unrecognized and untreated for many years.

Key Points to Remember

- The typical Adrenal Fatigue Syndrome sufferer goes through multiple crashes and recovery cycles over decades as the body slowly decompensates.

- In each stage of Adrenal Fatigue Syndrome, crash and recovery takes on different characteristics, durations, and intensities.

- Precipitating events often act as major triggers for each crash.

- Most AFS sufferers can look back at their history and see a progression of symptoms.

- Generally speaking, as AFS progresses, crashes become more frequent and more intense. The trigger needed to precipitate a crash reduces. Recovery also becomes less strong and takes longer as AFS advances.

Chapter 14

Mary's Story—Illustrating the Problem

The narrative that follows is a mini-case history of a woman named Mary, but her story matches that of millions of women. We've included it because in Mary's story, we see a woman pass through early stages of Adrenal Fatigue Syndrome and through Adrenal Exhaustion to near failure. The numbered graph included at the end of this chapter will help you follow along and see the progression of Adrenal Fatigue Syndrome in one typical sufferer.

Mary's adult life started much like many normal teenager's after a healthy childhood. As with many young people, Mary began to test—and stretch—the limits of her body around the time she went off to college. For the first time in her life, Mary independently arranged her own schedule and social life. Wanting to embrace everything in her new life, she stayed up late studying and socializing with her new friends and exploring the exciting city where her college was located, while also working as a waitress a few hours a week.

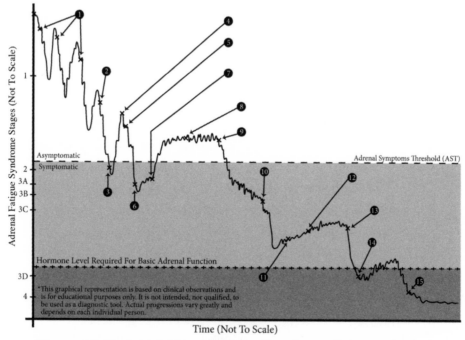

Figure 15. Typical Adrenal Fatigue Syndrome Progression
(See Figure 14 for notes in Figure on each point in progression.
They are absent in Figure 15 but explained in the text.)

When she first noted feeling tired in the morning and dragging through her day, she revved herself up with coffee drinks and sweets to keep going until the weekend when she could sleep in until noon. (Point 1 in the diagram.) By Monday, she would feel fine again. Since her roommate and other friends lived the same way, Mary saw nothing unusual about her college lifestyle.

During these young adult years, her menstrual period occasionally was a little slow in coming, and she noted with frustration her stubborn premenstrual acne, but here, too, she saw nothing out of the ordinary. As long as Mary could stay up late, but still manage the extra fatigue, she believed everything was normal.

Mary had no idea she was already in Stage 1 of AFS Syndrome, and even early Stage 2.

Approaching her senior year in college, her family experienced some financial problems, which meant they could no longer help out with her school expenses. Mary increased her student loans and found a second part-time job. Throughout that year, she felt especially pressured to strike out on her own and find a job soon after graduation.

During her senior year, a friend noted that Mary seemed stressed out and suggested that running would help her cope. Once she started running, Mary enjoyed challenging herself and pushed past the fatigue she felt after a mile or two. She didn't think there was anything unusual about being so tired at the end of each run. Rather, she believed she had let herself become out of shape, and therefore, continued to treat her fatigue with coffee and quick energy sugary foods. On a few occasions she was so tired after a run that she was forced to take a nap, but neither she nor her friends considered her extra fatigue unusual. (Point 2)

At this point, Mary was in an environment that was, in a sense, self-reinforcing. Other students lived much the same way, and Mary herself saw that many of her friends faced challenges far more daunting and intense than her own. Older professors and Mary's parents would not have seen anything of note in Mary's student lifestyle. However, Mary lived with Stage 1 AFS, experiencing small crashes from which she quickly recovered. It would never have occurred to her to call these episodes adrenal crashes.

After Mary graduated, she returned home. She took a waitressing job while she did an extended job search, which took almost six months. Finally, she found an entry level corporate job in a suburb not far from her hometown. She launched into an independent life and was determined to do well as she climbed the corporate ladder. Mary brushed off the periodic crashes and minor fatigue that began to be part of her daily life. Being young and strong and ready to embrace life, she pushed through the week, relying on snacks and coffee. Sometimes she'd overeat at lunch and feel mentally foggy through the afternoon—a sign of a food coma. Like others in her office, she drank coffee or tea and ate chocolate to help her stay awake during late-afternoon meetings. She also had energy drinks with her so she could keep her energy up and found an herbal formula at a health food store to fend off fatigue. (Point 3)

Always in the back of Mary's mind were her family's financial problems, which eventually forced her parents to move from the family home to a small apartment. The first year on her job, Mary used her vacation days to help with the move, which wore her out. Again, here, she was experiencing the crashes of Stage 1, but for the most part, her body bounced back. Later, with each recovery, however, she felt less well and never fully renewed, despite periods of rest. (Point 4)

Her father had developed heart disease, which worried Mary and her siblings, and motivated Mary to stay physically fit, even entering races. She was disturbed that she could barely finish a 10K road race, but she was too busy to give it much attention. Around this time, Mary found herself taking over-the-counter pain medication to ease her menstrual cramps, she also developed benign lumps (fibrocystic changes) in her breasts, which made her breasts tender and painful during the week or ten days prior to her premenstrual period. When she asked her doctor about these symptoms and her irregular periods, she was told that these were not serious—many women experience the same cluster of menstrual complaints.

Here we see Mary developing *estrogen dominance*. We also see what happens when symptoms that are *common* are confused with being just a *normal* part of being a woman.

Mary's doctor gave her a standard answer but failed to link these signs of estrogen dominance to potential health problems down the road. True enough, millions of women develop these symptoms and they are considered by many a normal part of women's menstrual cycles. When something is considered normal, that usually means it isn't taken seriously and is rarely linked with the big picture of health or declining health. Mary continued to try to catch up on sleep during her weekends, much as she had in college, but she never quite came back as strong as she had before. These adrenal crashes were taking a toll, but her body still had reserves.

As is common, Mary remained in Stage 1 and early Stage 2 throughout her twenties and early thirties, but nothing seemed particularly unusual about her symptoms. Plus, she was always grateful each time she bounced back from bouts of fatigue and mental exhaustion. Like so many people who lead hectic lives, Mary brushed off her intermittent symptoms as the normal peaks and valleys of modern life. She read magazine articles about women who were determined to get ahead and have it all, and while that described her, she tried to take care of herself and avoid the pitfalls of this strenuous life journey.

Mary advanced in her career, eventually being hired by another company at a higher salary and a more impressive title. She married and was soon pregnant with her first child. As much as she wanted children, she confided in friends that she found pregnancy quite stressful, especially when she had to go away on a couple of business trips during her second trimester. Although she continued to manage, her overall energy level continued to drop. (Point 5)

Mary continued working until a couple of weeks before delivering her baby and returned to her job a few months later. Two years later, she had her second child, and admitted to her husband that she was relieved to have their two healthy children, but certainly wouldn't have more. Her childbearing years were over.

The two pregnancies changed Mary's hormonal patterns, and although only in her late thirties, she began complaining to her friends about putting on extra pounds, pointing out, too, that her skin was especially dry. Like many women in Mary's generation, she felt anxious about both her family and her job. When she was home, she thought about work, and when she was at work, she thought about home. She resented her husband's lack of willingness to do his fair share of childrearing or the chores necessary to keep their home going. Eventually, this resentment and other difficulties whittled away at their relationship, but Mary put on a united, happy front to family and friends. She only confided to one close friend about her dissatisfaction with her married life.

When her father died suddenly, Mary unsuccessfully attempted to keep going through her continuing exhaustion (Point 6), but her grief was so deep that she sought counseling to help her cope. Meanwhile, her menstrual difficulties continued, and she experienced symptoms like brain fog and fitful sleep. Mary understood that her life was stressful, but she didn't have information to connect her symptoms to Adrenal Fatigue Syndrome.

At forty, Mary had crossed the threshold from Stages 1 and 2 of AFS and into Stage 3, Adrenal Exhaustion. She had symptoms all the time, meaning that she no longer snapped back from bouts of fatigue; sleep didn't renew her energy, as it had during her college years and during her twenties and into her thirties. She always found reasons for her symptoms, though, so she could tell herself that soon the stressful times would ease. Unfortunately, her life took twists and turns over the next years, including a nasty divorce, the source of ongoing stress.

Although she no longer ran, Mary walked to maintain her fitness level and to keep extra pounds off. She also spoke with her doctor about the array of symptoms that were her daily companions—anxiety and constant mild depression, and fatigue that never completely went away. Her doctor eventually ordered various tests, including thyroid function, but the results fell into the so-called normal range. Still, Mary's doctor believed that she was suffering symptoms of a stressful life and prescribed antidepressants and sleeping pills, which became hallmarks of life in her forties. (Point 7)

Being highly intelligent, Mary read about stress and its effects on health, and she embarked on a self-guided journey to get a handle on her life. Despite disappointments in her personal life, she was proud of her professional accomplishments. However, she felt anxious about continuing her progress and had a nagging sense that the unrelenting pressures at work had taken a toll.

Like many women approaching midlife, she tried to reassess, but fatigue itself sometimes prevented her from fully taking stock. In addition, as a single parent, she had a tremendous amount on her plate. Mary began to rely on nutritional supplements, and she tried various herbal formulations guaranteed to boost energy. In fact, she became an avid consumer of health information and natural food store "cures." When these OTC remedies, plus antidepressants, seemed to work, Mary again felt optimistic and believed she'd turned a corner toward well-being. (Point 8)

Mary's happiness, unfortunately, did not last. While her health and energy levels stabilized for a while, she needed more supplements to sustain the same energy level. This worked for a while. One day, she received news that her best friend had died in a car accident. This was a major stressful event (Point 9), and Mary's symptoms came crashing back—literally. Fatigue returned, even worse than before, along with thinning hair and continued dry skin. Supplements seemed to be less effective than before. She also had many food cravings and steadily added pounds. Mary's doctor ordered more thyroid tests and added a synthetic thyroid hormone replacement to an already long list of medications. Again, she seemed to improve a bit, and friends encouraged her to get back to the gym and join a weight loss program to shed the extra pounds. Mary continued to have regular minor crashes that went on for a few years. Her body gradually weakened over time as fatigue became more prominent with each crash.

By this time, Mary had fallen deep into Stage 3C (Point 10), and she struggled to keep up with her job and children and turn her life around. By her mid-forties, even she realized that she was living a marginal life, barely hanging on. Almost all her non-work hours were spent recovering her strength, which meant she seldom saw friends and used all her energy to keep up with her children's activities.

Odd and new symptoms appeared as Mary's chronic symptoms steadily worsened. She developed allergies and sensitivities to fluorescent light, and she was on edge and anxious most of the time, even startling when her phone rang. In addition, she took periodic courses of steroid medications to treat bouts of bursitis, and she also suffered constant muscle and joint pain.

Adrenal crashes became more frequent, with longer, slower recovery periods. As she approached menopause, Mary felt hopeless and disappointed in her efforts to improve her health. Her periods were irregular and heavy, and her doctor warned that a hysterectomy was in her future, as uterine fibroids had developed and were growing in size. This was another sign of estrogen dominance, but her doctor was not familiar with that connection. With increasing fatigue, she had to take time off from work to get more rest, and her body slowly recovered. (Point 11)

Mary lived—uncomfortably—in Stage 3C for many years. During this time (Point 12), she began experiencing paradoxical reactions to medications and nutritional supplements. Tired all the time, she also felt wired when she took vitamins and adrenal glandular recommended by a nutritionist. Instead of helping her, she felt odd and what she called wired-and-tired. (Point 13) Eventually, Mary's efforts to cope with the symptoms and still function, even marginally, gave way when a major crash hit that landed her in Stage 3D. (Point 14)

Looking back to her college years, if anyone had told Mary that she'd need to take an extended medical leave of absence from her job, she wouldn't have believed it. However, even Mary's psychiatrist recommended this step, explaining that depression and stress had weakened her. As a precaution, Mary's doctor again tested her adrenal function to rule out Addison's disease, but again, the results fell into the normal range. Because she felt lightheaded and experienced blood sugar drops and surges, Mary was tested for diabetes, and was considered pre-diabetic, though her serum fasting glucose was invariably normal. Her frequent hypoglycemia was clinically confusing. Finally, she was told that conventional medicine could do no more for her.

Mary decided to use her medical leave to work hard at getting well. This started with a detoxification program she'd read about; she even tried coffee enemas. She tried, again, to meditate and she sought spiritual direction, but she couldn't shake the mental fog and confusion that dominated her days. The detoxification plan backfired, intensifying the symptoms and sending Mary to bed rest days at a time.

This time was also marked by numerous trips to the ER with heart palpitations, extreme dizziness, and weakness. These symptoms reminded Mary of her father and his premature death. On each trip to the ER, she was told that it was likely she'd had a panic attack or had eaten something that produced allergic symptoms.

Going back to work was out of the question, and by this time Mary was already living off the proceeds of the sale of her house. Her midlife years turned out to be nothing like she'd expected.

At this point, Mary was incapacitated, and in addition, she felt very much alone. (Point 14) Mary had turned into a patient for whom no diagnosis quite fit and no treatment worked over an extended period of time. By the time she found an integrative doctor, Mary couldn't tolerate most of her medications, including even the low dose of hydrocortisone meant to help correct her symptoms which were consistent with low cortisol seen in AFS. Her new doctor eventually gave up.

Having little other choice, Mary spent the better part of three months in bed. She gradually regained some strength, although she experienced periodic crashes throughout her recovery and she was always at risk for crashes. She now took a basket of more than ten different nutritional supplements every day with little effect. She spent hours online visiting various forums on fatigue and trying out different modalities as suggested by fellow sufferers. The harder she tried, the worse she became. She finally realized that her damaged body needed personalized attention and guidance as she was at the end of her road. Further trial and error was only making her worse. In her early fifties by this time, Mary had many signs of aging, from dry, wrinkled skin to thinning bones and arthritis. Most of all, she realized that she felt old and tired, and also sad that, starting in her late thirties, she'd begun missing out on the joy of life.

How Mary Recovered

Every day, countless individuals like Mary are in desperate search of a way to regain their life and vitality. Mary was fortunate because her body, though severely damaged, managed to recover with time and a proper recovery program.

Eventually, Mary was able to return to work close to her home. By this time, Mary had reconnected to what mattered most to her. She no longer felt the need to strive and get ahead. She felt a sense of calm and peace as she returned to a lifestyle that matched her body's capacities and ability to handle stress in a creative fashion. She built a life rich in quality, which is a blissful place to be. Mary emerged from the long nightmare, regretting the time she lost feeling tired and unhappy, but grateful for her life and the recovery she achieved. She also hoped that her example would influence her children's lives and inspire them to find greater balance.

The key to Mary's story was her persistence. She took responsibility for her health and her care. After multiple false starts that stretched over years, Mary finally found a nutritional program through the *Dr.Lam.com* web site. Mary's story is meant to inform, not alarm, but it provides the kind of narrative that reflects the path many walk. Of course, many women and men will continue to pursue active lives and big goals. Our hope is that with the knowledge of Adrenal Fatigue Syndrome, adults will live more thoughtfully and pay attention to the symptoms of stress and adjust their lives accordingly.

Mary's story describes the problem, a summary of sorts of a typical long term progression of AFS. It pulls together, in the story of one person, the information you have read thus far. In the next section, we discuss the kinds of things Mary did to gain a good degree of recovery and find balance in her life.

Key Points to Remember

- Mary typifies many women and men who ignore the signs of AFS for too long while they pursue their careers, raise families, and try to manage hectic schedules that simply can't be sustained.

- Mary's symptoms are typical of someone who advances through the various stages of Adrenal Fatigue Syndrome.

- Fortunately, Mary took corrective action with the right professional in the nick of time and recovered well.

Part 2
THE SOLUTION

The Approach

In the previous 14 chapters, Adrenal Fatigue Syndrome was described as a condition that befalls most everyone at one time or another over a lifetime. Now it is time to bring your understanding of the condition together with information about recovery.

We begin with a discussion of Adrenal Fatigue Syndrome and the mind-body connection. As you have already seen, components within the body are fully integrated and intimately intertwined. While the predominant symptoms of AFS appear to be physical, mediated largely by cortisol dysregulation, such as fatigue, hypoglycemia, and low blood pressure, inevitably, we see mental components such as anxiety, depression, and irritability when AFS reaches the advanced stages. In other words, the entire neuroendocrine system is involved, starting at the brain and eventually encompassing every other system. Complete healing, therefore, necessarily needs to integrate a thorough understanding of both the mind and the body.

The chapters that follow include the mind-body discussion to explain our approach to supporting adrenal recovery through a variety of natural remedies, diet, exercise, and lifestyle suggestions. Although Adrenal Fatigue Syndrome *is not a disease*, recovery can be a long and complex journey that includes trial and error and no single clear recovery path.

Chapter 15

Adrenal Fatigue Syndrome and the Mind-Body Connection

Until the seventeenth century, the body and mind were considered as one inseparable unit. At that time, our understanding of physiology was in its infancy; and in the West, the Roman Catholic Church was powerful and influential. When Rene Descartes, a philosopher and scientist, delved into a study of metaphysics, historians tell us that he made a pact with the church: As a man of science, Descartes would restrict himself to the study of human anatomy and the realm of the material—the physical—and leave the mind and soul to the care of the church.

From that time on, separating studies of the mind and body, treating them as distinct and separate entities, became the trend in western philosophy and science. This is why we still see scientists restricting their work to what they can observe and quantify. The body is broken down into its components, and in general, the function of the mind is not considered as important.

Since the mid-twentieth century, the many specialties of western medicine have moved increasingly further away from the idea that the mind can physically alter the body, and therefore, they do not believe that mind-body disorders exist. The current concept of evidence-based medicine, which usually refers to large double-blind studies, evolved from the thesis that considered the mind and body separately. Meanwhile, those in religious life lifted thought, reason, and emotion out of the body, into the realm of the spiritual, thereby reinforcing the idea that health is a material concern, grounded in what we can see and measure and not connected with the world of the unseen.

The hypothesis of splitting a human being into two distinct and unrelated units has not proven to have significant scientific standing, although modern medicine has accepted this premise on face value and hasn't engaged in a philosophical debate or questioned the foundation of this thesis. Modern medicine is so preoccupied with physical medicine and treatments that tend to slice the body into pieces, that it's often considered quackery to venture into the influence of the mind. In fact, when conventional medicine fails to provide answers to patients' problems, these individuals are often told, "It's all in your mind," as if the patient is imagining symptoms. These patients are often sent home and worsen as they are left to self-navigate.

Mind-Body Connection Proven

Fortunately, eastern medicine has never forgotten that the body is indeed one whole and cannot be separated. Holistic practice, a relatively new concept in western thought, has not changed significantly in the east over centuries, and today, we see it increasingly becoming validated through neuroscience research. We now have irrefutable data that our minds and bodies are indeed connected and intertwined.

In the 1970s, we saw firm, documented evidence of a physiological link between the mind and body. The earliest research focused on psychological well-being and its relationship to physical health. This research involved those whose survival depended on organ transplants, and repeatedly showed that organ transplant recipients living the longest tended to be those with the strongest will to survive. In fact, as part of the organ recipient selection process, candidates routinely undergo psychological testing to evaluate their will to live. Since the 1970s, many additional studies have shown similar conclusions relating to survival among cancer patients and other terminal illnesses. Clearly, the mind's role, though not completely understood or defined, cannot be ignored and cast aside. Ongoing advances in neuroscience continue to confirm that the mind and body are truly inseparable.

Obviously, we don't need to be neuroscientists to appreciate the mind-body connection in everyday life. For example, imagine biting into a chilled pickle. Most people immediately begin salivating and perhaps have a tingling sensation at the very thought of the chilled pickle. This occurs because the mental image triggers a cascade of chemical messengers released by the brain that within seconds reach the target organ, the mouth.

Now imagine taking a deep breath when under stress and feel the calm return. Imagine yourself in a scene of peace and calm to help you fall asleep. Imagine having butterflies in your stomach when you are nervous. What is the common phenomenon of stage fright, with its symptoms of shaky hands, sweaty palms, and upset stomach, if not a mind-body reaction? These are simple reminders of how many of our daily activities are already embedded in this mind-body connection, which is to our advantage and provides awareness of our feeling states. Unfortunately, modern conventional medicine has largely ignored physical manifestations of stress, except, for example, to prescribe medications with a sedative effect.

Obviously, the state of our mental health counts, and if it declines, physical health can wear down. The converse is also true; as physical health declines, most of us feel mentally down, too.

Deepening Our Understanding

Even given the clear mind-body connection, we are still left with the central—and unanswered—question of how they are connected. Advances in orthomolecular medicine and neuroendocrinology have provided the answers. In fact, in many situations we can put the mind-body connection in the context of evidence based physiology. The immune system gives us a good example. Providing irrefutable proof of the mind-body connection, researchers found receptors on the surface of immune system cells that act as keyholes, and as such, they accept chemical neuro-transmitters released by the nervous system and the brain, such as norepinephrine. Hormones mediated by the autonomic nervous system (ANS) are a major transporter of messengers along this mind-body highway.

In addition, researchers have identified new neurotransmitters that talk to immune system cells. A stimulus such as emotional stress can trigger the release of a variety of chemicals, which then tell the immune system cells in a distant organ what actions to take. Throughout the day, a large number of chemical messengers, including adrenaline and norepinephrine, are mediated through various branches of the ANS. We now have established evidence that the brain has the ability to send signals to immune system cells, thus controlling the immune system. This is the science behind what most people have observed:

> **Individuals under stress and mental strain are more emotionally fragile and tend to fall sick more frequently than usual.**

The reverse also is true: Chemicals released by immune system cells affect the brain. The body's super highway of communication and influence is a two-way street, with multiple connection points to various other organs. It is a virtual network of servers, transmitters, nodes, and receptors.

More Evidence of the Mind-Body Connection

- Stress may lead to an increased output of pro-inflammatory cytokine from the brain and from the immune system, which in turn leads to the release of norepinephrine from the sympathetic nervous system.

- Excessive pro-inflammatory cytokine signaling may trigger automatic defensive mechanisms in the brain. Behavioral changes such as reduced interest in social activities, a depressed mood, and a change in sleep patterns including the desire to sleep more than usual, may be the result.

- Excessive pro-inflammatory cytokine may lead to a loss of energy and hence increase fatigue. The exact pathway is not fully known. Some researchers have speculated that thyroid dysregulation may be involved.

- Many mental illnesses, including depression, bipolar disorder, and anxiety disorders, are strongly associated with depressed cortisol production. Clearly the HPA axis is involved, but the adrenal glands themselves are structurally intact.

- Most under prolonged stress have a lower than normal serum cortisol level. This is a common and valid finding in those with post-traumatic stress disorder (PTSD) as well. However, their serum cortisol level is not low enough to meet the criteria for adrenal insufficiency. But, chronically, they do not have adequate output of cortisol in response to stress. Clearly, the adrenal glands are dysregulated, but the cause lies outside the adrenal glands themselves, most likely in the brain.

- The primary stress signaling agent in the brain is norepinephrine. It is in a positive feedback loop with corticotropin releasing hormone (CRH) which activates the HPA axis starting at the hypothalamus. That is, the more brain norepinephrine secretion, the more CRH is released, and the more is the HPA axis activity.

- Neurotransmitters that promote norepinephrine signaling include serotonin, dopamine, and GABA. Low serotonin output is associated with depression, a common finding in AFS. During times of stress, we need to increase production of these chemicals in order to boost norepinephrine output. It comes as no surprise that many of the antidepressants and antianxiety agents belong to a class of psychotropic drugs called *selective serotonin reuptake inhibitors* (SSRI), whose job is to increase extracellular serotonin by blocking the inactivation pathway.

- Histamine has long had a central role in the mediation of allergic reactions. Research evidence also supports a role for histamine (pro-inflammatory) as a central neurotransmitter. It has been implicated in the regulation of numerous and important activities of the central nervous system, such as arousal, cognition, circadian rhythms, and neuroendocrine regulation. Brain histamine levels are decreased in Alzheimer's disease patients, whereas abnormally high histamine concentrations are found in the brains of Parkinson's disease and schizophrenic patients. Low histamine levels are associated with convulsions and seizures. It's been speculated that stress increases histamine from brain mast cells.

Psychological Studies Reaffirm the Mind-Body Connection

In addition to scientific research, clinical psychological studies also show that the mind and body are strongly linked. A positive mental outlook can help keep you healthy. Consider the following:

- The National Survey of Drug Use and Health finds that one in five American adults experienced a form of mental illness (a diagnosed mental, behavioral or emotional disorder) in the past 12 months.

- The World Health Organization (WHO) finds in developed countries, mental illness accounts for more disability than any other illness, including heart disease and cancer.

- Forty-three percent of all adults suffer adverse health effects from stress.

- Ninety-three percent of Americans say their thoughts, perceptions, and choices affect their physical health—how they feel on a day-to-day basis.

- Fifty-eight percent of Americans believe that good mental health goes hand-in-hand with good physical health.

- High levels of anxiety can cause up to seven times the risk of cardiovascular disease.

- On any given day, workplace stress causes approximately one million employees in the United States to miss work.

- More than one in four workers has taken a so-called mental health day off to cope with stress and its side effects.

Those who continue to divide the mind and body and set up artificial boundaries between them *are clinging to circumstances that ruled western society three centuries ago.* The body has not changed. The mind and body have always been part of the same whole, just as the head and tail of a coin are inseparable, but merely different points of the same coin.

Neurological and other research has exponentially increased our understanding of how the mind controls the body. Some illnesses have always been defined by anatomical systems, but now we must view them concurrently from many angles. If we don't, we lack a complete clinical picture, which must incorporate the direct physical pathology plus the less obvious but equally important mental component. The reason is simple: The universe appears to be essentially inseparable, and everything interconnects with everything else.

Despite the evidence, modern medicine has not fully embraced the mind-body connection, with grave consequences. This can lead to incomplete and mistaken diagnoses that prolong suffering and confusion. Even putting aside the harm to individuals, consider the social and economic costs of failing to understand or accept the mind-body connection. The consequences ripple through every institution in our society.

Denise (age 38) shows us that even those with the most severe cases of AFS can recover:

I suffered a lifetime of physical abuse from my mother, and then spent too many years in an abusive marriage. I am now a single mother of girls ages six and seven. My ex-husband relinquished parental rights and refuses to pay child support, so I struggle to support them. While I was still married, I had three major surgeries. My uterus and one ovary were removed, and then I had a bowel resection resulting from mistakes made during the first surgery. My remaining ovary has recurring cysts, and the other ovary was removed because it became encased in a cyst.

Although I had symptoms of adrenal fatigue before these surgeries, they became increasingly extreme two weeks after the second surgery. As I got worse and worse, I saw over ten different doctors, two of whom were endocrinologists who told me my tests indicated that there was nothing wrong with me. The rest of the doctors concluded my symptoms were caused by psychological problems, thus, they prescribed psychiatric medications. I went to two different psychologists who told me to push through it and that I was being overdramatic.

About a year and a half ago, I suffered a severe ear infection which left me with vertigo.

Since then, I heard about an integrative MD in my town. When I saw him, he agreed with my assessment that my symptoms were likely caused by hormonal deficiency, and the saliva test he ordered showed significant hormonal imbalances including cortisol deficiency.

Then, before I had a chance to begin recovering, my right knee retained large amounts of water for the second time in a year, and the orthopedic specialist injected my knee with steroids. At that point, I crashed big time and was bedridden. I eventually recovered some strength, but my health declined even more from that point on. I've been diagnosed with degenerative bone loss in my jaw, which also causes my right ear drum to bulge. Already severe chemical sensitivities increased, too. My MD attempted to regulate my hormones, including taking a low dose of cortisol, which was all I could handle. This doctor realized he didn't know enough about Adrenal Fatigue Syndrome, and I was referred to Dr. Lam for nutritional coaching.

It's taken a year to feel optimistic about the future for myself and my girls, but the time has been worth it because I have so much physical and emotional strength back. It was tough to face the fact that much of my life has been traumatic—constant abuse or the fear of abuse is traumatic and has physical and emotional consequences. The fact that I would develop Adrenal Fatigue Syndrome makes sense to me. My physical symptoms were real, of course, but so was the constant stress I experienced.

Mind-Body Confusion

In patients of all ages, many disorders labeled as psychiatric or mental in origin may actually be caused by hormonal imbalances or insufficiencies. For example, *clinical or subclinical cortisol* deficiency is seldom part of the differential diagnosis in a medical or psychiatric workup.

(Differential diagnosis is a method used to consider a patient's symptoms with a group of possible conditions or diseases, and then systematically narrowing the possibilities until, presumably, the problem can be correctly identified.)

> However, hypocortisolemia (low levels of cortisol) is easily misdiagnosed as depression when the patient suffers from subclinical cortisol insufficiency. In addition, many symptoms of AFS and cortisol insufficiency closely parallel and may be confused with psychiatric disorders such as PTSD (post-traumatic stress disorder), addictions, and complex somatic symptom disorder (CSSD).

As if this situation isn't confusing enough, research shows that patients with a variety of psychiatric disorders, including addiction, have increased prevalence of signs and symptoms of mild to moderate low cortisol. Such symptoms can be reversed, however, after proper evaluation that takes into account the mind-body component that should be an essential part of every diagnosis.

Mind-Body—Psychosomatic—Medicine

The emerging field of mind-body medicine is also referred to as psychosomatic medicine, which links symptoms with psychological states. At one time, menstrual cramps and headaches, to name but two examples, were considered psychosomatic conditions, thereby stigmatizing sufferers. Labeling certain conditions as psychosomatic tended to be dismissive, implying that they weren't quite real. In a sense, this lets the medical community off the hook. Menstrual cramps and headaches were not taken particularly seriously, and we saw a lack of effective preventive measures and/or treatments. This situation has changed, however, because of a greater understanding of the realities of the mind-body entity.

On the other hand, hundreds of conditions appear to be purely physical disorders, but their origin is in unconscious emotions. Therefore, in addition to their training in traditional western medicine, mind-body physicians need a thorough knowledge of psychoneuroimmunology, psychoneuroendocrinology, and psychogenics.

In mind-body medicine, the thesis is that the mind contains the root cause of the physical distress. Further, the mind can make decisions outside of conscious awareness, and symptoms are part of that picture. Unfortunately, many in the medical arena still perpetuate the stigma of a psychosomatic diagnosis, which makes it difficult for patients to acknowledge its reality. In fact, 90 percent of adults will not acknowledge its presence, because of the implications of saying that an illness is "all in your mind." Most people are still insulted by that attitude and equate it with being told they are mentally ill. This is unfortunate, because the symptoms are very real, the result of a *physical* process.

Sometimes, patients' fears are well founded. For example, many in conventional medicine reinforce skeptical attitudes about mind-body therapy. When AFS patients do not recover in expected ways and on certain timetables, i.e., thyroid medication doesn't bring about improvement and antidepressants don't help energy or sleep, then some doctors eventually throw up their hands and tell patients they're out of options. Some doctors may suggest that if patients aren't already being treated for psychological disorders, then perhaps it's time to see a psychiatrist. These are the patients who feel abandoned and left to self navigate, all the while struggling to understand what has happened to them.

In an attempt to justify a diagnosis of mental disorders, physicians often prescribe psychotropic medications, including antidepressants, sleeping pills, or antianxiety drugs. When patients don't improve, they are eventually referred to psychiatrists for further adjustments to the medications. In the United States and elsewhere in the west, physicians and patients prefer the quick fix of prescription drugs that suppress symptoms. So, rather than dealing with the root cause of the physical and mental dysfunctions and symptoms, patients come to believe the mistaken notion that drugs effectively treat most conditions.

The range of mind-body disorders is wide and includes mildly bothersome back pain, for example, to severe pain of unknown origin. Because physicians often focus on symptoms rather than causes, they end up with a skewed frame of reference and thus incorrect diagnoses. Let's look in greater detail at the way the brain works.

The Unconscious and Conscious Mind

We can broadly divide the brain into the unconscious and conscious mind, and the two work together. Think of an iceberg floating in water. The conscious mind is what we see and notice above the surface; the unconscious mind, the largest and most powerful part, remains unseen below the surface.

When we talk about "my mind," we're referring to the conscious mind. We associate the conscious mind with what we learn growing up—thinking, analyzing, forming evaluations and judgments, and making choices and decisions. The unconscious mind holds awareness going back to childhood that is not presently in the conscious mind; all memories, feelings, and thoughts outside of conscious awareness are by definition unconscious or subconscious. We use our unconscious mind all the time, but don't realize it. For example, once we consciously learn to drive, our unconscious mind keeps us alert and helps us react and respond without conscious effort to second-by-second changing road conditions.

Our intuition and insight comes from the unconscious mind. When the conscious mind stops working and goes to sleep, our unconscious mind continues, producing the obvious dreams we create, but also suggesting solutions to problems that elude us. Think of how often we fail to immediately solve a problem only to have a sudden flash of insight in the middle of the night while sleeping, or while focusing on something else. This is how we see the unconscious mind working.

The unconscious mind can be injured or traumatized, especially during childhood. Consider the much too common traumas of sexual and physical abuse. Such early childhood trauma can carry into adulthood and influence personality traits and produce symptoms, including dysfunctional behaviors such as being obsessive-compulsive, aggressive, dependent, childish, showing the capacity for cruel and antisocial behavior, intensity of thought and behavior, and the drive for perfectionism. As we become adults, we often overlook and suppress these dysfunctional traits because we learn that it's socially unacceptable to release such inner discontent that arises from an injured unconscious mind. Sadly, such suppression only makes things worse, as repressed feelings can turn into anger and rage that can wreck havoc internally over time.

A deeply injured unconscious mind is unable to mend itself, and injuries become cumulative over time and continue to rest unhappily within our unconscious mind. Like a cancer, this discontent grows slowly but surely and does not go away until it is brought into consciousness, acknowledged, and properly dealt with. For example, dreams arising from the unconscious speak to us in symbolic language. When analyzed or pondered, these dreams can shed light on conflicts, thus bringing forward the needed information into consciousness.

Imbalanced personality traits, such as those mentioned above, become compensatory and defensive mechanisms that cover up the injured unconscious mind. As time goes on, however, physical symptoms can surface as the body *de*compensates, often when we encounter additional stress or advancing age. This is when mind-body disorders become fully integrated. Patients will report physical symptoms such as pain of unknown origin when the underlying root cause has a strong mental cause or association. Physicians not alert to this mental component will be easily misled by treating the physical symptoms without healing the mind. The result can be devastating.

Disorders Induced by Unconscious Emotions

Here's a sample list of physical disorders that can be directly induced by unconscious emotions:

- tension myositis syndrome (TMS)
- fibromyalgia
- carpal tunnel syndrome triggered by non-repetitive action
- gastric reflux
- irritable bowel syndrome (IBS)
- gastric ulcers of nonbacterial cause
- spastic colitis
- skin disorders, such as eczema, hives, angioedema (swelling beneath the skin), acne, and psoriasis
- esophageal spasms
- hiatal hernia
- allergic phenomena (e.g. allergic reactions triggered by allergens such as pollen, but the immune system is weakened by direction of the unconscious mind)
- rhinitis, commonly called a stuffy nose or congestion, asthma, sinusitis (inflammation of the sinuses, usually difficult to treat and often developing into a chronic condition)
- conjunctivitis
- tension and migraine headaches
- sexual dysfunction
- tinnitus (chronic ringing or buzzing noises in the ears)

In addition, the unconscious mind can play an important role in some conditions, but not be the main or only cause. These include autoimmune conditions such as rheumatoid arthritis and lupus, and certain heart arrhythmias. In mind-body disorders, the pain symptoms are meant to be protective distractions. In other words, pain, anxiety, and depression are not symptomatic of the underlying illness or disease, but they may appear so on the surface. Rather, these symptoms are part of a normal reaction to the frightened unconscious, the content of which is not allowed to surface and be recognized and dealt with. In other words, if we suppress childhood trauma and discomforting experiences, the body may produce symptoms such as pain or depression.

Those who research mind-body medicine embrace the idea that symptoms can be a manifestation of the struggle between the conscious and unconscious mind. According to some, the mind advances pain as a strategy of avoidance, distracting us from dealing with the many unresolved dysfunctions at the unconscious level. Such unconscious dysfunction can include pain, anger, rage, and long standing disappointments that have accumulated from early childhood events. Perhaps it is easier to deal with bodily pain than the deeply rooted emotional pain within. This is especially true when it's not socially acceptable to express these suppressed emotions, a situation that varies from culture to culture and family to family.

Recognizing the unconscious mind is an important milestone in recovering from mind-body conditions, because once the internal dysfunction is recognized, the conditions can often greatly improve. Specifically, we often see symptoms of pain of unknown origin drastically subside once patients acknowledge internal anger and rage.

For example, those with TMS often report a reduction in pain by simply writing down their discomfort at the onset of pain. This is an amazing testament to the healing power of allowing the suppressed voice of the unconscious to be heard. Once acknowledged, the need for pain as a tool to divert attention away from the unconscious hurt ceases to be productive, and pain symptoms no longer serve a purpose. Thus, pain spontaneously subsides and the patient improves. However, for maximum healing, deep-seated psychological issues need mind-body coaching and psychotherapy.

Adrenal Fatigue Syndrome and the Mind-Body Connection

We see more than a casual association between Adrenal Fatigue Syndrome and mind-body conditions. Simply go back and consider the list of common symptoms of AFS—everything from reduced energy and muscle and joint pain of unknown origin, to heart palpitations and depression. Many patients report insomnia, low immune system function, multiple chemical sensitivities, and poor GI assimilation. Many other symptoms exist as well.

Those in Stage 3 Adrenal Fatigue Syndrome are particularly vulnerable to additional symptoms such as anxiety and depression, myositis, neuropathy (degeneration of nerves), gastric ulcers, dysbiosis (imbalance in intestinal flora), and low immune function. We commonly see this group of symptoms when a patient progresses through the phases of Stage 3. Obviously, the list resembles previously mentioned mind-body conditions.

So, is there a connection between Adrenal Fatigue Syndrome and the mind? Based on clinical observation, the answer is a resounding yes, and especially among those in advanced stages.

> It remains to be determined if Adrenal Fatigue Syndrome is the end result of mental dysfunction, or if the mental imbalance is caused by AFS. In all likelihood, there are many factors, and the "which comes first" question may not be relevant at this point. However, the close connection between the adrenals and the mind is increasingly clear. Neurotransmitters, our important chemical messengers, and autonomic nervous system hormones are greatly involved in this connection. Clearly AFS in the broadest sense is part of a continuum of the body's neuroendocrine response to stress.

We see this when we look at particular clinical scenarios. Advanced AFS sufferers commonly complain of muscle pain of unknown origin, similar to the pain reported in fibromyalgia and myositis. Multiple pathways exist that can lead to the same symptoms. For example, myositis can result when the body enters a catabolic (breakdown) state during AFS, mediated by cortisol. The breakdown of muscle, along with the lack of timely repair and rebuilding, leads to pain when muscles are palpitated or stretched as the overall muscle mass is reduced.

We also can link myositis to a low metabolic state, whereby normal chemical metabolites are unable to be promptly cleared from the body, and instead, these metabolic byproducts are deposited in joints and muscles and act as inflammatory agents. Finally, myositis can be linked to mind-body disorders occurring as tension increases. Those with advanced AFS often have all three causes intertwined, and it's not easy to separate them.

When we factor in secondary symptoms, the clinical picture can seem quite complex and confusing. For example, myositis is often very painful, which in turn both contributes to and exacerbates depression and insomnia, both of which are symptoms in mind-body disorders. As insomnia sets in and sleep patterns are disturbed, the body doesn't receive the right amount of nighttime rest to recharge itself, which leads to less energy during the day.

In a continued downward cycle, reduced energy makes it difficult to maintain a fulltime job or business, which might quickly lead to financial problems, which then add to the stress. When an already compromised body accumulates an increasing amount of stress, that person may feel even more anxiety, depression, anger, rage, and loss of self confidence. (We see this in Mary's Story, Chapter 14, *Mary's Story—Illustrating the Problem.*) This is a vicious cycle of cascading pain and compromised daily activity. Clinically, we see a convoluted picture of multisystem dysfunction that defies conventional medical logic. The only path to clarity is to step back and carefully look at the overall state of the body and assess what's occurring.

The common wisdom is to assign much of the blame for the Adrenal Fatigue Syndrome symptoms to cortisol dysregulation, and rightly so, at least in many cases. We can't discount the wide ranging negative effects in various systems of the body when optimum cortisol levels are not maintained on an ongoing basis. That said, many situations exist in which cortisol alone cannot be held responsible for all the symptoms. We often see individuals with normal cortisol levels, but their symptoms are consistent with Adrenal Fatigue Syndrome. In addition, we need to be alert when those with adrenal weakness either fail to improve over time, or we can't find a good reason for slow recovery. In these specific situations, we must consider other organ system dysfunctions, including infection, metal toxicity, mineral deficiency, and mind-body imbalance.

To complicate matters further, unresolved anger and rage are the most common underlying traits associated with mind-body conditions. Many with advanced AFS, harbor long standing anger and thus have similar root issues. The anger could be from a variety of sources, including from the condition itself. By that we mean that many patients experience stress because the conventional medical practitioners they count on for help fail to adequately acknowledge what they are going through. They also may experience stress as they fail to improve over time and from their inability to work. Perhaps they are harboring anger and rage from a childhood traumatic emotional injury to the unconscious mind. It's nearly impossible to separate the entire emotional state of mind into components, because they are all intertwined. Surely, if individuals can reduce anger and rage, that will help the adrenal's healing process, regardless of the root cause. The question is *how,* and for that, we need to look at the physiology of how the mind and body are connected.

In Chapter 9, *Stage 3C—Disequilibrium,* we mentioned the autonomic nervous system (ANS), which is the primary physical conduit between the unconscious mind and the body. Simply put, dysregulation of the ANS, mediated by the key hormones epinephrine and norepinephrine, is the hallmark of Stage 3C AFS. We also see the prominent psychological expression of the unconscious mind, including irritability, anxiety, insomnia, and depression throughout Adrenal Exhaustion. Clearly, the role played by the ANS in connecting the mind and body is critical.

What Does this Mean For You?

Whether or not you feel there is a significant mind-body component in your situation, maintaining proper mind-body balance is important for general good health and recovery from AFS. The key is to rebalance ANS hormones, bearing in mind the following:

- A healthy mind contributes to faster recovery.
- A healthy mind doesn't contribute to getting sick.
- The adrenals are in constant communication with the mind.
- This communication benefits both the physical and mental aspects of well-being.

Perhaps most important, we see no downside or harm in understanding the mind-body component, but the benefits are numerous and significant.

When considering the mind-body connection, take care not to view this through a personal lens, as in blaming yourself for problems. These mind-body issues are universal and part of human life.

A variety of calming and empowering mind-body strategies have been proven successful to help rebalance the mind-body state, resulting in a more balanced body with less adrenaline release. You will read in detail about some of these strategies, including Adrenal Breathing and Adrenal Restoration Exercises (Chapter 27, *Adrenal Fatigue Syndrome and Healing Exercise*). These can bring the following results:

- Decreased anxiety and depression.
- Decreased pain, especially myositis.
- Enhanced sleep and elimination of insomnia.
- Strengthened immune system and reduced infection.
- Increased sense of control, peace, and well-being.
- Decreased fatigue and increased energy.

Therapeutic Mind-Body Balancing Tools

Breathing as a therapeutic tool has been overlooked for centuries, yet it remains one of the best and most powerful ways to harness the body's internal energy toward a proper mind-body balance. The best way to accomplish this is by doing our Adrenal Breathing Exercise. We designed this special breathing exercise to rebalance the autonomic nervous system dysfunction seen in advanced Adrenal Fatigue Syndrome. Special techniques are employed to produce a calming effect without over-stimulating the mind. A balanced reconnection of the mind and body allow hormonal flow that is favorable to AFS recovery. Those with heart palpitations, anxiety, depression, irritability, strong heart rate, and insomnia will benefit most. Whether or not you have a mind-body component, this is an excellent way to optimize bodily function. We say much more about this in Chapter 27, *Adrenal Fatigue Syndrome and Healing Exercise.*

What It Means to You

As we move more deeply into the twenty-first century, we see many more healthcare professionals coalescing around now proven mind-body connections. We now understand that the mental and the physical are simply different aspects of the larger whole, and furthermore, the mental and physical planes penetrate and overlap one another. We can see in the manifestation of illness that an impact in one plane immeasurably influences the other. This is clearly seen in advanced AFS, where symptoms of mind-body dysfunction cover considerable ground, from pain and skin conditions to anxiety and depression.

> **It is our hope that as you expand your understanding of the mind-body connection, you will find ways to balance your life and move toward greater healing and fulfillment in your life. We place special emphasis on this because successful, holistic recovery from AFS must start with the recognition that the mind and the body are intricately connected, and that can't be ignored.**

From a physiological perspective, the key in restoring the proper mind-body balance rests with rebalancing the autonomic nervous system. As you will soon realize, Adrenal Breathing, Adrenal Restorative Exercises, and Adrenal Yoga (not associated with any spiritual practice) are excellent tools to promote Adrenal Fatigue Syndrome recovery.

The more advanced the AFS, the more significant is the role of the mind, not only in the cause, but in the recovery as well. In the next chapter, we specifically discuss the ways we approach recovery from Adrenal Fatigue Syndrome.

Key Points to Remember

- Any AFS recovery must start with the understanding that our body is an integrated whole. What happens to one part affects the other. Many of the symptoms of advanced AFS are triggered from the central nervous system and mediated through chemical messengers of the mind. Knowing how the mind and body are connected in AFS is the logical starting point of any recovery process.

- Ample scientific evidence from neuroscience points to the mind-body integrated relationship. This is no longer an area of debate.

- Mind-body medicine is a new medical specialty with the thesis that physical disorders have a strong mental component, or originate from the mind but are mediated by hormones and other chemical messengers. Mind-body conditions include irritable bowel syndrome (IBS), tension myositis syndrome (TMS), gastric reflux, spastic colitis, rhinitis, carpal tunnel syndrome triggered by non-repetitive actions, etc.

- Many symptoms of advanced Adrenal Fatigue Syndrome are similar to symptoms of mind-body dysfunction.

- Cortisol output imbalances alone cannot explain all symptoms of advanced AFS. A mind-body connection, mediated by the ANS, the autonomic nervous system, clearly exists.

- Maintaining proper mind-body balance, regardless of whether AFS is present, is good for health. The key is to reduce sympathetic and enhance parasympathetic tone. This is best done through our Adrenal Breathing Exercise.

Chapter 16

A Total Body Approach to Adrenal Fatigue Syndrome

M edical knowledge of Adrenal Fatigue Syndrome is still in its infancy, and most individuals with the problem are unaware that their symptoms are attributable to AFS. Symptoms of AFS vary so much, and no standardized recovery protocol exists, both of which complicate our understanding of the condition. For these reasons, we see great confusion about how to help those in need.

As practitioners, we have gained clinical expertise over time by handling many severe cases of AFS. Fortunately, the recovery toolbox contains many tools, including a variety of medications, hormones, glandulars, herbs, vitamins, dietary guidelines, and combinations thereof, plus lifestyle tools, including exercise regimens, achieving optimal sleep, and so forth. Despite this comprehensive arsenal of recovery tools, *complete* Adrenal Fatigue Syndrome recovery remains elusive and for many unattainable. This has led to a common misconception that once seriously afflicted with AFS, it is virtually impossible to overcome.

As we've said, AFS as a condition is under investigated. In addition, mild AFS often goes undetected because symptoms arise intermittently and lack a consistent pattern. However, if properly guided, sufferers usually recover within a relatively short time. Even some self navigation efforts can be effective, as long as the body still has reserves and is able to tolerate trial and error recovery attempts without crashes or setbacks. On the other hand, advanced Adrenal Fatigue Syndrome may leave many individuals housebound and even bedridden. In these cases, proper recovery requires extensive clinical experience and patience, taking into account the body's depleted reserves and high levels of sensitivity.

We see many women and men with severe AFS because they come to us for nutritional coaching as a last resort, usually because conventional medicine and traditional naturopathic ways have failed. Some had never heard of AFS when they found their way to us, and these advanced cases served to educate us about the best ways to help those afflicted.

Our philosophical approach to AFS involves four foundational principles, which we incorporate into a systematic personalized program. What works for patient X might be wrong for patient Y. In any case, our program integrates conventional and holistic strategies into a comprehensive natural healing strategy we call the *Total Body Approach.*

The Four Principles of the Total Body Approach

FIRST: We believe the body is a closed ecosystem capable of self-maintenance and self-healing under normal circumstances.

When stressors overwhelm our internal repair mechanism, breakdown occurs. These stressors can be acute or chronic, physical or emotional, but they are excessive and cause the body to decompensate. Symptoms surface as warning signs of internal disturbances in normal functions; the weakest organ system often is the first one to give way. For example, those with constitutionally weak adrenals relative to other, stronger organ systems may manifest Adrenal Fatigue Syndrome. Likewise, those with weaker cardiovascular systems may develop heart problems, and those with a weak gastric system might develop gastric ulcers. This explains why some people can have severe stress but no Adrenal Fatigue Syndrome.

That said, once severe stress triggers the decompensation cascade of one system, many other systems become sequentially affected. This occurs because the body is not a collection of separate organ systems. Rather, they are all linked internally through many hormonal axes. A disturbance in one system starts a domino effect that results in a potentially overwhelming convolution of symptoms concurrently involving many body systems. This is why in those with advanced AFS we often see symptoms like insomnia, depression, arrhythmia, hypoglycemia, irregular menses, and hypothyroidism. In general, the weaker the adrenals, the more prevalent the symptoms. Although some symptoms such as salt cravings and hypoglycemia are principally caused by adrenal dysfunction, many other symptoms such as arrhythmia and depression are due to the breakdown of other organ systems that had been normal.

SECOND: Mild Adrenal Fatigue Syndrome generally manifests as lack of physical energy, but advanced AFS usually manifests as a mind-body condition rather than solely a physical dysfunction.

The brain ultimately controls the adrenal function by way of the hypothalamic-pituitary-adrenal (HPA) axis and a variety of chemical messengers. Our emotional states have a big impact on adrenal function. Common organ systems that are targets of mind-body disturbances include components of the nervous system, plus the endocrine and metabolic systems. Because knowledge of these systems helps us understand the connection between symptoms, we discuss them throughout this book. Our scientific perspective calls for evaluating each person's unique history, constitution, environment, emotions and mental state, and nutritional status, plus the often convoluted and pressing symptoms, as a whole unit rather than as unrelated parts. This provides a complete picture of the overall clinical state. Ultimately, the best nutritional solution provides both physical and mental health support.

THIRD: We view symptoms as our friends, not our enemies.

Symptoms are the only way the body can tell us what it wants us to do. In our view, we need to allow symptoms to manifest in a controlled environment with minimal discomfort. For example, many symptoms of AFS, such as salt cravings, hypotension (low blood pressure), palpitations, adrenaline rush, anxiety, and hypoglycemia tend to improve when the adrenals are returned to health.

> As long as the body is not in acute crisis, we should gently support it while giving it a chance to heal itself. At the same time, we gain insight into the body by observing symptoms during recovery.
>
> This does not mean that we allow unpleasant symptoms to continue unchecked, but we consciously avoid the trap of focusing only on alleviating symptoms. We keep our eyes on the big picture and use symptoms to guide us and support the adrenal's internal healing process nutritionally. The goal is to strengthen the adrenals and prevent future problems.

We seldom see long term success with overzealous recovery strategies based on addressing symptoms rather than nurturing the body back to health, and for good reason. Since symptoms are signs of underlying dysfunction, suppressing symptoms in one system might trigger dysfunction in another system, but often subclinically.

Symptoms soon become even more convoluted and overwhelming when one dysfunction is superimposed on another. We often see this as a side effect of the recovery effort, particularly when conventionally trained physicians prescribe medications that produce side effects. This is a major problem, and the more medications prescribed, the greater the risk of side effects.

• **FOURTH: We let our body educate us at every opportunity so we know what it wants.**

We closely monitor the side effects and potential harm coming from well intentioned nutritional strategy to which each body reacts differently. Our body teaches us every day of its likes and dislikes, if only we listen closely. The more we learn, the better we are able to effectively self navigate. Most of us are not in tune enough with our body. We therefore focus on educating sufferers about their individual body types and what factors they must adjust to in order to return to health and maintain health. We teach them how to listen to and interpret the body's signs, and we educate them to live harmoniously with their body as they take control of their health. We also make sure they understand the pros and cons of each tool in the toolbox, the reasons to use the tool, and what possible negative side effects to look for. As you can see, we devote our energy to *educating* rather than *medicating*.

The Seven Steps of the Total Body Approach

Using the four guiding principles, here are seven specific steps we use to formulate and personalize our Total Body Approach.

Step 1: Know the Body

We take the time to develop an in-depth understanding of the body and its constitutional state, and no shortcut exists to establish this foundation. We confirm this qualitatively through our customized nutritional plan that gently tests and challenges the body while simultaneously nurturing it. By noting each body's unique response, we are able to further personalize a plan specific to that body's needs. In this way, we facilitate recovery.

Although a painstaking and time-consuming process, we've found it the fastest way to facilitate overall recovery. The insights we gain help us avoid the risk of future crashes, which are major setbacks for any recovery program. Overall, we reduce total recovery time, and the healing process is more pleasant.

Step 2: Establish the Dominant Dysfunction

To fully anticipate the body's reaction to any single component of our Total Body Approach, whether it is a nutrient or the diet, *we identify each person's major intrinsic root weakness.* The body as one unit is only as strong as the weakest organ system. The weakest system is also usually the first system to be symptomatic, and thus, the dominant dysfunction. Each person usually has one weakness that is uniquely more susceptible to insult, comparatively speaking. For some, the thyroid may be the weakness, and hypothyroidism may be the first sign of internal weakness. For others, it may be gastric discomfort. For some, it may be the cardiac system, with hypertension as the first sign. The organ system with the most dominant dysfunction is also the weakest link to the entire recovery effort. Therefore, it is important to identify and help the body—naturally and nutritionally—deal with the dominant root cause. Knowing the prominent dysfunction helps us to personalize a recovery program with maximum chances of success.

For example, the natural compound *GABA* (a neurotransmitter that regulates anxiety and sleep) is generally a good sleep aid for those who are adrenal dominant, but it's not as effective for the thyroid dominant. Thyroid dominant individuals generally do well taking 5-HTP (an amino acid that's a precursor to serotonin, a neurotransmitter) to help them sleep. Each nutrient has its own best-use pathway, and for maximum effectiveness, it must be matched to the correct condition.

> As for diet, thyroid dominant types benefit most from a vegetarian diet with increased fiber load to enhance gastric assimilation. On the other hand, the ovarian dominant type usually benefits from a diet high in protein relative to carbohydrates. The adrenal dominant type usually does best on a balanced diet with a slight bias toward more protein and fat, along with higher meal frequency to overcome hypoglycemia. Those with a mixed type require a combination of the above.

In terms of exercise, thyroid dominant types usually do best with rhythmic exercise like running/walking, bicycling, or swimming. Ovarian dominant types do best with more gentle and mentally focused exercise such as yoga. The adrenal dominant type is trickier because we can divide them into two main categories: those with high adrenal function and those with low adrenal function. Strenuous exercise often helps the high adrenal type burn off the excess adrenaline. Those with low adrenal function should usually not exercise until the body regains its footing through nutritional and diet support. When the body's reserve is increased, a gradual scaling up of isometric and isotonic exercises can be considered.

Step 3: Determine the Severity

Adrenal Fatigue Syndrome in its mild form is clinically very different from its more advanced stages. Symptoms of mild and early stage AFS may include insomnia, lack of energy, irritability, high blood pressure, salt craving, anxiety, and weight gain. Additional symptoms of advanced Adrenal Fatigue Syndrome, however, can include hypoglycemia, *low* blood pressure, heart palpitations, weight loss, severe depression, and menstrual irregularities. Using the same recovery tools that were successful for mild AFS to treat those in more advanced stages might backfire. In other words, the right tools for early stage AFS can lead to worsening symptoms in those with advanced AFS. Misunderstanding this principle is a common mistake.

We use the tools to reach our goals, and choose the tools based on our underlying strategic concept. Without this clear conceptual strategy that guides how and when to use the tools, they easily can be misused and produce undesirable results. Evaluating and knowing each sufferer's clinical state helps us choose the tools to use, but we also understand that no single tool works all the time. As the body changes, the choice of tools must also change. Clearly, what is nutritionally beneficial for one person may be toxic for another. However, what was beneficial for a person at a particular stage could be negative for that same person during the course of recovery.

Step 4: Prioritize and Personalize

We prioritize and time our nutritional therapeutic recommendations to match the body's readiness. Most people in advanced AFS have many problems involving other organ systems. By prioritizing our approach, we can systematically create a plan while not losing sight of what is important at any point in time. For example, some with both ovarian and adrenal dysregulation improve fastest and do best if we deal with the ovarian dysfunction first. The opposite may apply for others. Still, for some, we need to approach both simultaneously.

We facilitate sustained recovery by taking a one-step-at-a-time approach. We prefer a gradual and enjoyable steady path to recovery rather than one dominated by periods of euphoria followed by setbacks. Such a pattern can worsen the overall condition and slow down the entire recovery process.

Step 5: Challenge the Body

In order to give the body the most gentle and valuable nutrients possible, we use qualitative nutritional challenges, which are specific protocols we follow in order to prove or disprove the underlying hypothesis. A challenge helps us gain insight into the body's response before we choose the tools from the recovery toolbox. For example, we can gain insight into the body's aldosterone regulation by drinking salt water and seeing how the body reacts. It's essential that we understand the purpose of each challenge, and both positive as well as negative responses provide valuable information. Well planned challenges in various forms help us to understand the body's readiness before embarking on a nutritional therapeutic course.

Step 6: Monitor Closely

We carefully monitor the body's reactions by using a listening-focused, narrative approach with close follow up. This means we listen to what is being reported to us. Currently, we don't have objective and quantitative tests to assess adrenal function in real time. Our Total Body Approach calls for taking small steps, and we constantly evaluate and update, getting as close to real-time body reaction as possible. We do this by paying attention to the various signs and symptoms the body exhibits every day. We are especially attentive to how a body performs under challenges and how it reacts under stress.

For many centuries, medical practices used this listening-focused, narrative-based approach—it was the norm. However, it's now an endangered art form because modern clinical medicine relies heavily on investigative tools. Certainly, astute health practitioners use the many investigative tools at their disposal, but final recommendations are usually based on an extensive patient history, clinical insight, and experience. This is even more important with AFS because we lack complete understanding, and laboratory results are not very reliable.

Step 7: Patience

Biological repair takes time. The body isn't like a light switch that we turn on and off at will. Our use of gentle nutrients facilitates internal, sustainable, and long-term change at the cellular level. Many do show signs of improvement within a reasonable period of time, but severe cases can take much longer.

Bear in mind that proper adrenal recoveries usually take a series of steps resembling going up a flight of stairs, with lots of pauses in between each step. The first few steps up are usually fast, with short pauses. By the end of this stage, most are overjoyed as they rediscover and reclaim their lost energy. While the total energy state of the body is still far below that of someone whose health is optimal, most AFS sufferers are happy to have the energy for a balanced social, work, and family life. As we progress further up the recovery stairway, pauses become longer, and the incremental increases in energy become fewer. This is normal. With proper planning, a steady and sustained recovery can usually be achieved, provided we have patience and allow the body to rest when called for.

If no improvement is noted for a sustained period of time, we often find a very good, but hidden, reason. No amount of water can put out a fire if oil is quietly added on the side. Those in this category need patience in order to initiate a systematic approach to discovering the underlying cause. Most of the time, if we look deep enough we can find the hidden reason. Those who focus on understanding the body will likely find it, and in our role as clinicians we facilitate that process. We usually have to say goodbye to those who are too focused on quick recovery or are unrealistic in their recovery goals. Granted, it's relatively easy to stimulate the body and drive energy output. However, that approach eventually backfires and AFS worsens because the root cause is never uncovered and dealt with.

If we look at recovery as a race to the finish line in a track meet, our Total Body Approach is akin to running at a steady pace and feeling fresh at the end line. It's about enjoying the race along the way, rather than sprinting, only to collapse well before the finish line.

Many with AFS tend to have Type A personalities, defined as intense, compulsive, and always inquisitive. They often want to understand the science of AFS, which can be beneficial. However, we discourage patients from *excessive* focus on trying to explain every single symptom or physiological pathway, because this tends to increase anxiety and further drains the body of its already limited reserves. Overall, it slows recovery. We find that those who recover completely at a relatively fast pace trust and listen to our recommendations and follow them carefully. We encourage everyone to use their energy doing what they enjoy in life in a balanced way, stopping to smell the flowers along the way.

Being Mindful of Limitations

Our Total Body Approach can facilitate, but not mandate what the body does. We can affect recovery only as fast as the body allows a long term, sustained return to health. Some do well in a short time; with others, the preparation period may be longer. Those who are older or constitutionally weaker often face the biggest challenges. Therefore, we remain constantly on the lookout and open to alternative methodology.

The Big Picture

Our Total Body Approach integrates the best of conventional and natural healing processes nutritionally. Our focus is deploying natural compounds to satisfy what the body is crying out for, and we believe in accommodating the body's requests whenever possible. We teach those who seek our help to listen to the body, which is something many of us do not know how to do.

Given the right tools, the body is capable of bringing about its own healing, at least in most cases. We are facilitators of this process. In addition, our Total Body Approach calls for a focus on the whole person by integrating a holistic approach.

Along with recovery, our goal is to teach each person how to live post-recovery, and how to prevent recurrence in the future. Finally, to give the body ample time to recover, patience is a hallmark of our approach. We do not force the body into functions for which it is not prepared.

Key Points to Remember

- The AFS recovery tool box contains many tools. Knowing what to use and when, are signs of clinical excellence.

- Our Total Body Approach comes after years of helping those with AFS recover. It is a comprehensive and nutritionally oriented program designed to give the adrenal glands the right gentle tools for it to self-heal instead of forcing it to perform with stimulants.

- The approach is formulated based on four basic foundational principals and contains seven specific steps.

Chapter 17

Seven Adrenal Recovery Mistakes

By this time, you know that most cases of Adrenal Fatigue Syndrome are mild (Stages 1 and 2), lasting a few days or weeks, with eventual full recovery. This generally occurs without awareness that AFS is involved. A minority of people find recovery a challenge. Their symptoms last longer than usual; they eventually improve, but never fully recover. Still, a smaller number of people slowly decompensate and their condition gets worse with time. These are the individuals who slowly slip into advanced stages of AFS (Stage 3 and beyond).

When sufferers experience frequent episodes of Adrenal Fatigue Syndrome symptoms that increase in severity and duration, we consider this a sign of recovery failure. The body has a built in, self repair system, but it is often not fully engaged in the recovery process. We see many reasons for this failure, and we discuss seven of the most common below. Keep these in mind as you embark on your search for help.

Mistake 1: Following Advice from Inexperienced Healthcare Providers

As they embark on a journey of recovery, most patients quickly realize that most mainstream physicians are not well educated about AFS. On top of this, modern medicine has a tendency to lean heavily toward laboratory-based approaches to healing, rather than narrative, body-based approaches. In addition, we do not yet have accurate and foolproof laboratory testing for Adrenal Fatigue Syndrome. *Paradoxically, the more advanced the adrenal weakness, the lower the clinical correlation with laboratory results.*

> To untrained physicians, the maze of complaints is a challenge. Dysfunctional adrenals affect virtually every system of the body including the central nervous system, cardiovascular system, peripheral nervous system, hormonal system, and gastric system, just to mention a few. Therefore, practitioners need a thorough understanding of neurology, cardiology, endocrinology, and psychiatry. Since most physicians specialize today, their training is on a narrow, clinical focus, and they often lack experience in the multiple disciplines necessary to fully comprehend AFS in its broadest sense.

Unfortunately, treating symptoms becomes the standard of care instead of focusing on the root problem. This is why patients often end up with myriad prescriptions, including antidepressants and antianxiety medications, along with other agents that treat symptoms. Many different specialists often treat sufferers separately for digestive disorders, gynecologic disorders, psychological symptoms, allergies, and so forth.

The number of physicians with true expertise in advanced Adrenal Fatigue Syndrome invariably gained their expertise from years of clinical experience. In severe cases, full recovery can easily take a year or more. Inexperienced practitioners are often misled by laboratory tests and preoccupied with treating symptoms. These practitioners find it difficult to handle other than the most mild and straightforward cases of AFS and usually give up when it comes to advanced cases. Unfortunately, sufferers are unaware of these limitations and are misled into thinking they're on the right track. Disappointed, they eventually self-navigate as their symptoms get worse. Finding the right healthcare professional is your greatest challenge and task. Appendix A offers some tips on how to find the right physician for you.

Mistake 2: Excessive Use of Prescription Drugs and Medications

We live in a world where *symptoms are often classified as diseases.* Therefore, controlling symptoms is often confused with "curing" the disease, even when the condition is chronic. In the case of AFS, this common approach frequently ends in disaster. Masking pain, for example, is not the same as curing the condition that causes the pain. The symptoms of AFS are like pain, they're signals that something is amiss. But suppressing symptoms doesn't work and only punishes the body. The body responds by punishing with worsening symptoms.

The logical approach is to give the body the tools to heal itself, while monitoring the symptoms and using them as a barometer to evaluate progress toward healing. Sadly, this method is rarely deployed. Suppressing symptoms with various prescription medications is the norm. Unfortunately, most medications have side effects. For example, the dozens of common side effects of antidepressants alone include dry mouth, blurred vision, constipation, sleep disruption, headaches, nausea, loss of libido, and agitation. We can multiply this by the number of medications many individuals take simultaneously. Needless to say, this practice stresses the liver and the adrenals, and many with Adrenal Fatigue Syndrome never fully recover when their treatments are based on prescription medications, which can range from steroids to antianxiety drugs to sleep medications.

Mistake 3: Over Reliance on Laboratory Testing

As we learned in Chapter 11, *Diagnostic Tests—What You Need to Know*, diagnostic testing is severely limited when it comes to Adrenal Fatigue Syndrome. It is common to have significant AFS symptoms, but the lab tests are within the normal range. We often see lab results that confuse and mislead. Laboratory interpretation is challenging even for experienced clinicians. Physicians often find themselves chasing a moving target. In advanced AFS, the more we rely on laboratory tests, the more confused we get because of multiple inconsistencies in the correlation between test results and symptoms. As a result, patients are often subjected to numerous trial and error protocols undertaken by physicians with the best intentions but who were clinically misled by laboratory tests. This approach further weakens the body's already low adrenal function. Many come to us confused and frustrated as a result.

The body's signs and symptoms are far superior in gauging adrenal weakness than laboratory test results performed with current technology. The gold standard remains a good and comprehensive narrative history of the sufferer taken by an experienced clinician. Laboratory tests can be helpful when properly used.

Mistake 4: Improper Use of Nutritional Supplements

You likely know that natural compounds differ from prescription drugs in many ways. Prescription drugs usually follow a well defined and highly predictable efficacy curve, meaning that the desired response is usually generated within a predetermined range of therapeutic dosing. The body does not have a natural, built-in system of metabolizing non-natural compounds such as synthetic drugs, so with high dosages, toxicity results. Similarly, when natural compounds are used inappropriately, recovery is not only impeded, but the condition worsens over time. In these situations the compounds do more harm than good. This is one of the greatest mistakes made among those who embark on self-guided and nonprofessionally guided programs, especially if the Adrenal Fatigue Syndrome is advanced. (See Chapter 19, *Nutritional Supplements for Nutritional Fatigue: An Introduction*) for more detailed information about the use of natural compounds.)

Mistake 5: Failure to Recognize Paradoxical and Unusual Reactions

When medical treatments, usually with a drug, have the opposite effect of what we expect, we call that a paradoxical reaction. For example, if a sleep medication causes worsening insomnia, we call it a paradoxical reaction. Likewise, if a sedative causes hyperactivity, that's a paradoxical reaction. We see this when steroid drugs worsen AFS instead of helping. Experienced clinicians watch for these abnormalities.

Although we don't know the reason, paradoxical reactions are generally more prevalent with natural compounds. We do know that one person's beneficial natural compound can be toxic to another person. This can occur over time. In some cases, however, the body rejects these nutrients from the beginning. Instead of feeling better with an energy boost, the person feels worse and an adrenal crash could result.

The more advanced the AFS, the more paradoxical and unusual reactions tend to surface. The body is caught in a cascading downward state, with exaggerated responses mediated by hormonal imbalances in a positive feedback loop platform, along with its own violent attempt to rebalance itself. Such paradoxical reactions include:

- Severe fatigue but feeling wired at the same time.
- Fragile blood pressure that fails to normalize in quiet times.
- Reactive hypoglycemia despite metabolic medications to stabilize blood sugar.
- Palpitations made worse with cardiac medication designed to reduce irregular heart beat.
- Sudden anxiety attacks while on sedatives.
- Worsening fatigue with natural compounds that helped before.

While some of these symptoms can be due to drug intolerance, liver clearance problems, autonomic nervous system dysregulation, and side effects of natural compounds, many paradoxical reactions occur with no apparent medical logic. However, these paradoxical reactions are important warning signs of our body we need to take heed of. Failure to recognize such reactions can contribute to delayed or failed recovery.

Mistake 6: Failure to Recognize Multi-organ Involvement

Failure to recognize the multi-organ involvement associated with Adrenal Fatigue Syndrome often leads to a narrow focus that makes the condition worse off over time. As previously explained, the adrenal glands are regulated through the hypothalamic-pituitary-adrenal (HPA) axis. The adrenals themselves are then intricately connected to many other organs in a variety of axes. In women, one such intricate relationship is called the ovarian adrenal and thyroid (OAT) axis (Chapter 8, *Stage 3B—Hormonal Axis Imbalances*). These three organs are intimately code-pendent on each other for optimal function. In men, the adrenal and thyroid are connected.

In the case of the OAT axis, when a medication alters one of the organs' functions, it will invariably lead to an often unrecognized change in the other two organs. For example, if thyroid medication is administered, it is not uncommon to see concurrent menstrual irregularities, a function of the ovarian hormones, and reduced ability to deal with stress and worsening fatigue, a function of the adrenals.

When multiple organs are involved and decompensate concurrently, the body's ability to recover is made much harder. For example, processing and assimilating nutrients becomes compromised, leading to reduced absorption of nutrients in the GI track, producing digestive symptoms. Liver function is reduced, although laboratory test results might be in the normal range. If not processed and metabolized properly, good nutrients become toxic, producing toxic metabolites that circulate in the body. If not properly cleared, these toxic metabolites can lead to brain fog, joint pain, skin rashes, allergies, muscle discomfort, and multiple chemical sensitivities among many other symptoms.

When the adrenals are not in optimal condition, no organ system is spared dysfunction. Therefore, an adrenal recovery program that does not factor in other organ involvement invariably fails as the condition worsens.

Mistake 7: Lack of a Comprehensive Recovery Program

The body is a closed ecosystem with a built in capability to self repair. If given a chance, it normally can recover on its own with the proper nutrients, lifestyle, dietary changes, and time. Recovery strategies focusing on this comprehensive approach often produce excellent results, even in severe cases, in a short time. By contrast, strategies that focus on controlling the symptoms and getting quick results often fail. For maximum recovery speed, the root cause, such as removal of stressors, improper dietary habits, and improper use of nutritional supplements, needs to be addressed through a comprehensive program.

The most effective recovery program should incorporate the following (which we discuss in detail later in this book):

- A customized nutritional supplementation program based on the person's internal needs and sensitivities.

- A customized dietary program based on the sufferer's metabolic needs.

- A customized lifestyle program including exercise based on the person's constitution and energy reserve.

The above three-pronged approach can produce dramatic and quick results if carried out under the supervision of an experienced clinician.

By now you realize that AFS is much more complicated and debilitating than you might have thought. Fortunately, with an individualized recovery plan, most patients can and do recover.

Key Points to Remember

The 7 most common recovery mistakes are:

- Following advice from an inexperienced healthcare provider.

- Excessive use of prescription drugs and medications.

- Over reliance on laboratory testing.

- Improper use of nutritional supplements.

- Failure to recognize paradoxical reactions.

- Failure to recognize multi-organ involvement.

- Lack of a comprehensive recovery program.

Recovery and the Body's Constitution—What You Can Expect

We are each born with a unique inner body type or *biological constitution*, although we can't measure it with a lab test or see it with a CT scan or an MRI. Given today's focus on standardizing treatments, the issue of constitution is rarely discussed in medical literature or considered in recovery plans. The body constitution reflects our genetic makeup. For example, three adults with strep throat will receive prescriptions for antibiotics and told to take them for a certain number of days. They expect to start feeling better after two or three days on the medication. Patient X fully recovers in a week, patient Y recovers in ten days to two weeks, but Patient Z not only needs three weeks to feel well again, but needs more rest than either Patient X or Y. Although many factors can contribute to shorter or longer recovery, the varying constitutions of the three adults likely play an important role.

Individual constitution plays an important role in everything, from back pain to surgery to the common cold. It's an extremely important concept for all those with Adrenal Fatigue Syndrome, because constitution plays a role in *all* stages and features of AFS. Identifying and understanding our patients' constitution helps us formulate, customize, and manage individual recovery plans. This is why we have devoted a chapter to AFS and body constitution.

When we talk about body type, we're usually describing the body's physical shape, especially as it relates to athletic ability or attractiveness. However, in the context of holistic healing, your body type, or biological constitution, refers to the inner makeup and your ability to deal with illness.

Even the most skilled conventionally trained physicians are unable to physically examine their patients and definitively determine their biological constitution. The biological constitution is a subtle concept and whether we are aware of it or not, it plays an important role in everyday life. For our purposes, we're using the terms "constitution" and "body type" interchangeably, but by any name, our constitution influences the way we metabolize nutrients, digest food, think and process information, both work and play, and sleep.

No two individuals experience the condition in exactly the same way—which is one reason it's difficult to study Adrenal Fatigue Syndrome. The wide varying experience of AFS comes back to body type. We can trace the confusion about AFS back to the variation in response to the same stressors, which influences the level of Adrenal Fatigue Syndrome in a way that often defies medical logic. Some people can be under severe stress and perform well, while others crash under what to some seems like only the slightest stress. Certain individuals with AFS progress slowly but steadily from Stage 1 to Stage 3 over time; others quickly deteriorate and never fully recover. In large part, we can attribute these differences to constitution.

What about Genetics?

We're born with a particular genetic makeup, or *genome*, which determines elements of our body from the obvious anatomical components such as blood, muscle, and organs, to the more subtle internal hormonal and metabolic systems. In fact, anti-aging research has found that about 30 percent of our longevity is determined by our genes, while 70 percent is determined by our diet and lifestyle. Under normal circumstances, the individual genome plays an important role in determining, for example, who gets cancer and who does not. We all know of lifelong chain smokers who never develop lung cancer while nonsmokers in perfect health may develop the disease and die quickly.

Weak parts exist in everyone's constitution because none of us are born perfect. Moreover, some have more weak parts, some less. For example, those with relatively weaker immune systems tend to get sick easily and more frequently. Others might have metabolic weakness, and for them, weight management is a lifelong issue. We have no control over the body type we're born with, but we can nurture our weak parts in order to restore and strengthen them as much as possible.

Recent genetic research illuminates this situation. Although our basic genome does not change over time, its expression does. In other words, as you age, your genes do not change, but your *epigenome* (the biochemical mechanism that turns genes on and off) changes dramatically. Today, epigeneticism has emerged as a factor with primary influence on the way environmental factors such as diet, lifestyle, and stress influence the expression of your genes. In other words, the expression of your genes, not the genes themselves, dictates whether you develop certain diseases.

In the case of the adrenal glands, certain factors can amplify constitutional weakness, including: aging, obesity, excessive childhood illness, prolonged stress, and overuse of antibiotics, just to name a few. The same is true for emotional trauma such as death of a loved one, physical trauma such as a car accident, relational difficulties such as divorce, and psychosomatic illnesses.

> If you were born with weak adrenal glands, it's likely that this weakness will be expressed when you're under stress, and this might lead to AFS. On the other hand, the absence of significant stress can delay the expression of this weakness for an indefinite period of time.

If you were born with constitutionally strong adrenal glands, you might not develop AFS despite severe stress. Those with weak adrenal functions might experience symptoms when exposed to stress, even as teenagers. Throughout your life, your genome, along with the epigenome, determines your body's weakest link and subsequent expression of illness.

A Different View: East versus West

Western medicine doesn't have a good understanding of the concept of the body constitution, and therefore, tends to treat all bodies alike, with the exception of certain identified genetic markers such as the genes linked with breast cancer. On the other hand, eastern medical philosophy emphasizes the forces of nature that govern the human body and are responsible for regulating all systemic, endocrine, metabolic, and functional changes in the body. These forces of nature are enveloped in the five vital elements:

- Air, the vital force behind all functions.

- Fire, the source of energy and heat and responsible for transformation, such as metabolism, hormones, and saliva production.

- Earth, the element of strength and anabolism (building up), such as collagen, ligaments, and muscles.

- Water, that which binds structures together, such as urine, sweat, and gastric enzymes.

- Space, where all factors exist, such as the oral cavity, and the respiratory and reproductive system.

For the body to feel good and function normally, all five elements must be in perfect balance. In ayurvedic medicine, the ancient philosophy of health and healing developed in India, the prakriti is the name for the individual biological constitution that remains constant throughout life. The prakriti manifests as individual physical attributes and physiological and psychological responses in line with universal laws. In eastern philosophical thinking, universal laws rule the formation, existence, and destruction of all objects on a space and time continuum of consciousness. Within these laws, every individual is a unique entity, and the prakriti, therefore, is one-of-a-kind.

Whether we look at it from the eastern or western medical perspective, AFS is an expression of how the body deals with stress. The degree of damage and subsequent recovery pattern depends largely on the body's biological constitution. Those with strong adrenal constitutions recover faster and have a longer sustained recovery when compared to those who have weak adrenals. This is in part the reason that many individuals never advance beyond Stages 1 and 2 with severe stress. However, those with weak adrenals might never fully recover after crashes, and these individuals might continue a downward path of decompensation over time.

> Unfortunately, no routine laboratory test exists to determine the body's constitution. The best assessment comes from a good narrative history that astute clinicians examine and interpret.

Since advanced AFS generally develops over a period of years, the body usually sends out many signals. However, most people pay little attention to these signals and choose to ignore them or write them off as normal in one context or another. When AFS finally triggers crashes and the body fails to recover, we're at a loss to explain what's happened. Most in advanced AFS can look back at their life retrospectively, and see that invariably their symptoms had been evident for a long time if they only paid attention.

Your Constitution

The pattern of recovery from AFS and the kind of nutrients required differ depending on the type of body constitution. This is why it's important to know from the start if you have a strong, normal, or weak body constitution if you think you have AFS.

You can see from the chart below, constitutions can range from very strong to very weak, with 68 percent falling into the normal range, as shown on a bell curve. The rest of the population falls in the remaining smaller distributions: 14 percent weak, 14 percent strong, 2 percent very weak, 2 percent very strong. (These ranges should not be taken as absolute.)

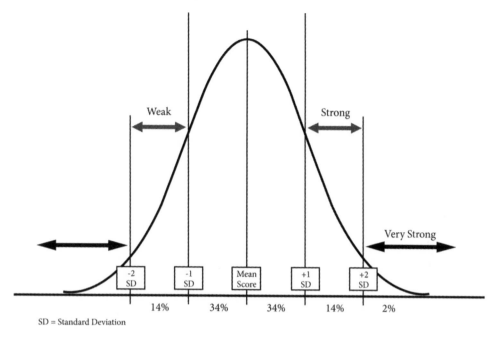

SD = Standard Deviation

Figure 16. Percentage Distribution of Strong, Normal and Weak Constitutions in the Population

Percentages alone don't tell us much, so we're better off attempting to describe what it means to have a strong or weak constitution.

The constitutionally *very weak* in overall health tend to get minor illnesses frequently and take a long time to get well. They frequently develop seasonal rhinitis or sensitivity to pollen during the spring. They tend to be intolerant to heat during the summer, experience rolling colds and flu during the fall, and are intolerant to cold in the winter. They often have multiple food sensitivities, especially for wheat, dairy, and corn products, and are highly sensitive to both over-the-counter (OTC) or prescription medications. Their gastric system seems to be sensitive to the environment, so they are often more susceptible than normal travelers to travelers' gastroenteritis. Despite these symptoms that affect them most of the time, their routine laboratory tests usually look normal. They frequently visit physicians for one ailment or another, and seem to be always struggling to stay healthy.

On the opposite end of the spectrum, those who are constitutionally *very strong* seem to never get sick, even for one day. They are often described as strong as an ox. They stand up better to viruses and stay healthy when others fall prey. Routine laboratory tests are also within the normal range.

Those who have *strong* overall constitutions are less likely to develop AFS, and if they do, the progression tends to be slower, the adrenal crashes are less intense, and they can recover faster and sustain their recovery.

Those with weak constitutions have a higher propensity to develop AFS, even when they're exposed only to the stresses of normal daily living. In addition, they have higher chances of deteriorating to advanced stages, and their adrenal crashes tend to be more intense, with delayed and protracted recoveries that are difficult to sustain.

Looking back on their lives, most adults can surmise their overall constitutional status. The majority of us fall into the normal range, with our share of common colds, stress, and strain.

Aside from the general biological constitution of the body, each organ has its own constitution too, which explains why many who are constitutionally weak have strong adrenals. The opposite is also true. Therefore, determining the biological constitution of the adrenal glands depends on a host of factors, many of which remain unknown, but these factors certainly include the adrenals' intrinsic constitution and that of other closely related organ systems such as the thyroid and ovarian systems.

Body Constitution and Advanced AFS

Nowhere is the constitution's effect on Adrenal Fatigue Syndrome recovery more prominent than in Stage 3C, the state of disequilibrium (see Chapter 9, *Stage 3C—Disequilibrium*). You will recall that we also refer to Stage 3 and its phases as Adrenal Exhaustion. At this stage we often see concurrent ovarian, adrenal, and thyroid dysfunction (OAT axis imbalance, see Chapter 8, *Stage 3B—Hormonal Axis Imbalances*), along with dysregulation of hormones such as cortisol, adrenaline, norepinephrine, thyroid, insulin, and estrogen. Symptoms include hypoglycemia, moderate to severe fatigue, low blood pressure, anxiety, insomnia, adrenaline rush, heart palpitations, low libido, POTS (postural orthostatic tachycardia syndrome), PMS (premenstrual syndrome), menstrual irregularities, and hypothyroidism.

During this time, the emergency backup system is activated to maintain homeostasis. The autonomic nervous system is on full alert, and the body can be flooded in a sea of adrenaline. For many, this is a wakeup call that their adrenal glands are in deep trouble, with rapidly declining adrenal function.

Being aware of the body's constitution allows for an optimized recovery program for Stage 3C, and is also important because the weaker the constitution, the faster the decline and the slower the recovery.

> **Failing to factor the weaker constitution into a recovery plan is a common mistake that might delay or worsen the recovery outcome.**

The following graph illustrates how the body's constitution affects the recovery phase of Stage 3C Adrenal Fatigue Syndrome recovery:

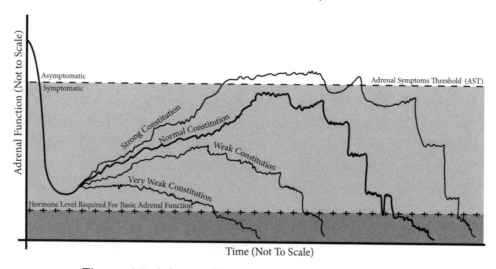

Figure 17. Adrenal Exhaustion Recovery Pattern
Based on Body Constitution

It is evident from the above graph that the degree and speed of recovery varies greatly depending on one's constitution. Below, we look in detail at each recovery pattern in relation to the constitution. Refer to the graph above to follow the line.

Very Weak Constitution

Only a small percentage of the general population has a very weak body constitution, but these individuals are the most desperate when afflicted with AFS and no noticeable recovery occurs after an adrenal crash. The body may go through a period of stabilization, but even this is marred with multiple minor crashes along with intermittent major ones where energy drops 30 percent or more compared to the immediate pre-crash level.

Severe symptoms such as hypoglycemia, low blood pressure, and insomnia continue to persist and get worse over time, and normal daily activities are severely disrupted. It is not unusual for these individuals to spend much of their time in bed or on the couch. Many become completely bedridden. Not only has recovery failed, but energy levels continue on a sloping downhill path. Ultimately, some form of crash will occur that pushes the key adrenal hormones and functions below that which is necessary for basic normal adrenal function. The timeframe varies, but we're usually looking at a matter of months, that is, if we fail to make it a priority to quickly nurture the adrenals back to health. Once this crash has occurred, the body declares a state of emergency that keeps only the most basic functions going, but compromises others, such as gastrointestinal and reproductive functions.

Weak Constitution

Those with weak constitutions are likely to experience a noticeable but mild recovery after a major crash when they have progressed into Stage 3C.

We might see a sustained period of gradual improvement, but progress is generally slow. Minor crashes and setbacks are expected along the way. Eventually, the sufferer reaches a plateau in which the person doesn't improve, and more rest doesn't increase the body's energy level. On good days, normal activities can be carried out. However, bad days are quite frequent and extensive rest is needed. In Stage 3C, we can say that the body is marginally functional at best. When a new stressor hits, inevitable crashes follow which lower adrenal functions, much like a series of small downhill steps. A period of stabilization follows each crash; these periods might be accompanied by a gradual reduction in energy levels, or, a better situation, the same energy level is maintained.

Follow-up crashes tend to be increasingly intense and severe, with longer recovery times. If there is no intervention, the body likely will experience a major crash and enter into Stage 3D AFS. After a brief pause and declining stabilization period, adrenal failure may ensue. As compared to those with very weak constitutions, those in this category are more fortunate because the natural progression of the condition is somewhat slower, thereby allowing patients to experience intermittent periods where they function more normally. Unfortunately, if nothing is done to help the recovery process, a high risk exists for the ultimate outcome, adrenal failure.

Normal Constitution

Most of us find ourselves in this category, one in which Adrenal Fatigue Syndrome comes on slowly and gradually over years or decades. Those in this category are likely unaware they have developed AFS until they enter Stage 3. If a crash does occur, these individuals often are able to mount a reasonable and moderate level of recovery over time. Unfortunately, this cannot be sustained.

After a major crash into Stage 3C, the recovery pattern is characterized by significant energy improvement over time. The body might welcome rest, but it is not necessarily required, because the person's biological constitution is strong enough to sustain some setbacks. Minor crashes surface periodically, but are still manageable. The setbacks tend to be rhythmic in nature. Taking afternoon naps and going to sleep early helps tremendously.

Although a full recovery back to the asymptomatic level above the Adrenal Symptoms Threshold (AST) is usually not possible, recovery may be close to that level. Individuals remain symptomatic below the AST, but are far better than they were at the peak of the crash. Some discomfort is inevitable, but proper rest and lifestyle adjustments can bring about improvement.

Those with normal constitutions need to rest frequently in order to cope with fatigue. The problem is that these individuals are accustomed to full and active lifestyles, and they tend not to change their ways. In fact, most in this category are usually in denial for a long time, even when the body shows signs of being in trouble. Those who have been constitutionally weak all their lives are used to slowing down and taking frequent naps, but those in the normal constitutional range live as fully productive individuals and they generally consider resting only at the end of the day.

The vast majority of us who have normal constitutions struggle to balance work and rest, and even when we seek professional help, we don't necessarily comply with the advice we're given. However, if we don't allow sufficient time to nurture the body back to health, we are creating a setup for subsequent crashes, and with each crash the body tries to mount a recovery effort, which brings relief at first. However, over time, continued crashes weaken the adrenals and influence the recovery curve, which tends to be stable at best.

Ultimately, many crashes followed by flat stabilizations resemble downward stair steps, a process that can last for months and even years. Eventually, the body's reserve is so low that it crashes and likely will enter into Stage 3D Adrenal Fatigue Syndrome. After a final stabilization period, the risk of adrenal failure becomes high.

Strong and Very Strong Constitutions

Those with a strong adrenal constitution usually are able to mount a steady and significant recovery from Stage 3C. The recovery curve is smoother than those with a normal constitution because the body is better able to cope with setbacks. Eventually, the body returns to the level of function above the AST and these individuals become asymptomatic. These fortunate people experience a sustained symptom-free period, but this changes over time.

Some individuals with a strong body constitution recover without intervention and do not experience interruptions in their normal daily functioning. Moreover, they might sustain this asymptomatic period for years. Externally, they appear cured and totally normal, but internally, the body is struggling to stay asymptomatic as it stays marginally above the AST. These individuals recover relatively quickly from occasional minor crashes, characterized by unpleasant but tolerable symptoms.

Stretching into decades, these individuals are usually able to continue their fulltime jobs, and when they are tired, they might try taking various natural compounds designed to boost energy. Because the symptoms are marginal, they don't see a need to visit their physician for help. Eventually, however, the years and decades add up if the chronic stressors are not removed. Then, one of the inevitable major stressful life events comes along, such as the death of a loved one or a major career or financial setback. Because we have a tendency to be ill prepared for this kind of event, it normally comes as a surprise. Sufferers often deny that AFS exists and they continue to push themselves past symptoms.

The Context of Recovery

Our society's Type A climate rewards aggressive personality styles. Generally, Type As also ignore symptoms. We have relied on the idea of quick fixes, such as antibiotics, to name one category of drugs. Until recently, we ignored the pros and cons of their use, their overall effectiveness, and the consequence of microbial resistance that ultimately renders them ineffective. Pharmaceutical companies are involved in a continuous scramble to find new antibiotics.

> In the process of finding quick cures, we have lost the concept of convalescence. By that we mean giving the body time to heal from infections and illnesses, like colds and flu.

Out of fear of losing their jobs, employees may be afraid to stay home when they are ill, and even if they do take a couple of days off, they often return too soon, thereby undermining the idea that the body needs rest to fully recover—what we used to call convalescence. Some parents go to work when they're ill in order to save their own sick days to stay home with their children.

Over the long term, this isn't beneficial for individuals or the society, but it's the situation that seems entrenched and is unlikely to change in the near future.

The result is the strain on the adrenals is overlooked when we push past the symptoms of illness that tell us the body needs rest.

Since Adrenal Fatigue Syndrome is not a well known condition, the situation tends to become even more complicated. Sufferers lose valuable time that should be used to nurture the body to rebuild the adrenal reserve that is slowly but surely dwindling. Eventually, crashes become more frequent and intense, and recovery becomes less successful and these individuals no longer stay asymptomatic. Unless the downward trend changes, the body may eventually crash into Adrenal Fatigue Syndrome Stage 3D and ultimately risk entering adrenal failure.

The following graph summarizes the various patterns based on constitutional types. As you can see, it shows seven recovery patterns:

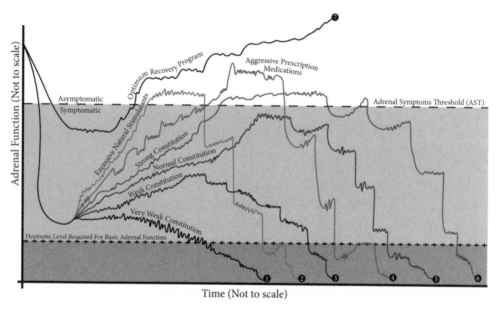

Figure 18. Adrenal Exhaustion Recovery Patterns

Pattern 5 is the most common. Here we see the slow deterioration over time for those who have a normal constitution and suffer Adrenal Fatigue Syndrome.

In Pattern 6, we see that the time can be lengthened if the intrinsic body constitution is strong. It is clear that the stronger you are constitutionally, the slower your overall decline.

In Pattern 3, we see that those with a weak constitution do poorly. Their recovery is often suboptimal, and their decline over time tends to be accelerated when compared to the natural progression.

In Pattern 1, we see clearly that those with a very weak constitution do the worst. Their recovery is characterized by rolling crashes that they never seem to recover from.

In *Pattern 2*, we also see what happens when those who self-navigate use natural stimulatory compounds excessively or inappropriately. This practice compromises the normal recovery process for most. In *Pattern 4*, we see that aggressive use of prescription medications can worsen the outcome, especially in the presence of a weak constitution. Both Patterns 2 and 4 could leave the sufferer worse off than if nothing is done and nature is allowed to take its course, which we see in Pattern 5. In other words, the person becomes worse, and if this occurs in an individual who has a weak or very weak constitution, then we can expect disastrous results.

In *Pattern 7*, we see what happens with a correctly formulated and personalized recovery program. Any good recovery program attempts to reduce crash intensity, bring about a sustained, robust recovery that is asymptomatic, and reduce the risk of subsequent crashes. So, regardless of constitutional type, we want to mimic the Pattern 7 recovery curve as much as possible.

Barrier to Recovery: Excessive Use of Natural Stimulatory Compounds (*Pattern 2*)

Using natural compounds such as certain herbs and glandulars can be of great help in mild Adrenal Fatigue Syndrome (Stages 1 and 2). However, results can be dangerous for those in Stage 3, Adrenal Exhaustion, if they pursue this strategy without professional guidance. Unfortunately, some in this stage embark on aggressive self-guided programs, exemplified by Pattern 2 in the above graph. Unfortunately, the results can be perilous for the individual in such a program.

After the initial adrenal crash into Stage 3C Adrenal Fatigue Syndrome, recovery results may be promising at first. Recovery is fast and furious as the body's energy level is propped up and sustained with natural compounds. The adrenals are put into overdrive to increase their hormone output and energy returns. Sometimes, the energy level may even return to that above the AST and the sufferer becomes asymptomatic. While the overall energy level may not be the same as pre-crash, unpleasant symptoms are at least not prevalent. The sufferer is misled into thinking that his problem is resolved.

The adrenal glands have a blunted response over time to such a continued stimulation strategy. More natural compounds are needed to have the same sustained energy level. In time, the overall energy level plateaus and fails to increase even with higher dosages. Soon the maximum stimulatory level is reached, at which time the body starts to decompensate. Eventually, the adrenals start to fail, usually precipitated by a stressor triggering the first major crash after a plateau is reached.

After the first major follow up crash, those doing self-guided programs begin to use even more stimulants, believing they need more to avoid another crash. There again may be a period of recovery, but the duration is shorter, and the level of recovery is mild at best, and more crashes follow. With each subsequent crash, the crash intensity is increased. The body's ability to mount a recovery is blunted, and in fact, may slowly decompensate and roll into subsequent crashes, with one crash followed by another. This progression can happen quickly, not far behind those with the very weak constitution mentioned earlier.

Needless to say, this is an undesirable recovery pattern even for those with a normal or strong constitution. Over time, this is a recipe for failure. What the adrenals need are gentle nutrients to nurture themselves back to health, not to be continually put on overdrive without rest, which is what some of these natural compounds may do in those suffering with advanced Adrenal Fatigue Syndrome. It comes as no surprise that this undesirable recovery pattern can only get worse if the constitutional state is weak or very weak.

Barrier to Recovery: Aggressive Use of Prescription Medications (*Pattern 4*)

Physicians commonly prescribe thyroid and/or steroid medications to treat fatigue and low metabolic rates. While these potent drugs have their roles to play, their aggressive use over time can pose a significant risk and, in some, worsen Adrenal Exhaustion. In these situations, recovery tends to progress steadily at first. With each increase in medication potency, dosage, or delivery system, a corresponding increase in energy level appears to immediately follow. This is exemplified in Pattern 4 within Figure 18 on page 229.

Patients and doctors usually are encouraged as fatigue improves and laboratory test results appear to be improving too. As long as the medicine is taken regularly, patients seem to be increasingly asymptomatic, often reaching a peak effect when patients feel as if their bodies are almost back to normal. This situation can continue for a few years. The only problem is that strong medication is needed to keep this energy level sustained. Over time, doctors may add steroid medications in ever increasing doses. However, eventually the adrenals simply cannot be stimulated any further and refuse to cooperate. Eventually a stressor will come, and a major crash follows.

In this situation, physicians unaware of AFS, miss the essential characteristics of the crash, and many doctors tend to increase the dosages of medications, but the response is blunted. At that point, the intensity of the crash increases and recovery efforts are marred, and more crashes follow. Doctors at this time may have exhausted their major arsenal of drugs, and some medications may have even backfired as the patient's symptoms worsened. Patients may be abandoned and may seek help elsewhere, or as often happens, they either go back to self-navigating or they start down that path. Either way, that path frequently ends disastrously at Adrenal Fatigue Syndrome Stage 3D. After a brief and heroic but ultimately unsuccessful attempt to reverse the situation, adrenal failure risk remains high.

> **Those who fail to improve with prescription medication need to be alert and seek further professional advice.**

As expected, those with strong constitutions tend to fair the best even under conditions of treatment error, but those with weak constitutions fair worse. Individuals with very weak constitutions, as described above, often can't tolerate prescription medications. They tend to decompensate the fastest and have the highest risk of adrenal failure.

Recovery Hopes and Complexities

By now, you should have a big picture perspective of Adrenal Fatigue Syndrome. We hope you can see that Mother Nature is always right, and the body does behave logically after all. With this clarity and our alignment with nature, recovery becomes an easier task. We no longer fight our body, but instead give it the tools to heal itself. From our experience, this is the way Mother Nature likes it, and we are wise to follow her lead. In the coming chapters, we examine how natural compounds are used in this quest.

Key Points to Remember

- We are each born with a unique inner type of biological constitution. This determines how strong we are in the presence of external insults. This constitution cannot be detected by laboratory tests, but is generally evident if one reviews the medical history carefully.

- Individual constitution plays an important role in AFS recovery, because those with stronger constitutions usually recover faster than those who are weaker.

- Excessive use of natural stimulatory compounds and aggressive use of prescription medications can be barriers to the recovery process, because they can worsen Adrenal Fatigue Syndrome if not done properly.

- Understanding your symptoms in the context of your constitution allows you to have an honest assessment of your recovery capacity.

Chapter 19

Nutritional Supplements for Adrenal Fatigue: An Introduction

When correctly used, nutritional supplements play a large role in adrenal support and recovery. In particular, they help to provide the necessary ingredients for the adrenals to produce the hormones required. They help to stabilize HPA axis dysregulation, rebalance the autonomic nervous system, enhance brain function, and reduce inflammation, just to name a few.

Consider the following:

- Vitamins C and B provide the necessary raw material for the adrenal glands to make a wide variety of hormones that may be deficient.

- Vitamins A and D are generally anti-inflammatory.

- Omega 3 vs. omega 6 balance helps determine the balance between inflammation and anti-inflammation.

- Vitamin D reduces insulin resistance which helps the body tolerate low blood sugar from cortisol dysregulation.

- Vitamin D increases serotonin and dopamine production.

- B vitamins are necessary cofactors for many of the processes involved in neurotransmitter signaling.

- Magnesium is a necessary cofactor in many enzymatic reactions.

- Glandulars and herbal compounds can help provide additional support when the adrenals are weak, while calming the adrenals when they are in overdrive. Hormonal therapies have their place, too, especially in times of acute stress.

Nutrient Recovery Toolbox

We can look at these three general categories of recovery tools on a continuum of potency:

- Vitamins, enzymes, probiotics, and minerals are generally the gentlest tools in the toolbox.

- Glandulars and herbal compounds tend to be mildly potent.

- Hormonal medications tend to be the most potent and, if not properly used, often produce undesirable side effects and potential addiction problems.

This broad classification provides only general rules. For specific outcomes, we need to look at the form, delivery system, and dosage of each. In that respect, the above categories are designed to give us a bird's eye view rather than a specific protocol. The following examples will clarify what we mean:

- High dose vitamin B5 (pantothenic acid) is more potent then low dose pantethine (explained in the next chapter) within the vitamin B category.

- Low dose hormones can be less potent than certain forms of glandular compounds when the body is sensitive.

- Sublingual vitamin B12 is a far more potent form than its capsule form.

- A cream form of natural progesterone is far gentler for the liver than oral forms of progesterone (called Prometrium®).

Using the right nutritional cocktail of vitamins, minerals, glandulars, and herbs at the right time can often be equally or more effective than using prescription steroids.

We tend to gauge supplements by their potency to help us compartmentalize them in our mind, but potency in and of itself should not be the sole yardstick used when evaluating and choosing the right supplements. One can easily bring about a higher level of energy with more potent supplements, but the energy coming from that strategy is often not natural. In other words, the person may feel a sense of being propped up, but that could bring with it a sense of anxiety. As a result, one can be energized and feel tired at the same time, which we've previously described as feeling artificially wired-and-tired, a classic sign of energizing the body in the wrong way. It's a misleading situation.

> A short term boost can often result in a longer term crash when the body finally rejects such ill fated attempts to heal the adrenals with compounds unwelcome by it. We can't forget that the body always wins these battles.

Caveats exist for the subjective classification we've designed for educational purposes. We don't want them to be taken literally as part of a structured protocol. Unfortunately, no one can offer a perfect cookbook supplement program because each person is unique. Most individuals with Adrenal Fatigue Syndrome do better with a well designed cocktail of supplements, but some do better with single supplements. As we've said, paradoxical reactions occur, and in extreme cases, supplements may be contraindicated.

> The best supplement programs match the individual needs with the characteristics of each compound, and usually use the best of each class as needed, along with various forms and delivery systems. The proper blend of supplements facilitates the body's absorption capacity to match clearance capability, meaning that unwanted metabolites are excreted out of the body on a timely basis, thus avoiding toxic built up.

The key to selecting the right supplement cocktail involves thorough knowledge of the unique properties and effects of each compound, along with the individual's detailed nutritional history. Each person is different in terms of constitution, body sensitivity, stage of adrenal weakness, and reaction, so a nutrient beneficial to one person can be toxic to another. Even in the best of hands, some trial and error is required.

Natural compounds have a variety of properties to keep in mind:

- First, the way many natural compounds behave at one dose can be very different from how they behave at another dose.

- Second, what is considered an optimal dose is not well known or established. The RDA (Recommended Dietary Allowance) was set up for vitamins and minerals (primarily) as a guide to prevent recognized vitamin deficiency diseases such as scurvy or rickets. The prevailing view among many in holistic and nutritional medicine is that the RDAs for many vitamins and minerals are insufficient to maintain optimum health, and are irrelevant to the concept of therapeutic uses.

- Third, most natural compounds have few or no recognizable side effects at doses many times higher than the RDA, because the body has a built in mechanism to metabolize them effectively.

- Fourth, we have few studies about possible toxic consequences of many of the natural compounds at high doses, primarily because it's difficult to fund studies on non-patentable natural compounds. As a result, we lack standardization of these compounds.

- Fifth, the same natural compounds (such as certain herbs) have adaptogenic properties. This means they can behave differently in the same person, depending on that person's state of dysfunction. The same compound can be beneficial to those with mild AFS, but can become stimulatory when the fatigue is severe.

- Sixth, the optimum therapeutic dosage required for recovery is body specific. The right dosage for one person can be very different for another person, even if the degree of adrenal weakness is similar.

- Seventh, depending on the delivery system, we see a drastic difference in the bioavailability of nutrients to the cells. For example, the absorption rate of high dose orally delivered vitamin C by capsule or powder is far less than that achieved with the liposomalized form (discussed in the next chapter and in Appendix C).

- Eighth, manufacturers of natural compounds use different grades and purities, but this is not disclosed to the consumer on the bottle labels. Low quality nutritional supplements are usually less effective than higher quality supplements.

Nutritional supplements are widely used by consumers, but because the average consumer doesn't know much about them in detail, they often misuse these products. In addition, incompletely informed consumers don't know what compound to take, how much of it, or what form to use. It is no surprise that therapeutic failure is common.

When natural compounds are used inappropriately, recovery is not only impeded, but the condition often worsens over time. In these situations the compounds do more harm than good. This is one of the most common mistakes made among those who embark on self guided and nonprofessionally guided programs, especially if the Adrenal Fatigue Syndrome is advanced. Therefore, it is impossible to provide anything but general guidelines about nutritional supplements, leaving the precise dosage, delivery system, form, and the ultimate cocktail to a qualified healthcare practitioner.

Why We Recommend a Nutritional Cocktail

Through the years we have found that a well structured nutritional cocktail promotes AFS recovery far better than any other approach. This is why:

- First, different nutrients work at different parts of the cell. Vitamin C, for example, is water soluble and protects us from free radical attacks outside the cell. Vitamin E, on the other hand, is fat soluble. It is able to penetrate the cell wall easily and combat oxidative damage intracellularly.

- Second, different nutrients complement each other in their duties. Numerous studies have shown that taking multiple nutrients in their optimal dosages is better than taking single vitamins. No magic bullet exists in nutritional supplementation. It is wise to obtain broad coverage. Glutathione, for example, complements vitamin C, and vice versa.

- Third, different nutrients have different target organs. For example, saw palmetto focuses on the prostate gland, while milk thistle focuses on the liver, gingko has blood thinning properties, and vitamin E improves circulation to the brain.

- Fourth, by combining the synergistic effects of multiple nutrients, the dosage of any single nutrient is decreased. It has been shown, for example, that the oxidative effect of a combination of vitamins C, A, and E is much higher than when any one of these vitamins is used alone to achieve the same effect.

In the next three chapters, we introduce some of the tools we use. We have organized them to closely match how they are used in our daily practice, reflecting the clinical approach we take by using the gentlest nutrients as the first line of defense.

Group 1: First Line of Defense

Key compounds in this group include vitamins C, D, E, B12, B6, B5, magnesium, digestive enzymes, iodine, glutathione, lecithin, NADH, inosital, pantethine/pantothenic acid, D-ribose, collagen, fish oil, and CoQ10, just to mention a few. We have found that even with advanced Adrenal Fatigue Syndrome, these nutrients are of great benefit. Not all are needed at the same time. In fact, most of the time, we use only a select few. The key is using the *right* tools. Even a damaged body can heal if we only give it the right tools with the right delivery system at the right time. Indeed, we are saddened when sufferers come to us with a long list of potent supplements (sometimes twenty or more). They can't stop taking them because many have potential unpleasant withdrawal symptoms, but they can't continue them either because they are wired-and-tired. Before one embarks on any nutritional program, the exit strategy must be considered.

When properly combined, this group of gentle compounds facilitates a smooth recovery process, including a sense of calm and natural revitalization with few withdrawal or addiction issues when the time comes to discontinue.

Sometimes, however, this group may not be enough. In such cases, we can consider and slowly move our way up to Group 2 as needed.

Group 2: Used Only as Needed and with Great Care

The second group of compounds, glandulars and herbs, are considered more potent than those in Group 1. Again, this is a rule of thumb only. Ultimate clinical efficacy depends very much on dosage, delivery system, and the body's acceptance. This group includes adrenal and thyroid glandulars, licorice, rhodiola rosea, maca root, ashawandgha, and ginseng. These have good adrenal adaptogenic properties and are particularly suited for mild Adrenal Fatigue Syndrome.

As a general rule, they also tend to be increasingly stimulatory as adrenal weakness progresses. This is, however, not universally true. Those with advanced Adrenal Fatigue Syndrome (Stage 3 and beyond) should exercise great care. Many individuals have a false sense of complacency after starting these compounds because they feel energized. Unfortunately, in the long run they find themselves addicted and unable to stop taking them, or they may need increasingly larger doses to maintain the same energy. Invariably, the dosage eventually reaches the maximum stimulatory level and devastating crashes follow.

Group 3: Used As a Last Resort

This last group consists of hormones, including pro-hormones such as pregnenolone, weak hormones such as DHEA, and strong hormones such as testosterone and hydrocortisone. Hormones are the ultimate chemical messengers that control the body. While useful in managing acute AFS in a crisis situation, we're sad to see so many individuals on long term steroid use and unable to get off.

> **As you have surmised, our philosophy is to use the gentlest compounds possible, moving to more potent nutrients when all less potent avenues have been exhausted. The reason is simple: The higher the potency, the more side effects, and the harder it is to discontinue due to addiction and withdrawal problems.**

Once adrenal function normalizes, nutritional supplements should be reduced or eliminated. As mentioned before, we are always mindful to keep this important exit strategy in mind as we design the right protocol, because we want the body ultimately to be on its own, and if possible, without dependence on any external support.

Where to Buy Supplements?

As you can see, the nutritional toolbox for AFS easily contains hundreds of natural compounds. Each has its place. The task of selecting the proper nutrients, dosage, and delivery system is a clinical art that takes decades to master. Because wrong nutrients can actually makes matter worse, we recommend seeking professional help, especially if you are in the advance stages of Adrenal Fatigue Syndrome. Those, however, who are in early stages, or those who are healthy and wishing to prevent AFS, have more latitude and self-navigation is acceptable.

From our experience, nutritional cocktail blends work the best because most nutrients work synergistically and potentially affect each other when properly compounded. Furthermore, with the blends, one can reduce the number of nutrients needed. Remember that more is not necessarily better in AFS. See Appendix G for the specific line of supplements we recommend.

Key Points to Remember

- Nutritional supplements are generally very important and useful in Adrenal Fatigue Syndrome recovery.

- The proper characteristic, dosage, form, delivery system, and timing are critical factors to consider.

- Because each person is different, what works for one person may be toxic for another. For best results, a customized program works best.

- Nutritional compounds administered in the form of a cocktail usually work best.

- There are three major groups of nutritional supplements, from the most gentle to the most potent:
  - Group 1: Gentle nutrients—vitamins, enzymes, and minerals
  - Group 2: glandulars and herbs
  - Group 3: Hormones, used as a last resort

Chapter 20

First Line of Defense— Gentle Nutrients

We use a group of first line nutrients we consider the most useful in helping the adrenals recover. Most with Adrenal Fatigue Syndrome, especially those with Adrenal Exhaustion, are internally over-stimulated due to an overactive sympathetic nervous system. That's why we believe in having the right non-stimulating natural supplements, those that help with recovery without further stimulating the already weak and tired adrenals.

Key members of this group possess common characteristics; in particular, they are intrinsically gentle and nurturing to the adrenal glands. It should be remembered, however, that no matter how intrinsically weak or gentle a compound is, the end result may differ significantly depending on the stage of adrenal weakness. It is not unusual for those with Stage 3D AFS to be intolerant to all supplements, even at extremely low doses. When individuals come to us for help, we teach them how to listen to the body's inner voice and correctly interpret the body's response to supplements.

Vitamin C: A Gentle Nutrient

Adrenal Fatigue Syndrome sufferers usually have an inadequate supply of many key nutrients. Out of these, subclinical vitamin C deficiency is the most prevalent. While no outward symptom of scurvy is seen, as happens in clinical vitamin C deficiency, the body's need and appetite for vitamin C go up tremendously when the adrenals are weak.

Vitamin C is so gentle that most healthy people taking it would hardly notice any difference physically and mentally. This is, in fact, a hallmark of good health. Those with AFS, however, may have a different experience, depending on the level of weakness. Generally, the more advanced the adrenal weakness, the more vitamin C is needed. However, one can be more sensitive to vitamin C as well, due to a variety of reasons, thus it is not universally positive for everyone.

www.DrLam.com   243

The adrenals contain one of the highest concentrations of vitamin C in the body, and this is where it is most needed, because it's a key catalyst of adrenal hormone production, including cortisol. Its antioxidant effects are particularly important in the presence of tissue-destroying oxidants in periodontal disease and other stealth infections that trigger AFS.

In addition to its critical adrenal support function, vitamin C is perhaps the best electron donor because of its water soluble properties and, thus, is readily bioavailable to the cells. Toxins deplete electron stores in the cell. Having sufficient electrons inside the body reverses potential cell death brought on by bacterial, environmental, and industrial toxins. In addition to its adrenal support function, vitamin C helps in the formation of critical collagens responsible for keeping the vascular and musculoskeletal systems pliable and healthy.

In times of stress, the body's requirement for vitamin C increases many fold. Having a sufficient level of vitamin C in the body is critical to help:

- make anti-inflammatory hormones, including cortisol
- prevent a catabolic state from worsening
- boost immune function to fight infection
- prevent heart disease
- overcome opportunistic infections, and
- neutralize systemic toxins from environmental and periodontal diseases

Proper vitamin C fortification should therefore be a cornerstone of any adrenal recovery program if tolerated.

Since humans are one of the few animals that cannot produce vitamin C, we are fortunate it is found abundantly in fruits and vegetables such as papayas, tomatoes, and Brussels sprouts, to name only three. However, relying on food sources alone for vitamin C is seldom sufficient in healing the adrenals, and much higher doses are needed. Remember, one orange delivers only about 65 mg of vitamin C. This is why nutritional supplements are recommended.

Most commercially available vitamin C is derived from corn sources. Those who are highly sensitive or allergic to corn can consider vitamin C derived from other food sources such as tapioca and acai berry instead.

Vitamin C is readily available, but it is also widely misused due to lack of knowledge. Choosing the proper combination of forms and delivery systems of vitamin C cocktails is an important clinical challenge for those with advanced adrenal weakness. It takes extensive clinical experience to create a personalized vitamin C cocktail that incorporates key attributes of each form and delivery system into a well designed, custom, nutritional cocktail to ensure sustained delivery without overstimulation.

Forms of Vitamin C

Vitamin C comes in many forms, each with its own properties and characteristics. Ascorbic acid, the most common form, is water soluble. It dissolves quickly in water and is excreted out of the body quickly, too. Because of its relative fast action, once absorbed, ascorbic acid tends to act quickly and therefore is described as "spiky." Effervescent forms of vitamin C are particularly prone to this characteristic. Those with a sensitive stomach or advanced AFS may find ascorbic acid hard to tolerate, especially in high doses.

Natural (from food) and synthetic ascorbic acid (from a tablet) are chemically identical. There appears to be no clinically significant difference in the bioavailability and bioactivity of natural and synthetic ascorbic acid.

The gastrointestinal absorption of ascorbic acid occurs through an active transport process, as well as through passive diffusion. At low gastrointestinal concentrations of ascorbic acid, active transport predominates, while at high gastrointestinal concentrations active transport becomes saturated, leaving only passive diffusion. This is where vitamin C is being absorbed without expanding energy from an area of high concentration to an area of low concentration passively. This form of transport is generally less efficient. As the amount of vitamin C intake increases, the overall absorption efficiency decreases. For example, a vitamin C intake of 180 mg is about 80-90 percent absorbed, but an intake of five grams is only 20 percent or less absorbed by most. Fortunately, this problem can be overcome with the liposomalized form of vitamin C discussed later and in Appendix C. Much of the excess vitamin C is removed from the body in the urine.

Mineral Ascorbates

These ascorbic acids are chemically bound or, in scientific terms, chelated to minerals as one unit. Commonly used minerals include calcium, sodium, and magnesium. These units, also called mineral salts of ascorbic acid, or commonly known as mineral ascorbates, are buffered and, therefore, less acidic. Thus, mineral ascorbates are often recommended to people who experience gastrointestinal problems (abdominal pain or diarrhea) with plain ascorbic acid. When taking large doses of mineral ascorbates, it is important to consider the dose of the mineral accompanying the ascorbic acid. Some minerals are more desirable than others.

Sodium ascorbate: 1,000 mg of sodium ascorbate contains 889 mg of ascorbic acid and 111 mg of sodium. Individuals following low-sodium diets (e.g., for high blood pressure) are generally advised to keep their total dietary sodium intake to less than 2,500 mg/day. However, most with advancing AFS develop low blood pressure due to inadequate sodium store. Administration of sodium ascorbate could significantly increase sodium intake and help blood pressure normalize. It is therefore the preferred form for Adrenal Fatigue Syndrome.

Calcium ascorbate: 1,000 mg of calcium ascorbate generally provides 890-910 mg of ascorbic acid and 90-110 mg of calcium. Calcium in this form appears to be reasonably well absorbed. Excessive calcium intake can sometimes worsen cardiac arrhythmia. Therefore, we don't recommend excessive intake. Ester-C® (a popular form of vitamin C) contains mainly calcium ascorbate, but also contains small amounts of the vitamin C metabolites: dehydroascorbic acid (oxidized ascorbic acid), calcium threonate, and trace levels of xylonate and lyxonate.

Potassium ascorbate: This form is not recommended for Adrenal Fatigue Syndrome in large amounts as most AFS sufferers already have high levels of potassium relative to sodium, though lab tests usually show both as normal.

Magnesium ascorbate: The recommended dietary allowance (RDA) for magnesium is 400-420 mg/day for adult men and 310-320 mg/day for adult women. Magnesium helps to relieve tense muscles and acts as nature's powerful relaxant, making it a wonderful sleep aid.

Mineral Ascorbate Cocktail

For AFS, mineral ascorbates are best taken in a blend (such as Quantamax® discussed in Appendix G) including sodium, calcium, and magnesium ascorbates along with bioflavonoids and a small amount of ascorbic acid. They work well together. Not to be forgotten are important cofactors such as L-lysine, L-proline, malic acid, and citrus bioflavonoid. L-proline, L-lysine, and mineral ascorbates support collagen synthesis. Malic acid helps to increase energy, and along with magnesium, helps to stabilize gastric intestinal irritation and relax tense muscles. *Citrus* bioflavonoids help vitamin C to be made more bioavailable to the cell. *Potassium* ascorbates should be avoided in AFS.

Ascorbyl Palmitate

Ascorbyl palmitate is a fat soluble form of vitamin C. It is used as an antioxidant and preservative in foods, vitamins, drugs, and cosmetics. It is an amphipathic molecule. One end is water soluble and the other end is fat soluble. This dual solubility allows it to be incorporated into cell membranes. When incorporated into the membranes of human red blood cells, ascorbyl palmitate has been found to offer protection against oxidative damage and to protect vitamin E (a fat-soluble antioxidant) from destruction by free radicals.

Being fat soluble, it is absorbed into the cell membrane where ascorbic acid is unable to reach. Therefore, it is retained in the body for a longer period of time. Those with sensitivity to ascorbic acid will find this form particularly useful because of its gentleness.

Ascorbyl palmitate works best in a blend (such as C-Support detailed in Appendix G) with mineral ascorbates and citrus bioflavonoids as synergistic cofactors. Ascorbyl palmitate also acts synergistically with other antioxidants such as vitamin E.

Delivery Systems

The advance of nanotechnology and liposomal encapsulation technology offers a significantly enhanced oral liquid delivery system with superior absorption from the small intestine rather than from the stomach. The liposomal delivery system dramatically improves bioavailability and is by far the best oral form of vitamin C delivery if tolerated. A large amount of vitamin C can be delivered by liquid orally with a very high rate of absorption with this system, if used properly. Care should be taken to avoid any formula that contains alcohol as a preservative. (See Appendix C for a detailed discussion of this technology and ingredients to avoid.)

This system is ideally suited for Adrenal Fatigue Syndrome because high doses can be administered easily by mouth. Because absorption occurs at the small intestine and the stomach is bypassed, gastric irritation is minimal if any. Diarrhea is also significantly reduced because most is absorbed and does not remain in the GI tract where it triggers water retention at the large bowel. Nutritional cocktail blends (such as LipoNano® C detailed in Appendix G) rather than mono-therapy works best. Important synergistic co-factors that enhance effectiveness include alpha lipoic acid, and grape seed extract / polygonum cuspidatum.

While the bioavailability of vitamin C delivered by liposome is far superior to other forms of vitamin C, ascorbic acid in its various forms still has its place and should not be ignored. The absorption tends to be faster and the results more immediate. Because each body reacts differently to vitamin C, no one-size-fits-all protocol exists. A thorough knowledge of these forms is important. Various forms of ascorbates, including regular and liposomal vitamin C, should be used together in a nutritional blend or cocktail mix for maximum and sustained effect. Taking the right combination can go a long ways toward AFS recovery. Well formulated vitamin C blends tend to be more expensive compared to plain ascorbic acid, but well worth the cost, especially for those with advancing AFS.

Vitamin C Safety

Over the years, many research studies have concluded that vitamin C is one of the safest and most nontoxic natural nutrients we can take. Both long term and high oral intake of up to 20,000 mg and intravenous doses of up to 300,000 mg of vitamin C are safe and have no side effects. Likewise, studies show no evidence of toxicity or side effects when late-stage cancer patients are given up to 50,000 mg of intravenous vitamin C daily for up to eight weeks. Moreover, AIDS patients were given anywhere between 25,000 to 125,000 mg of vitamin C on a regular basis based on bowel tolerance without any side effects. Vitamin C is undeniably a safe supplement even when given in high doses over a long period of time in healthy adults.

We have seen reports of heartburn in some people (primarily in those with a sensitive gastric lining) while using vitamin C. Diarrhea is also a common occurrence when the intake of vitamin C exceeds the body's bowl tolerance level (BTL). This is a temporary effect and subsides once vitamin C dosage is reduced. This is not considered a side effect but rather a sign of maximum saturation from oral ingestion.

Those with Adrenal Fatigue Syndrome, especially in the advanced stage, may experience increased anxiety and or fatigue when taking vitamin C. This is generally due to a clearance problem related to the liver and not the vitamin itself. Vitamin C is broken down into metabolites prior to its excretion from the body. If this breakdown process is dysfunctional or functions sub-optimally (as we frequently see in advanced adrenal weakness), the speed of clearance is reduced. As a result, metabolites accumulate and circulate in the body for a longer period of time. These excessive circulating metabolites can trigger a wide variety of re-toxification reactions, with symptoms including malaise, joint pain, anxiety, fatigue, heart palpitations, and so forth, which are not side effects of vitamin C. We usually see these symptoms reverse by themselves as liver function improves.

Vitamin C and Iron

Vitamin C enhances iron absorption many fold, but it must be taken simultaneously with the iron so both vitamin C and iron are present together in the intestine. If additional iron absorption is not desired, then vitamin C and iron can be taken two hours apart.

Note: Those with *hemochromatosis*, a disorder in which high amounts of iron build up in the body, should take only moderate levels of vitamin C.

Vitamin C and Kidney Stones

Since studies have shown that vitamin C contributes to the increased production of oxalates in the body, it is commonly linked with a buildup of kidney stones. However, no evidence has surfaced to pinpoint vitamin C as the sole culprit in the increase in kidney stones, and other factors exist that contribute to oxalate development.

When ingested, vitamin C is broken down into dehydroascorbic acid (DHAA) and further metabolized and converted into diketogulonic acid. Finally, it is broken down and metabolized into lyxonic, xylose, threonic acid, or oxalic acid (oxalate). Oxalate is the metabolic end product after the human body breaks down vitamin C. The body cannot break oxalates down into smaller compounds. Confusion arises because of the presence of calcium oxalate, the primary component of kidney stones. Moreover, some suggest that the intake of vitamin C promotes the development of these kidney stones due to the oxalates produced when vitamin C is broken down by the human body. However, studies have shown that these theories are not well supported.

A number of factors cause a buildup of calcium oxalate stones in the kidney. High vitamin C intake when certain medical conditions are present is just one of many. Kidney stones are linked to the presence of heavy metal chelating agents such as DMPS and EDTA. Taking vitamin C may increase the oxalate level in the urine, which is why many believe prolonged use of the vitamin increases calcium oxalates in the body. However, other research shows a leveling of oxalate production even though vitamin C dosing was continued. Furthermore, the human body excretes significant amounts of oral vitamin C without being metabolized. In addition, in order for the body to use vitamin C, it doesn't need to be broken down to oxalates. As much as 89 percent of vitamin C administered is eliminated as DHAA.

Dietary sources of oxalates include: spinach, rhubarb, parsley, citrus fruits, and especially tea. Likewise, Swiss chard, cocoa, chocolate, pepper, wheat germ, peanuts, refried beans, lime peel, and various soy-based foods also have high oxalate content. High protein foods such as sardines and herring roe also increase oxalate secretion in the body.

Those who take excessive calcium supplements, especially the elderly, may need to be more careful. Excess calcium from supplements finds its way to other compounds in the body. For example, the calcium combines with oxalates already present in high concentrations. However, studies show that vitamin C taken with calcium carbonate and other oxalate sources can facilitate stone formation. Therefore, individuals who have kidney stones should take sodium ascorbate as a vitamin C supplement and should reduce calcium ascorbate as well as regular calcium supplements.

For patients with kidney problems, it's necessary to monitor vitamin C therapy as well as other oxalate sources as a safety precaution. Totally avoiding vitamin C is not a sound recommendation since the human body still needs this vitamin, whether AFS is present or not. In normal individuals, no conclusive evidence has pinpointed vitamin C as the sole cause of renal and kidney failure caused by excess calcium oxalate crystal formation. In some people, the decline in kidney function after vitamin C therapy is more likely related to dehydration and pre-existing kidney disease. In fact, these are two major causes of the decline in kidney function, not vitamin C therapy. Before blaming vitamin C for decline in kidney function, we need to study the person's medical history. When using any medication or nutrient, proper hydration is always necessary and helps prevent crystallization as well as concentration of precipitates (solid substances made from liquids) in the human body, which includes kidney stone crystals.

Vitamin C and G6PD Deficiency

Likewise, the same caution about vitamin C is necessary for those with G6PD deficiency (glucose-6-phosphate dehydrogenase deficiency, a genetic disorder affecting red blood cells). Iron levels in G6PD deficient cells detrimentally interact with vitamin C, and G6PD deficient cells rupture due to the presence of vitamin C. Vitamin C, in rare cases, can promote a hemolytic (related to red blood cells) crisis in individuals with G6PD, although this is difficult to predict. If using vitamin C, this group of patients should be supervised.

Vitamin C and Thyroid Medication

Some with hypothyroidism take thyroid medication but aren't able to achieve their target serum TSH level. However, research has found that vitamin C, along with levothyroxine (a thyroid hormone), decreases TSH levels substantially, by as much as 27 percent. Studies have shown that over a period of six weeks, taking levothyroxine along with 1 gram of vitamin C mixed with water was able to help the majority of patients achieve their TSH target level. Taking vitamin C along with levothyroxine medications should be considered in patients with difficulties in the absorption of levothyroxine. Those recovering from Adrenal Fatigue Syndrome with vitamin C support are likely to find their need for thyroid medication reduces as their recovery continues.

Vitamin C Tolerance and Withdrawal

As you take more vitamin C, your body adapts and gets used to higher levels. This tolerance is normal, but if you reduce vitamin C intake, do so gradually. A 300-500 mg reduction every week is usually safe. A sudden drop in vitamin C intake can trigger symptoms of scurvy, such as bleeding gums and easy bruising. If you experience these symptoms as you reduce vitamin C intake, slow down the rate of reduction. If your fatigue returns and worsens, it may be a sign that your body needs more vitamin C. Always consult your healthcare professional for guidance if you have such experiences. The body will adapt to the lower dosage over time, though the adaptation to lower doses is usually slower than adaptation to higher doses.

Dosage Consideration: **The current RDA for vitamin C is 75 mg for women and 90 mg for men. We believe that those with AFS require much more.**

- **Commercially available oral liposomal vitamin C, such as LipoNano® C, is the preferred delivery system. The dosage varies greatly from person to person, but most do well with 200 to 3,000 mg a day. Because this is a high potency form, always start at very low doses to ensure tolerance.**

- **Mineral ascorbates (preferably a proper blend of sodium, calcium, and magnesium ascorbate) dosage ranges from 200 to 2,000 mg a day.**

- **For fat soluble vitamin C with bioflavonoid, the dosages range from 200-1000 mg a day.**

- **Avoid effervescent and chewable forms of vitamin C.**

Those whose fatigue becomes significantly worse, or experience increased anxiety upon intake of vitamin C, should stop and seek professional advice. These paradoxical reactions are more prevalent as AFS advances.

As we've said, we see significant individual differences in the way the body accepts the various forms of vitamin C, which makes it critical that those with moderate and severe Adrenal Fatigue Syndrome consult a healthcare professional rather than embarking on a self-navigation program. Only those with very mild Adrenal Fatigue should self-navigate. The more advanced the AFS, the more critical it is to properly adjust the dosage to fit the body's weakened state. Otherwise, we risk worsening AFS.

Vitamin C is a wonderful natural tool. Most therapeutic failures arise from improper use or lack of knowledge about how to deliver this important nutrient in a cocktail to the cells through various forms and delivery systems.

Glutathione (GSH)

Excessive oxidative stress is implicated in premature aging, chronic degenerative disease, cancer, and diseases such as Alzheimer's. As you breathe, your body constantly reacts with oxygen as your cells generate energy, and consequently, produce free radicals, which are highly reactive molecules. These free radicals interact with other molecules in the cells, resulting in what we call oxidative stress that damages proteins and other cell components.

Oxidative stress also contributes to a host of *subclinical* dysfunctions, such as chronic fatigue, fibromyalgia, and Adrenal Fatigue Syndrome. The body has natural antioxidants available to neutralize undesirable effects of oxidative stress, one of which is glutathione.

When a person experiences an increase in oxidative stress, the levels of glutathione in the cells drop, which is a precursor to the death of cells. Unhealthy cells are compromised in their abilities to produce adequate amounts of glutathione to protect the body against harmful external toxins or free radicals. These cellular level battles within the body go on without our knowledge, of course, and can have catastrophic effects if the process is hampered in any way.

Glutathione detoxifies harmful chemicals such as lead, mercury, xenobiotics (a chemical present, but not normally produced or expected to be found in an organism), toxic metabolites, and pesticides that have accumulated in the cell. Maintaining sufficient intracellular glutathione levels is one of the key and most powerful lines of defense against cellular death. Glutathione is also considered a powerful detoxifier in the body.

Glutathione supports and protects the immune system and neutralizes oxidative damage caused by toxins and pathogens. Aside from these protective functions, glutathione also maintains the transport of amino acids. It also sustains the synthesis of DNA, protein, and prostaglandin (a family of hormones). These functions rely on glutathione to fight against degenerative diseases, cancer, infections, and in Adrenal Fatigue Syndrome, a situation in which the body is rapidly decompensating.

Electron Flow

Glutathione promotes the healthy flow of electrons and maintains their steady supply in the body's cells. This is the source of its effectiveness. Simply put, hindering the flow of electrons or robbing the cells of electrons is detrimental for health. The opposite also is true. When electron flow is abundant and smooth, cells are healthy and live longer. Poor flow of electrons corresponds to low energy, higher disease rates, low cell integrity, and cell death.

Glutathione donates electrons to the body's antioxidant pool, including antioxidants such as vitamin C, vitamin E, alpha-lipoic acid, and superoxide dismutase (SOD). In addition, glutathione neutralizes disease-causing oxidants and is capable of eliminating heavy metals. By protecting the body from free radicals and pathogenic attacks, it is keeping the cellular structure intact.

The Master Recycler

Glutathione is the most powerful antioxidant at the intracellular level and works synergistically with vitamin C, a key antioxidant in the extracellular level. Glutathione also recharges nutrients such as carnitine, vitamin E, and alpha-lipoic acid. After performing its antioxidant function, vitamin C is recycled and is accompanied by glutathione. This makes glutathione a part of the recycling chain in the body that allows it to reuse natural compounds without decreasing the benefits derived by the body. Glutathione is called the *master recycler*, and as such it keeps vitamin C in an electron donating state and plays a role in recharging vitamin C. To reciprocate, vitamin C alleviates the effect of glutathione deficiency and cellular death. In other words, vitamin C and glutathione mutually support and enhance the functions of each other.

Almost all diseases and toxins cause death and sickness by stealing electrons at the cellular level. This is why we know depleted electrons are part of chronic disease. Conditions such as Adrenal Fatigue Syndrome are part of a spectrum of low energy states where the body's energy output is reduced. The body's electrons are the fuel of life and are responsible for generating energy necessary to sustain life. To achieve optimum health and reverse this low energy state, a good flow of electrons is necessary. To achieve this, principal antioxidants, including glutathione, vitamin C, and vitamin E, work synergistically to replenish cells depleted of electrons. By helping each other supply and recycle electrons to the cells, the body can recover at the cellular level.

Dosage Consideration: Glutathione is a free amino acid peptide (substances derived from combinations of amino acids). The regular form of glutathione breaks down in the stomach before entering the blood stream. For best results, consider oral liposomal forms such as LipoNano® Glutathione (detailed in Appendix G).

Oral liposomal technology dramatically improves the bioavailability of glutathione. Bypassing the stomach, such liposomal encapsulated glutathione is absorbed in the small intestine and transported to the circulatory system directly. Consider 100-800 mg per day via liposomal encapsulation technology, such as LipoNano® Glutathione.

Pantethine/Pantothenic Acid

Few natural compounds are more powerful than pantethine and its relative, pantothenic acid. For decades, we've known that pantothenic acid is one of the essential nutrients we can use to help adrenal function. In fact, it is a good substitute for prednisone, a drug with serious and awful side effects, although it effectively treats autoimmune diseases including arthritis, allergies, and colitis.

Once inside the body, pantothenic acid forms a substance called pantethine, which is further converted into an enzyme called *co-enzyme A*. An extremely important compound, co-enzyme A is essential in the metabolism of protein, fat, and carbohydrates. It is also the starting point for the body's production of adrenal steroids, cholesterol, bile, and hemoglobin.

While pantothenic acid ultimately leads to coenzyme A, using pantethine is a much faster way to achieve the same effect as pantothenic acid and with intense potency. Pantethine allows the adrenal glands to generate more of the anti-stress hormone, cortisol, thereby reducing the body's inflammatory response. For maximum effect, it should be used in conjunction with a nutritional cocktail of vitamin C; bioflavonoids (substances found in plants and plant pigments that act as antioxidants); other antioxidants such as pine bark extract, ascorbyl palmitate (a fat soluble form of a type of vitamin C); and cofactors such as lysine, proline, glutamine, glycine, and carnitine (a derivative of lysine).

Pantethine helps reduce blood levels of triglycerides and promotes healthy cholesterol levels as well. A daily dose of 900 mg has been shown to reduce triglycerides by up to 32 percent, along with a 19 percent drop in total cholesterol and a 21 percent drop in LDL cholesterol (low density lipoprotein, the type of cholesterol considered bad). At the same time, HDL cholesterol (the good cholesterol) rose by 23 percent. Pantethine also protects the heart and arteries and acts synergistically with vitamin E against cholesterol build up.

Pantethine also helps increase the production of omega-3 fatty acids in the body (EPA, DHA, and other essential fats). Omega-3 fatty acids have powerful anti-inflammatory effects and reduce the clot promoting fats in cell membranes. Most spectacularly, pantethine produces no side effects.

Pantethine is furthermore an excellent nutrient to use with two major gastrointestinal problems, colitis, and Crohn's disease. A daily dose of 900-1200 mg of pantethine matched with 900-1200 mg of pantothenic acid drastically improves the two conditions. Improvement usually kicks in four to eight weeks after starting this combination, but many have reported benefits in much shorter time. Pantethine also helps promote the growth of beneficial intestinal bacteria. Further, it helps the body combat the overgrowth of yeast in the body and the accumulation of other toxic substances such as formaldehyde. Therefore, pantethine is a gentle, natural detoxifier.

Pantothenic acid, while not as strong as pantethine, has its own role. For example, in high doses (up to 10 grams a day), it can help with acne. Some people have reported reduced inflammation and improved symptoms of burning foot syndrome. It is also used in conjunction with non-steroidal anti-inflammatory drugs for arthritis.

Overall, pantethine is a remarkably safe and extremely valuable natural dietary supplement that is used for Adrenal Fatigue Syndrome, along with supporting normal cholesterol and triglyceride levels.

Dosage Consideration: Consider 300-1200 mg a day of pantethine along with pantothenic acid in a blend, such as Pandrenal® (discussed in Appendix G). Combination therapy offers the best clinical efficacy as both components are needed and they work well together unless a person is very sensitive. Much higher doses may be needed in AFS with the supervision of a healthcare professional.

Phosphatidylcholine (Lecithin)

Phosphatidylcholine (PC) is an excellent cell protector, especially for those in our nervous system. Soybeans and eggs are good sources. PC also serves as the main source of choline, which in turn is essential to form acetylcholine, an important neurotransmitter of the ANS mentioned earlier in Chapter 8, *Stage 3B—Hormonal Axis Imbalances.* Choline, on the other hand, is essential for our bodies to manufacture our own lecithin. When you buy lecithin from the health food store, you are buying a natural concentrate containing PC plus a mixture of other similar compounds, called phospholipids.

PC is a key nutrient in the health of the nerve, as it protects the inner cell from external insult. It is therefore good for a variety of nerve disorders, including tingling, memory impairment, Alzheimer's disease, and strokes. Remember that those with advanced AFS are invariably afflicted with some form of ANS, autonomic nervous system, dysregulation. Having the proper amount of PC in the body helps cushion that dysfunction. It also fights heart disease and enhances liver function to process fats. It has been shown to retard fatty liver progression. PC is also an important component of female hormone balancing. It helps the liver to convert estradiol, the form of estrogen with great cancer causing potential, into estriol, a safer, less potent, but less carcinogenic form of the hormone. Estrogen dominance, as we have already seen, is a major problem in those with advanced AFS, and PC can help.

Dosage Consideration: Lecithin granules are easily available and can be used in everyday meal preparation. They are great additions to recipes and a great salad garnish. PC supplementation in pill form is most convenient for most. Bear in mind that these contain usually only about 50 percent of PC by weight. Up to 35 grams per day has been used safely and well tolerated. Additional vitamin C should be included because vitamin C serves to protect us from the nitrosamines (a group of potentially harmful chemicals), which can be generated as choline is metabolized.

NADH

NAD (nicotinamide adenine dinucleotide) plays an important role in the energy production pathway of our body. The reduced form (with a hydrogen added) of NAD, called NADH or coenzyme 1, is the specific way by which all our cells get their energy. The body normally makes its own NADH from niacinamide (a form of niacin, vitamin B3), but aging and chronic diseases slow this conversion.

NADH is the quintessential energy giving compound, but not everyone can tolerate it. In the brain, NADH helps neurons make dopamine, a catecholamine neurotransmitter. Recall that dopamine is the chemical precursor of norepinephrine and epinephrine. Too much dopamine can therefore enhance catecholamine flow. This can worsen those who already have reactive sympathoadrenal response, as in Stage 3C Adrenal Exhaustion. Those who are constitutionally weak or sensitive may find this nutrient too spiky, with the potential of worsening anxiety and insomnia. In extreme cases, adrenal crashes may be precipitated. Fortunately, this is usually due to inappropriate dosage, usually a dosage that's too high.
Dosage Consideration: 2.5-20 mg as tolerated.

Vitamin E

Vitamin E is a great antioxidant. Free radicals generated internally by the adrenal glands during hormone synthesis need to be neutralized. Vitamin E performs this function inside the adrenal glands and throughout the body. It also helps to recycle vitamin C. High amounts of vitamin E are therefore needed for the adrenals to maintain optimal steroid production. This is particularly important during the recovery process. Because vitamin E is fat soluble, excessive amounts are not indicated. In addition, because it is metabolized through the liver, those with the low clearance issue we see so often in advanced Adrenal Exhaustion should use caution.

Vitamin E comes in many forms. The d-alpha-tocopherol form is natural and the preferred form, though a cocktail of mixed tocopherols is best for AFS. Because vitamin E is not a direct ingredient in hormone synthesis within the adrenal glands, its actions are slow. Allow three months of consistent intake to enjoy the benefit.

Dosage Consideration: 400-800 IU of mixed tocopherol daily. Because vitamin E has blood thinning properties, those on blood thinning medications need to be monitored.

Inosital

While this compound does not directly support adrenal function, it is an excellent natural relative of the B-complex family. It relieves nervous tension and encourages sounder sleep. Specifically, inosital levels are often lower than average in people hospitalized for depression. Resupplying inosital can lift spirits. Those with anxiety and obsessive-compulsive disorders (OCDs) also benefit, though higher doses may be required.

Fresh produce, whole grains, and red meats are good sources of inosital, and these food sources could supply up to 1 gram a day. However, a large amount could be in the form of fiber, thus not well absorbed. For this reason we recommend supplements.

Dosage Consideration: For everyday uses such as temporary anxiety and insomnia, 500-2000 mg at bedtime. Clinical depression and OCDs require much higher doses, up to 18 grams, as shown in research studies. Because inosital is a chemical relative of glucose, those with sugar imbalances and carbohydrate intolerance may experience intolerance and must be careful.

D-ribose

Ribose is a sugar molecule made from the body's glucose and is a vital component of ATP (adenosine triphosphate). Scientists consider ATP to be the energy currency, in that it is a high energy molecule that stores the energy we need. We can also think of it as a rechargeable battery. Ribose, an essential of ATP, rapidly restores energy, especially in diseased hearts and other muscles that need energy. Until the 1940s, D-ribose was believed to be a structural component of DNA and RNA, but with very little physiological importance. However, subsequent studies in the 1950s concluded that D-ribose actually plays a significant role in the metabolic reaction known as *pentose phosphate pathway*. This pathway is pivotal in many functions, including synthesizing energy and producing genetic material (the components of a cell that determine its structure and the ability to regenerate). It also provides substances used by certain tissues that produce fatty acids and hormones.

We have a great deal of human and animal research showing positive results from D-ribose in terms of improving energy and the function of the heart and other muscles. In addition, using D-ribose does not negatively affect the action of common drugs used in the treatment of heart disease.

When D-ribose is used with two other nutrients, L-carnitine and CoQ10, and integrated into AFS protocol, energy delivery is nearly always helped. This is also a useful nutritional cocktail to support heart health and many more conditions related to cardiovascular disease.

D-ribose is not a well known nutrient, but in the right setting, it is an excellent nutrient to enhance energy output. For this reason, this nutrient is important in dealing with conditions such as chronic fatigue, Adrenal Fatigue Syndrome, and cardiac weakness.

Anyone wishing more energy, gently delivered, can consider D-ribose. Unlike other nutrients, we don't refer to deficiencies of D-ribose in the tissues, that is, a lower amount or quantity than what is normal. The liver, adrenal glands, and fat tissues produce the most D-ribose, while others produce very little. Tissues relying most on aerobic energy metabolism, meaning they are reliant on oxygen, such as the heart and muscles, are affected by ATP drain, meaning they are severely affected by any amount of energy deprivation. D-ribose supplementation is the solution to this, because it gives back the energy. This is one reason for the success of D-ribose in cardiac patients.

We use D-ribose to help increase energy reserves during adrenal crashes, restore energy stores before and after exercise in those with AFS, and for those whom we believe will benefit from replenishing energy.

In essence, D-ribose, a naturally occurring sugar in the body, is regularly produced by our various tissues. Taking D-ribose supplements gives your body a little bit more of it to prevent fatigue and weak functioning. However, it is important to remember that D-ribose supplement studies have limitations. For example, studies have not included a placebo group or included long term follow up.

D-ribose supplements are easily absorbed by the body—about 97 percent is absorbed. Some individuals need a high dosage, i.e. those with low energy states, such as we see in advanced Adrenal Fatigue Syndrome, fibromyalgia, and chronic fatigue, and others who have difficulty delivering oxygen to their tissues. Those with sugar imbalances or carbohydrate intolerance may experience adrenal crashes with this compound. Therefore, for best results, we use D-ribose only under appropriate clinical conditions, and we don't recommend self-navigating.

If your health provider recommends D-ribose, always eat some food when you take it. Even a handful of nuts will suffice, but do not take this on an empty stomach. Because it is a form of sugar, those who are prone to blood sugar imbalances or have insulin or sugar sensitivity may develop reactive hypoglycemia if the body is not used to this nutrient. At high doses, side effects can include lightheadedness and mild diarrhea.

Note: Although no known contraindications of D-ribose therapy exist, we recommend that pregnant women, nursing mothers, and young children do not take it. We also recommend that you ask your doctor to advise you before taking D-ribose supplements.

Dosage Consideration: 1-10 grams daily to prevent cardiovascular disease, for adrenal support, for athletes on maintenance, and for others engaged in strenuous activity.

D-ribose is available in various forms. The powder form is the most common and bioavailable. We recommend including cofactors such as L-carnitine, co-enzyme Q10, and alpha-lipoic acid in a supplement regimen because they also enhance energy production and work synergistically with D-ribose.

Collagen

Collagen is the most abundant protein in the human body. It is critical in maintaining the health of the connective tissues that line the blood vessels, and it also contributes to the supporting framework upon which skeletal muscles operate. It reduces the catabolic (breakdown) state typically experienced by advanced Adrenal

Fatigue Syndrome sufferers with symptoms of muscle wasting. As is obvious, for optimum health, we need proper collagen synthesis.

Collagen production occurs in several stages, and the three key components are vitamin C, and the amino acids lysine and proline. Over twenty types of collagen exist, but Type I collagen is the most abundant in the human body. It is present in the skin, scar tissue, artery walls, tendons, and the organic parts of bones and teeth. Type III collagen is the second most abundant collagen in human tissues and occurs particularly in tissues exhibiting elastic properties. It is the collagen of granulation tissue (fibrous connective tissue) and is produced quickly by young fibroblasts, which are involved in synthesizing collagen, before the tougher Type I collagen is synthesized.

Around age thirty-five, collagen Types I and III decline, which is when skin loses its elasticity and wrinkles form.

In advanced Adrenal Fatigue Syndrome, the body breaks down collagen and muscle for fuel, a process that weakens the skeletal system. This is why we see symptoms such as fibromyalgia, chronic muscular pain of unknown origin, joint pain, loss of muscle tone, and reduced muscle strength. In order for the body to heal, this collagen must be replaced with the main building blocks of collagen: glycine, proline, lysine, and vitamin C. Of these, the body can manufacture only proline (from the amino acid glutamine).

Fortunately, collagen is readily available as a nutritional supplement and can be taken orally. Types I and III collagen are particularly well suited for Adrenal Fatigue Syndrome. This strategy is particularly useful before and after exercise. Hydrolyzed powdered form of these two types are available and promote maximum absorption within the body. It is important to use 100 percent pure collagen.

Dosage Consideration: 3-15 grams of Type I and III blended as needed.

Note: Excessive intake may lead to constipation and gastric discomfort especially in those with advanced Adrenal Exhaustion.

Probiotics

A healthy intestinal track is of paramount importance because gastrointestinal function is invariably compromised in advancing AFS. Common GI symptoms include constipation, poor food assimilation, bloating, and irritable bowel. Optimal gastrointestinal health depends on the balance of microscopic interplay between billions of beneficial (good) and pathogenic (bad) bacteria; the body needs both for normal bowel functions.

About 400 species of these "good bugs" inhabit the intestines and their total population is about 100 times the number of cells in your body. Remarkably, these microorganisms coexist peacefully in a carefully balanced internal ecosystem. As long as they flourish, they prevent the pathogenic, disease causing bacteria and fungi from colonizing. In this way, beneficial bacteria help keep you healthy. If the delicate intestinal environment is disrupted, pathogenic bacteria, parasites, and fungi such as clostridia, salmonella, staphylococcus, *blastocystis hominis*, and *Candida albicans* often move in, multiply, and then attack the beneficial bacteria.

> **Considerable research shows us that good bacteria, otherwise known as *probiotics*, help defend our bodies from the disease causing species of bacteria and also detoxify toxic chemicals. Beneficial bacteria also produce valuable vitamins including biotin, folic acid, niacin, pantothenic acid, riboflavin, thiamin, vitamin B6, vitamin B12, and vitamin K. These bacteria also assist in breaking down dietary proteins into amino acids, which are then reconfigured into new proteins useful for the body. Good bacteria also ensure that toxins are excreted from the bowels (via the stool) rather than being absorbed into the bloodstream.**

Acidophilus is an example of a beneficial probiotic in that they stimulate activity in the thymus and spleen (key immune system glands). They prompt the body to manufacture natural antibodies. Certain acidophilus strains even protect against the formation of tumors and promote production of interferon, a hormone that protects against cancer. When probiotics are present, they secrete mediators in which the pathogenic forms cannot grow. However, in the absence of probiotics, the pathogenic micro-organic forms take over and their toxins exclude the probiotics. This is one reason replacing our natural flora and keeping our bowels healthy and populated with probiotics is vital in preventing disease. Probiotics containing Lactobacillus acidophilus and Bifida can help detoxification programs.

Numerous studies help us understand the way probiotics work and establish the many beneficial and therapeutic aspects of probiotics. These include:

- Increased enzyme production, such as proteases, which digest proteins and lipases that digest fats.

- Improved bowel transit time and texture of the stool.

- Increased synthesis of immune antibodies and augmentation of gamma-interferon production.

- Reduction of lactose intolerance caused by a deficiency of the enzyme lactase, which leads to reduced bloating, gas formation, and stomach discomfort after milk consumption.

- Acts as an antitoxin with anti-carcinogenic and antitumor agents.

- Relief of dermatitis and other skin disorders by improving the balance of gastrointestinal bacteria.

Many scientists at the forefront of probiotics research believe that the toxins secreted from the pathogens, rather than the pathogens, are responsible for diseases. Probiotics help reduce the amount of toxic chemicals in the body, namely pathogenic bacteria and fungi, which produce their own toxins. At a local level, this minimizes the risk of colon cancers, protects the entire body, and improves overall health on a larger scale.

We can repopulate the beneficial bacteria by regularly supplementing with probiotics such as acidophilus. These microorganisms restore and maintain balance within your internal ecosystem while displacing noxious bacteria and fungi at the same time. They also increase the acidity of the intestinal environment that probiotics thrive in and harmful bugs detest. (As an aside, acidophilus literally means "love of acid.")

Acidophilus supplements are widely available in health food stores and drugstores, although it can be a daunting task to select among the numerous "something-dophilus" products. However, if you examine the labels you will discover a variety of useful bugs including *Lactobacillus acidophilus, Bifidobacterium bifidum, Lactobacillus bulgaricus,* and *Streptococcus faecium.* Some products may contain fructooligosaccharides, which are sugars that nourish beneficial bacteria to make them colonize faster. All of these ingredients are acceptable and any combination of them works well.

Acidophilus supplements contain living organisms, so freshness is critical. Purchase a product well before its expiration date, which should be clearly displayed. Once the supplements are opened, keep them refrigerated.

Dosage Consideration: 1-4 tablets before meals. Potency varies greatly from one product to another. It is best to refer to the instructions on the product label. For those who don't want to use these supplements, certain yogurt products contains the friendly bacterium *Lactobacillus acidophilus*, which can help restore intestinal micro-flora balance and inhibit the growth of potentially harmful bacteria.

Digestive Enzymes

Found in abundance in the body (over 1300 types), enzymes are molecule catalysts; they are considered the construction workers that facilitate all the bodily functions. For example, raw fruits and vegetables contain a plentiful supply of enzymes, *but cooking and food processing can destroy them.* When enzymes are destroyed, this affects the body's ability to digest food, deliver nutrients, and optimally perform its functions. Thus, toxins build up and accumulate in the body.

Digestive enzymes are especially important, as poor food assimilation is one of the main symptoms of AFS. Because plant enzymes help digest our food directly through the intestinal tract, supplemental enzymes help prevent feelings of bloating and exhaustion after a big meal. We consume an average of two pounds of food per day or twenty tons over a lifetime. Smooth passage of food through the gastrointestinal tract is critical to avoid stasis of feces, which releases toxins. Together with a diet high in soluble fiber, digestive enzymes help digestion.

Digestive enzymes also help other vitamins and minerals. For example, the fat soluble vitamins A, D, E, and K require fat for absorption. Fat must be broken down by an enzyme known as lipase. If lipase is not present in sufficient quantities, the fat will not be broken down, and if that happens, the vitamins are not released. Therefore, you can spend a fortune on vitamin pills, *but in the absence of the proper enzymes to release the vitamins into the body, the body flushes the vitamins out rather than using them.*

If our organs start to degenerate and fail to function properly, the stress of this process most likely shows up on the face. However, after consuming digestive enzymes one of the early signs of better digestion is improvement in skin tone. Digestive enzymes can therefore play a key role in adrenal support among those with dysregulated gastric assimilation.

> *Dosage Consideration: 1-4 enzyme tablets before meal as tolerated.* **Potency varies greatly from one product to another. It is best to refer to the instructions on the product label.**

Phosphatidylserine

Phosphatidylserine is a major component of nerve cell production and is sometimes used to enhance memory. It also reduces cortisol levels, as shown in research studies of otherwise healthy men engaging in vigorous exercise. Vigorous exercise is expected to increase cortisol but in the subjects phosphaditylserine was found to reduce post-exercise cortisol. In addition, testosterone levels, normally expected to drop after intense exercise, were not reduced and their perceived level of well-being immediately following exercise was positive.

These experiments are important because they show that phosphaditylserine is able to reduce cortisol levels when the body experiences stress. These studies used exercise to produce the stress, but the same principle holds for other types of mental or physical stress. This makes phosphaditylserine a valuable tool for controlling cortisol levels.

Bear in mind, however, that not all exercise results in increased cortisol production. For example, short term, moderate exercise does not increase cortisol concentration in plasma at all, and only minor changes in cortisol concentration occur during more intensive exercise lasting less than one hour. In practical terms, this means we don't need to avoid exercise for fear of boosting our cortisol level, and a game of tennis, a bike ride, or a walk around the block will not increase cortisol production. In fact, the stress reducing benefits of moderate exercise help keep cortisol in check. Physical activity also promotes cardiovascular health and mental acuity, helping us maintain a higher quality of life as we age.

Dosage Consideration: 200-1000 mg. Those with high nighttime cortisol and sleep onset insomnia may find this particularly helpful. Beware of paradoxical reactions in those with advanced Adrenal Fatigue Syndrome for reasons not known.

Vitamin B12

Vitamin B12 helps maintain red blood cells and nerve cells as well as protecting against a variety of conditions. Vitamin B12 also boosts energy. It is also needed to make DNA. It reduces homocysteine, an amino acid now known to promote atherosclerosis. Vitamin B12 deficiency produces symptoms similar to Alzheimer's disease.

B12 is found in animal foods such as meat, poultry, and dairy products, most of which should be consumed in moderation by those with AFS. Those over age fifty might have decreased stomach acid, which makes it difficult to separate the B12 which is bound to protein. In addition, vegans, the type of vegetarian who does not consume dairy products or eggs, are especially vulnerable to B12 deficiency and should take supplements.

Dosage Consideration: 100-1000 mcg. Many forms are available. The sublingual form is the fastest acting. Those who are sensitive or weak need to be extra careful because of the potential for overstimulation. If you decide to stop taking vitamin B12 supplementation, do not do so abruptly.

Magnesium

Magnesium (Mg) is an ubiquitous element in nature. Both plants and animals have an absolute requirement for magnesium, a mineral that plays a central role in photosynthesis in plants and many of the metabolic reactions in animals. Magnesium is a cofactor in over 300 enzymatic reactions in human beings. It is required for sodium, potassium, and calcium homeostasis, as well as for the formation, transfer, storage, and utilization of ATP (mentioned earlier as the energy currency in the body) at the cellular level. You cannot live without magnesium. The lower the cellular level of magnesium, the faster energy flow is depleted. It's that simple. Therefore, we can't underestimate its importance in optimizing adrenal function.

Magnesium works synergistically with vitamin C and pantothenic acid in steroid synthesis. As important as magnesium is, only about 25 percent of Americans meet the Recommended Dietary Allowance (RDA) of 300-400 mg per day for magnesium. Most American women get only 175-225 mg per day; men get 220-260 mg. Current statistics show that only 25 percent of surveyed populations have a magnesium intake *at or greater* than the RDA. In addition, almost 40 percent consume less than 70 percent of the RDA. It is fair to say that the majority of the North American population has a suboptimal intake of magnesium.

To get enough magnesium from diet, one needs to consume about 2000 calories a day. Nuts, whole grains, and legumes are high in magnesium. There is a poor correlation between blood magnesium and intracellular levels. Total body magnesium levels may decrease 20 percent during a fast, with no change in blood levels. While low blood magnesium levels may correctly indicate serious disease, a "normal" magnesium blood level by traditional laboratory testing may exist concurrently with a deficit in intracellular magnesium.

Common symptoms of magnesium deficiency include:

- Musculoskeletal symptoms: osteoporosis, chronic fatigue and weakness, muscle spasms, tics, tremors, and restlessness.
- Cardiovascular symptoms: atherosclerosis, cardiac arrhythmias, sudden death, and vasospasms.

- Female issues: PMS (premenstrual syndrome) and eclampsia.
- Psychiatric symptoms: irritability, depression, and bipolar disorders.
- Neurological symptoms: migraine headaches, excessive noise and pain sensitivity.
- Endocrine symptoms: insulin resistance.

The RDA for magnesium is about 2 mg per pound of body weight. The American diet typically provides 1.2 -1.5 mg per pound of body weight. Many magnesium experts believe that an intake range of 2.7- 4.5 mg per pound (about 400-700 mg a day) is optimal. Some on the forefront of magnesium research are recommending up to 1000 mg per day for healthy people, using the clinical symptom of diarrhea as a target marker. Once the marker is achieved, magnesium intake can be reduced. Asians, for example, are already taking 3-4.5 mg of magnesium per pound of body weight.

> **Caution:** The above general recommendation for the *healthy* cannot be used for those with Adrenal Fatigue Syndrome. The diarrhea commonly experienced can be a welcome event for those with AFS and who are constipated. However, those with preexisting or borderline diarrhea (due to IBS and other conditions) may find their situation worsens. As nature's muscle relaxant, it also helps the body to relax under normal circumstances. In AFS, paradoxical reactions with magnesium are common, such as irritation, constipation, anxiety, and increased fatigue. As good as magnesium is, we must therefore be careful when using this nutrient for AFS.
>
> *Dosage Consideration:* 400-1000 mg a day.

Vitamin B Complex

The entire B complex is needed in small quantities to promote each other's functions, but it is also needed throughout the entire steroid synthesis pathway within the adrenal glands. Fortunately, only a small amount is needed, and most on a balanced diet will have no difficulty fulfilling this requirement. Food sources of the B vitamins include whole grains, brewer's yeast, and miso.

> *Dosage Consideration*: Those who are nutritionally depleted can consider a daily B complex formula supplying at least 50-100 mg of B6, 100-300 mcg of B12, and 60-120 mg of B3.

Trace Minerals

Trace minerals include manganese, selenium, chromium, iodine, copper, and zinc. We need these only in small amounts, and most of us received sufficient trace minerals in a balanced diet. Good natural sources of these trace minerals include sea vegetables, algae, and sprouts. We usually do not recommend taking a general trace mineral formula for Adrenal Fatigue Syndrome. Due to the body's sensitivity, many of these minerals tend to behave paradoxically. Instead of a general calming effect, zinc, iodine, and selenium in particular, can trigger anxiety for reasons not well understood. Prolonged intake of trace minerals is also generally not recommended because of their pro-oxidative effects.

In specific situations, individual minerals may be considered, and that usually is the best use of such trace minerals. For example, iodine may be considered for thyroid support, and chromium may be considered to stabilize blood sugar.

Dosage Consideration: Not recommended unless under guidance.

Quercetin

We can consider quercetin the king of flavonoids and an excellent natural antihistamine. It also interferes with the pain-promoting, inflammatory substances the body generates in many autoimmune diseases associated with AFS, including rheumatoid arthritis and colitis. This is of great importance in advanced Adrenal Fatigue Syndrome, where many suffer from food allergies, delayed food intolerance, and multiple chemical sensitivities. Having quercetin on hand can bring tremendous reduction of the inflammation triggered by allergens. Quercetin antihistaminic effect is non-sedating. That is, even if you take large amounts you won't become sleepy, which is a stark contrast to the drowsiness so common with over-the-counter antihistamine medications. Studies show that quercetin has the ability to fight off an enzyme that neutralizes cortisol, which as you recall, is a natural anti-inflammatory chemical the body produces.

We can get more quercetin by drinking unfermented green tea as well as red wine, but these foods are not recommended for those with AFS. Apples, onions, tomatoes, green peppers, and broccoli are excellent sources of quercetin. Since a large amount of quercetin is required to produce a positive effect, it's best to take it in supplements. Otherwise, most people miss the beneficial effect by not taking enough. Always take it along with the digestive enzyme, bromelain, for maximum effect.

Dosage Consideration: 600-6000mg per day (with bromelain) in divided doses on an empty stomach.

Bromelain

The primary activity of bromelain, an enzyme found in pineapple stems, is to reduce inflammation and promote healing, especially in the muscles and joints. As such, it is used widely in sports medicine and trauma management. Bromelain's anti-inflammatory property also plays a significant role in managing asthma, arthritis, colitis, and other allergic responses. Use only high potency and high quality supplements. Bromelain works best when taken along with quercetin.

Dosage Consideration: 600-4000 mg. Bromelain's potency is rated in terms of GDU units; the higher the GDU number, the more potent it is. The recommended GDU units should be at least 2500-3500. We recommend taking bromelain on an empty stomach with quercetin.

Additional Gentle Nutritional Supplements

As we've said, the decision to take nutritional supplements in advanced AFS can be problematic because of potential paradoxical reactions. However, working with your doctor, consider taking the following in addition to those discussed in detail above. We employ these where specific supports are required and only when the body is ready. To achieve therapeutic effects, we need to ensure proper timing and dosage.

We suggest dosages, but these are subject to judgment and your doctor might want to adjust them to fit your needs.

- Vitamin D, 1000 to 5000 IU helps in hormonal synthesis.
- Lysine (an amino acid), 1-2 gm supports collagen synthesis.
- Proline (an amino acid), 500 mg-1gm supports collagen synthesis.
- Glutamine (an amino acid), 1-5 gm helps to stabilize blood sugar and the GI track.
- Chromium polynicotinate, 400-1200 mcg helps to stabilize blood sugar.
- SOD or superoxide dismutase, 100-1000 mg for liver detoxification.
- CoQ10, 300-1,000 mg, helps support cardiac heath especially if one has irregular heartbeat or is on statin medications.
- High potency fish oil, 1000-5000 mg DHA/EPA helps to support anti-inflammatory action.

- Chlorella, 1-2 tsp helps the body eliminate toxic metals as a natural chelating agent.
- Betaine hydrochloride (HCL), helps restore normal gastric pH if acid is deficient.
- Zinc, 25-50 mg can help support body metabolism.
- Malic acid, 50-200 mg helps enhance energy flow.
- Calcium D-Glucarate, 200-1000 mg helps liver detoxification.
- Activated charcoal as a gentle detoxifying agent and to combat diarrhea.
- Lithium orotate (a dietary supplement), 5-15 mg can help to stabilize mood swings.
- Gaba, 200-1500 mg can help reduce anxiety and promote better sleep.
- Taurine, 200-2000 mg helps with water retention by its natural diuretic effect.
- Soluble fiber, helps stabilize blood sugar and intestinal motility.
- Colostrum, 100-500 mg helps strengthen the immune system.
- Iodine, 3-50 mg helps support thyroid function if used carefully under guidance.
- Lipoic Acid, 300-600 mg a day by mouth or IV to support liver function.

Intolerance vs. Toxicity

While the nutrients discussed above are considered the most gentle, this is just a general rule of thumb. Remember that the more advanced the AFS, the more sensitive a person is to *any* nutrient. In addition, most compounds in this group are naturally occurring in our body from the day we are born. They are not foreign substances like herbs or prescription medications. As such, the body already possesses intrinsic pathways to absorb, assimilate, transport, and metabolize them. Overdoses produce only mild, if any, after effects and side effects. Symptoms of intolerance usually subside once supplementation is discontinued.

For example, excessive magnesium intake can cause diarrhea, which resolves after discontinuation. Fat soluble vitamins are more of a risk, but even with these, we now know that the upper safe limit is many more times than the Recommended Dietary Allowance (RDA). For example, the current RDA of vitamin D for adults is 600 IU; however, physicians routinely recommend 1000 IU a day. Some recommend up to 5000 IU a day, especially for those living in an area where sunlight is less abundant. The same is true for vitamin C. While the RDA is 60-95 mg daily, most healthy people take upwards of 1000 mg a day as part of a program designed to maintain health and prevent illness. The national nonprofit Vitamin C Foundation currently recommends 3000 mg a day for healthy individuals, and much more in times of illness.

The more advanced the AFS, the more challenging is the task to select the right compounds from this group. Invariably, those who are in very weak condition also have a highly sensitive body and are constitutionally weak. Some in this group can't tolerate any supplements. Others appear to get better at first, but then develop a gradual intolerance to these compounds and show more fatigue and anxiety.

With magnesium and vitamin C, for example, some individuals with AFS even develop constipation instead of diarrhea at high doses as the bowel tolerance level is reached. We see this as a paradoxical reaction. Well-being returns as the dosage is reduced.

While these kinds of reactions are reported as "vitamin toxicity," it should be more accurately described as a form of intolerance. The difference is significant. The body's unpleasant symptoms in such a situation are likely to be a reflection of its inability to clear metabolites out of the body and are unlikely due to the intrinsic toxic property of the vitamin or mineral itself. Reactions can be overcome by adjusting the nutrient dosage, and we often see intolerances resolve spontaneously as adrenal health returns.

Unfortunately, many simply abandon a good nutrient the moment such intolerance develops, labeling these valuable nutrients toxic, and forever depriving themselves of such treasured tools in the recovery process. This is very different from some compounds within Groups 2 and 3 (discussed in the next chapters) in which intrinsic negative properties exist that are true toxicities. The signs of toxicity appear at high dosages and compound the body's already poor clearance in those with advanced AFS.

We hope you see how important it is to match nutrient dosages to an individual's specific state. This is of paramount importance throughout the recovery process if a consistent and sustained recovery is desired, rather than a rollercoaster ride. Blindly taking supplements based on what works for others, an incomplete understanding of the intrinsic property of nutrients involved, and lack of correlation to one's unique constitution, can worsen AFS and trigger adrenal crashes.

Key Points to Remember

- Gentle nutrients include vitamins C, D, E, A, B5, pantethine, B12, chlorella, D-ribose, bromelain, quercetin, probiotics, collagen, enzymes, magnesium, HCl, phosphatidylserine, CoQ10, iodine, fish oil, and so forth.

- Vitamin C is particularly important, provided the right dosages, delivery systems, and forms are properly chosen and taken in a blend.

- Vitamin C is very safe, although caution should be taken for those with kidney disease, G6PD deficiency, kidney stones, and iron overload.

- Magnesium is an important mineral that relaxes muscles and calms the nervous system.

- Glutathione is an intracellular antioxidant and electron donor. It is the master recycler.

- Pantethine /pantothenic acid are powerful B vitamins with strong adrenal support properties in addition to their lipid support effect.

- D-ribose is a natural nutrient that enhances energy directly within the ATP cycle.

- Collagen is an important building block for protein needed for those in a catabolic state.

- Probiotics and enzymes are important tools to normalize internal dysbiosis (imbalance of intestinal flora) commonly seen when gastric assimilation slows down.

- Quercetin and bromelain are important natural antihistaminic compounds useful for those with chemical or food sensitivities.

- Intolerance to Group 1 nutrients should not be confused with toxicity.

Chapter 21

Second Line of Defense—
Glandulars and Herbs

G landulars and herbs have a role in a treatment plan for Adrenal Fatigue Syndrome. They can be considered when first line defenders described in the last chapter have failed to bring about complete recovery or in special situations. When we talk about *glandulars*, we're referring to raw glandular or non-glandular tissue derived from animals. Glandular products are commonly derived from several organs, including: thyroid, adrenal, thymus, testis, and ovary. Less frequently used are the pituitary, kidney, liver, pancreas, spleen, lung, heart, brain, uterus, and prostate.

Herbs are plants valued for their flavor, scent, or other qualities. Across our planet, they are universally used in cooking, as medicines, and often in spiritual rituals, too. Certain herbs can be beneficial for recovery from Adrenal Fatigue Syndrome, while other herbs can be quite detrimental and delay or prevent healing.

Both glandular products and herbs are widely used for Adrenal Fatigue Syndrome, but because of the lack of standardization and research, information about them is often incorrect, which tends to lead to their misuse. Proper guidance is needed in order to avoid the pitfalls and side effects.

Glandulars enjoy widespread popularity, and one reason is their adaptogenic properties, that is, their ability to enhance or boost energy when it's low and to tone down energy when excessive. These compounds are well suited for those with mild Adrenal Fatigue Syndrome, when the body has sufficient internal reserve. When adrenal function is compromised and has advanced to Stage 3C, the adaptogenic properties of many of these compounds become less apparent. Instead, for reasons not well understood, they tend to behave more like stimulants. This might be detrimental to those unaware and can lead to overstimulation of an already weak adrenal system. The more advanced the Adrenal Fatigue Syndrome, the more prominent the negative stimulatory effects appear. For this reason, what seems to be harmless for one person can be toxic to another.

The Basics of Glandulars

Past and current healers have frequently used tissue extracts to fight various diseases. This practice goes back over 3000 years. For instance, bone marrow extracts have been used for the treatment of anemia. Pancreatic glandular was standard therapy prior to the discovery of insulin. Desiccated thyroid is still used by many alternative practitioners to manage hypothyroidism. Many people use glandulars as a source of natural hormones. In addition, glandular therapy is the foundation for elements and components of today's hormone therapies, including thyroid and estrogen replacement, and steroids such as prednisone.

Commercial glandular extract therapy began in the 1920s with the discoveries made by Swiss physician, Paul Niehans, at his clinic in Montreaux, Switzerland. Dr. Niehans went on to develop live cell therapy, and thousands of severely ill patients came to his clinic as a last resort. His therapies also became famous for rejuvenation, and those who flocked to his clinic included the wealthy, royalty, presidents and celebrities. Live cell therapy remains a popular practice in Europe today.

By the mid 1930s, several companies produced *adrenal* cell extracts in liquid and tablet forms and countless physicians used them for their patients. By the early 1940s, adrenal glandular extracts were widely prescribed by physicians as part of their adrenal support treatment. As recently as 1968, they were still made by some of the leading pharmaceutical companies. Adrenal extracts are used to replenish and eventually normalize adrenal function. Adrenal cortical extracts can be discontinued once they have done their job of repairing adrenal function, which is their advantage over cortisol hormone replacement.

Theoretically, glandulars can come from any animal, but most often they are derived from cow (bovine), while others come from pig (porcine) and sheep (ovine). Different glandulars and glandular extracts have various properties and uses. For example:

- Thymus and spleen extracts may influence the immune system.
- Thyroid extracts can help with low thyroid.
- Adrenal extracts may help support weak adrenals.
- Testis extracts may influence androgen levels.
- Ovarian extracts may influence estrogen levels.

The difficulty of standardized testing prevents research and represents one of the primary setbacks in current use of glandulars. Modern scientific studies involve isolating variables into one variable used in double-blind experimental settings.

Clearly, it isn't possible to test any glandular within the limited structure of a double-blind study because these substances contain enzymes, vitamins, fatty acids, amino acids, minerals, neurotransmitters, and a host of nutrients in addition to the tissues within the gland. We can't isolate any single substance or hormone, such as cortisol or thyroxine, because of the many different substances present within each glandular extract.

Since glandular products contain many substances, including hormones, a major problem is our lack of knowledge about how much of these hormones or other substances are available in these extracts, which vary from batch to batch and animal to animal. In addition, it's difficult to know which of the many substances has a therapeutic influence and how the specific glandular interacts with myriad other substances in the body. With so many substances occurring in a single glandular, it's difficult to measure the kind of effect they may have in the long run, especially when used as a nutritional supplement. Nevertheless, based on eighty years of anecdotal evidence, little doubt remains that glandulars, when used properly, possess healing properties. Since the advent of adrenocorticotropic hormones, the use of glandular extract has been neglected.

Generally, the best glandular products come from freeze dried extracts derived from animals raised using organic methods in New Zealand, where no bovine spongiform encephalopathy (mad cow disease) has appeared. Reputable glandular products are subject to in-process and finished product testing. These tests include microbial contamination tests to assure acceptable total bacteria counts and the absence of disease-causing bacteria.

We consider each popular glandular individually.

Desiccated Thyroid Glandular

Desiccated thyroid is the dried and powdered thyroid gland, with the fat and connective tissue removed during processing. Desiccated thyroid is often derived from hogs, but may also come from cows and sheep. Desiccated natural thyroid is often prescribed to manage hypothyroidism. Pharmaceutical preparation is standardized and contains both thyroxine and triiodothyronine. Natural desiccated thyroid drugs have been available since the late 1800s, but fell out of favor in the 1950s when synthetic levothyroxine (Synthroid®) was introduced. However, the natural desiccated thyroid has regained popularity among patients and practitioners, in part because many patients report feeling better on these drugs. Armour® thyroid (porcine), and Thyrolar® (bovine) are common FDA approved drugs in this class.

Note: Prescription desiccated thyroid drugs are *not* the same as over-the-counter (OTC) thyroid glandular supplements. Countless OTC thyroid extracts are marketed as dietary supplements; many likely do not contain any significant hormones, but many do. Therefore, choosing the right product can become the proverbial tale of trial and error.

Many with Adrenal Fatigue Syndrome take prescription thyroid medication, making over-the-counter thyroid glandular unnecessary. Concurrent use of thyroid glandular and prescription thyroid replacement may lead to *hyper*thyroidism. If indeed the thyroid needs support, many other more gentle nutrients (such as kelp, iodine, and the amino acid, tyrosine) can be considered. Low thyroid function associated or secondary to Adrenal Fatigue Syndrome usually improves by itself once adrenal function improves.

Adrenal Glandular

Adrenal glandular products are widely promoted and used for Adrenal Fatigue Syndrome. After taking adrenal glandular, many users report that increased energy replaces fatigue and a sense of calm replaces anxiety. However, these reports generally come from those with *mild* AFS, not those with advanced adrenal weakness, in whom adrenal glandular often has a stimulating effect. As energy returns, this could be considered a desirable outcome, but significant side effects can occur if taken long term. *Taking adrenal glandular habitually to sustain energy is one of the common reasons for recovery failure, because these compounds can become addictive and produce withdrawal side effects when individuals stop taking them.*

Here's a closer look at how this generally unfolds:

- First, as seen with other addictive substances, the body can develop a tolerance and then more glandular is needed to produce the same effect.

- Second, at high doses, the glandular may actually trigger an adrenal crisis as the body's ability to handle the stimulant reaches maximum tolerance level. A wired-and-tired feeling may result in insomnia and hyperirritability along with extreme fatigue.

- Third, withdrawal and rebound symptoms may surface when the glandular is stopped, evidenced by even greater fatigue.

- Fourth, adrenal glandular may trigger a series of paradoxical and undesirable effects, including among other things, panic attacks, heart palpitations, fast heart rate, and fragile blood pressure.

Given these potential side effects, most consumers should exercise care and use adrenal glandular on a short term basis, provided that the Adrenal Fatigue Syndrome is mild. The more advanced the AFS, the more one should be wary of adrenal glandular and leave advice about its use to experienced clinicians.

Due to the lack of standardization, many products are available to consumers, but not all are created equal.

Other Glandular Products

- Thymus glandular contains substances that influence the immune system, but it is very difficult to know the nature of both their short term and long term effects on the immune system. The body contains countless immune substances, and it is extremely difficult to predict all the potential interactions when taking a thymus glandular. Furthermore, there could be wide variations in responses among individuals.

- Testis and ovary glandular extracts may contain testosterone and estrogen, respectively. Some consumers have tried to use these glandulars for libido support. We usually don't recommend them because much better ways exist to support and closely monitor hormonal function.

- Pituitary and hypothalamus glandular extracts are usually stimulatory in nature and should be used with caution. They are usually found as part of a scattershot approach to adrenal healing which is highly undesirable.

Taking a Look at Herbs

Every established civilization in the world has some form of herb-based tonic used to support energy. We now know many of these tonics support adrenal function through their main mechanism of action. The following herbs are commonly used for Adrenal Fatigue Syndrome recovery.

Licorice Root (*Glycyrrhiza glabra*)

Highly prized in Chinese medicine, licorice is grown in Europe and Asia and is used in many Chinese patented herbal formulas. The most well known herb for adrenal support, licorice is an anti-stress herb that increases energy, endurance, and vitality, and acts as a mild tonic. Licorice naturally fortifies cortisone levels by blocking conversion of cortisol into cortisone through inhibition of the enzyme 11beta-hydroxysteriod dehydrogenase. It has been used to help decrease symptoms of hypoglycemia, a common side effect of decreased adrenal function.

Licorice causes increased production of aldosterone, a hormone frequently deficient in advanced AFS. The herb can raise blood pressure for those whose blood pressure is normal. Although licorice candy doesn't offer the same benefits as preparations made from the root, it too, can cause an increase in blood pressure in those who are sensitive. Licorice can also soothe nervous stomachs and stimulate blood circulation in the heart. Until the 1930s, physicians prescribed licorice to treat Addison's disease.

Deglycyrrhized licorice (DGL) is made by removing the glycyrrhizin, the part of the plant responsible for its bittersweet taste. However, for positive adrenal effects, only real licorice should be used, not DGL.

Note: *Pregnant women should not take licorice. In high doses (3-5 gm/day), it lowers testosterone in women. Excessive intake can raise blood pressure.*

Side effects of licorice include headaches, elevated blood pressure (hypertension), lethargy, upset stomach, diarrhea, facial puffiness, edema, increased fatigue, anxiety, irritability, and grogginess. It may increase (potentiate) the effect of the drugs warfarin (an anticoagulant) and digoxin, a drug commonly used to treat cardiac disease. Here, as with glandulars, these side effects are more prominent in those with advanced Adrenal Fatigue Syndrome. The weaker the adrenals, the more we can anticipate stimulatory side effects. Most of the side effects are associated with what appears to be the loss of adaptogenic properties, which results in a preponderance of stimulatory properties.

Ashwagandha Root and Leaf (*Withania Somnifera*)

Ashwagandha is an ancient Indian herb with a history of therapeutic uses. Known as a tonic for all kinds of weaknesses, ashwagandha is famous for its direct beneficial effects on adrenal function. Ashwagandha promotes strength and vigor and is regarded as a rejuvenator and mild aphrodisiac.

Ayurvedic physicians use ashwagandha as the treatment of choice for rheumatic pains, joint inflammation, and other related conditions. Ashwagandha is also considered an adaptogen.

It is considered an adaptogenic, cardiotropic, and cardioprotective herb. Studies have shown that a 30-day course produces a significant increase in super oxide dismutase (SOD), an important antioxidant. Under a normal therapeutic dosage, patients do not experience side effects from ashwagandha. This means the herb is used no more than a few months, with intermittent days off or "holidays" if a high dose is used. To date, no significant drug interactions have been found. Some people have complained of slight drowsiness after using ashwagandha, but a majority of people have had no trouble at all, providing they are constitutionally strong.

Those with advanced AFS may find that this herbal compound increases energy. Like licorice, the stimulatory properties tend to be exaggerated and may become *too* pronounced in those with advanced adrenal weakness. This can lead to anxiety and a sense of being wired. For this reason, we recommend close monitoring if using this herb. However, for reasons we don't know, a small number of people with advanced AFS who have problems with other nutritional therapy may tolerate ashwagandha.

Korean Ginseng Root (*Panax ginseng*)

Generally, Panax ginseng enhances energy flow. It is more suitable for men than women, and some women have experienced adverse side effects, such as facial hair and acne. In men, taking too much ginseng can lead to symptoms of aggressiveness, irritability, or sexual excess. That said, Korean ginseng is a natural remedy for Adrenal Fatigue Syndrome and men can start taking it in small doses and gradually increase the amount. (It's best for women to avoid its use altogether.) Side effects include insomnia, headaches, upset stomach, breast pain, diarrhea, vertigo, and anxiety, and as with other herbs, its stimulatory properties tend to be more pronounced in individuals with weak adrenals.

Siberian Ginseng Root (*Eleutherococus senticosus*)

Unlike Korean ginseng, Siberian ginseng root is good for both men and women. The main benefits of Siberian ginseng are increased resistance to stress, normalized metabolism, and neurotransmitter regulation. Siberian ginseng counteracts mental fatigue and is known to increase and sustain energy levels, physical stamina, and endurance. In addition, Siberian ginseng is also an antidepressant that helps improve sleep, diminishes lethargy, reduces irritability, and induces a feeling of well-being. However, in the presence of AFS, Siberian ginseng root should be used short term and limited to mild cases in order to avoid stimulatory side effects that invariably overwhelm the body, and over time, worsen the overall condition.

Ginger Root (*Zingiber officinale*)

An adaptogen for the adrenals, ginger root helps modulate cortisol levels, normalize blood pressure and heart rate, burn fat, and increase energy and the metabolic rate. Ginger also stimulates digestive enzyme secretions for proteins and fatty acids.

Ginger root may contain aristolochic acid, which can cause serious kidney/ urinary system disease (e.g., renal fibrosis or urinary tract cancer). Symptoms include an unusual change in the amount of urine or the presence of blood in the urine. Liquid preparations that feature ginger often contain sugar and/or alcohol, so those with diabetes, alcohol dependence, or liver disease must be cautious.

Ginger is not recommended for use during pregnancy. Since it isn't known if ginger is excreted into breast milk, we recommend consulting your doctor before taking ginger root products while breastfeeding. (The casual use of small amounts of ginger as found in everyday cooking and baking or in commercial ginger teas is not detrimental.)

Ginkgo Leaf (*Ginkgo biloba*)

The ginkgo tree is one of the oldest living tree species, and ginkgo biloba comes from this tree. The Chinese have used ginkgo for thousands of years to treat various ailments, including lung congestion, asthma, to support circulation and libido, and as an anti-aging substance. It is well recognized for its positive effects on brain functions including enhanced mental alertness, reduced brain fog, enhanced memory, and reduced mental fatigue.

The adrenals suffer from a tremendous amount of oxidative stress, especially when producing excess cortisol during the stress response. This leads to a significant increase in free radicals within the same adrenal cells that make the needed hormones. Ginkgo leaf possesses strong antioxidative properties to sequester free radical production, thereby protecting the adrenal glands, the brain, and the liver from free radical damage.

Ginkgo also contains several bioflavonoids that improve blood flow to the brain, ears, eyes, heart, and extremities. Its side effects include gastrointestinal discomfort, headache, increased risk of bleeding, diarrhea, nausea, vomiting, restlessness, anxiety, and increased fatigue.

Maca Root (*Lepidium meyenii*)

Maca root is an herb that grows high in the Andes mountains in South America at elevations up to 15,000 feet. It is one of the few plants that can be cultivated in the harsh climate of the Andes. For more than two thousand years, native Peruvians have used it as food and medicine, to promote endurance and improve energy, vitality, sexual virility and fertility. It is best known for its aphrodisiac properties. It also possesses adaptogenic qualities with glucose and cortisol. It has also been shown to reduce elevated glucose and stress-induced ulcers.

Active ingredients of maca root include free sugars, sterols, amino acids, alkaloids, tannins, and cardiotonic glycosidesuridine. The main physiological pathway of action is through stimulation of CNS, the central nervous system. Hormonal pathways do not appear to be involved. Studies show it does not influence hormonal blood levels of testosterone, for example. In addition to its aphrodisiac and energy boosting effects, this herb can also partially reverse sexual dysfunction that often occurs with the use of SSRI type antidepressants, such as Prozac®, Paxil®, and Zoloft®.

Being an herb of stimulatory nature, high doses can lead to anxiety and insomnia. Those with advanced Adrenal Fatigue Syndrome are particularly vulnerable. Possible side effects include insomnia, anxiety, sense of impending doom, and nervousness. In extreme cases, one can develop irregular heart rate. For mild AFS, this herb is best used in small doses as part of a nutritional cocktail rather than as a stand-alone nutrient.

Rhodiola Rosea

Rhodiola Rosea is found in the colder climates of Europe, where for centuries it has been used to cure most ailments. Historically, rhodiola tea is popular among Russians as an energy booster. This herb can help ease the symptoms and support the healing process of many conditions, including anxiety, depression, stomach problems, fibromyalgia, and other nervous system maladies. This plant contains dozens of substances and it's difficult to identify all the active ingredients, although we can name rosavin, salidroside, rosin, and rosarin.

This herb is classified as an adaptogen. It acts as a muscle relaxant and regulates blood flow, which help support cortisol production in the adrenal glands when more cortisol is needed. It is better used in stressed individuals with high cortisol level during early stages of AFS. In some people, especially those in Stage 2 of AFS, the adrenal glands secrete too much cortisol. Unfortunately, the release is not steady but sporadic. Rhodiola rosea is also used to help the adrenal gland slow the secretion. This results in a sense of calmness throughout the day instead of periodic spikes of well-being followed by emotional lows resembling a rollercoaster ride. This herb can also help those suffering from fibromyalgia to sleep through the night and function normally throughout the day.

Rhodiola has also been shown to improve mental awareness, physical strength and endurance, stress, memory, and anxiety in healthy people. In the case of anxiety, it is best used when combined with other herbs such as kava, passion flower, 5-HTP, tryptophan, and ashwagandha.

In the presence of AFS, especially in advanced stages, it is important to remember that high dosages of rhodiola rosea extract could cause overstimulation and insomnia, thus aggravating anxiety and leading to a wired-and-tired state. On the other hand, those with mild AFS may find this herb an excellent adjunct in the early stages.

> Caution: Herbs and glandulars are widely used and touted as possessing adaptogenic properties and marketed as tonics. Their stimulatory properties have made them popular among those with very mild AFS (who might not ever suspect they have it), because energy is increased and fatigue is reduced. Clinically, these stimulatory effects are more pronounced in those with weak adrenals. Stimulants are the equivalent of giving too much gas and flooding the engine in a car, thus putting additional stress on the adrenals to work harder and produce more energy. This finally further depletes the adrenal glands, and the short term sense of well-being tends to fail over time.

Short term use of herbal formulas and glandular products in mild cases of AFS is acceptable, but when adrenal weakness is pronounced, professional guidance should be considered. In addition, stay alert for the paradoxical or unusual reactions we have discussed elsewhere in this book, including:

- excessive fatigue
- panic attacks
- unstable blood pressure
- insomnia
- anxiety/irritability

Consider these warning signs of inappropriate use. Blended formulas are particularly convenient and effective, such as Adreno-Blast™ (see Appendix G). Glandulars and herbs have their place in adrenal recovery, and judicious use avoids over-stimulation, addiction, and withdrawal concerns.

Note: If you are already on high doses of herbs and glandulars, stopping abruptly can lead to withdrawal symptoms and may trigger adrenal crashes and is not recommended.

Dosage Consideration: Herbs and glandulars come in many forms, from raw powder to standardized extracts. Potency and purity also varies depending on the batch during harvest. It is not possible to give standard dosage recommendations. Always read the product label and consult your doctor prior to beginning such endeavors.

Key Points to Remember

- Glandulars and herbs are widely promoted as healing agents for Adrenal Fatigue Syndrome.

- Many of these have adaptogenic properties and are useful in early stages of AFS.

- Their predominant properties tend to become stimulatory for those in advanced stages of AFS.

- Adrenal and thyroid glandulars from porcine (pigs) sources are the most common form of non-standardized glandular support.

- Popular herbs include licorice root, ashwagandha, ginger root, maca root, rhodiola rosea, ginkgo, and ginseng.

- Standardized thyroid glandulars are prescription medications due to their high potency.

- Due to the lack of standardization, it's not possible to recommend dosages for non-standardized herbs or glandulars; they are specific to each product.

- The use of glandulars or herbs, whether standardized or not, should be done with care and only as needed. Long term use requires professional supervision.

- Under most situations, this group is not needed provided that Group 1 compounds are properly used.

Chapter 22

Tools of Last Resort—Hormones

A drenal hormones are essential for life and building and restoring health. Too much or too little threatens our well-being and prevents us living in optimal health. In the *early* days of adrenal hormone replacement, many decades ago, researchers had very little information about the proper dosage or the toxicity complications. Misled by improvement in their patients' symptoms, they gave patients many times more adrenal hormone, specifically, cortisol, than the normal amount. This sounds dramatic, but many patients died from the toxic effects.

Long term and excessive use of cortisol has negative side effects, too, so much so that cortisol is banned as a performance enhancing substance in competitive sports. Because of these bad experiences, researchers were scared off and avoided prescribing adrenal hormones such as cortisol whenever possible.

In Chapter 8, *Stage 3B—Hormonal Axis Imbalances*, we discussed the way some physicians use thyroid replacement to overcome the low energy brought on by Adrenal Fatigue Syndrome. This occurs because some practitioners assume patients with AFS suffer from primary hypothyroidism, and prescribe thyroid replacement. However, many individuals continue to suffer. Again, in the *early* days of thyroid hormone replacement, before synthetic hormones were available, patients received up to many times the usual dose of thyroid hormone, often resulting in severe toxic effects.

Clearly, hormone replacement therapy for AFS requires great care and its use must be put into perspective. In the right situation, with the right dose, hormone replacement can be of great benefit.

Medical science is just beginning to learn that even mild to moderate hormone deficiency, which remains undetected in routine blood tests, can nevertheless lead a person to feel awful and function poorly. We see this often in Adrenal Fatigue Syndrome.

To briefly review, adrenal hormones are under the control of the HPA axis, as well as the autonomic nervous system; over fifty hormones are involved. Dysregulation of any one can produce unpleasant symptoms. For example, low aldosterone levels can lead to blood pressure irregularities and fatigue; high estrogen can trigger

PMS and anxiety; imbalanced cortisol output can lead to sugar dysregulation, hypoglycemia, and sluggishness; and high epinephrine output can trigger heart palpitations such as atrial fibrillation and panic attacks. Those in the advanced stages of Adrenal Fatigue Syndrome are especially vulnerable.

Since routine laboratory testing is often unreliable, we believe paying close attention to the signs and symptoms of AFS is perhaps the most effective way to assess the need for hormone replacement. Further, treatment decisions about hormone replacement for AFS are best left to knowledgeable, experienced professionals. Because we still lack complete understanding of these many hormones and their mechanisms, we always expect some trial and error, even in the best of hands.

Premature use of adrenal hormonal replacement is a common mistake and can be a major cause of recovery delay or failure. In fact, improper use of corticosteroid such as hydrocortisone can make the condition worse due to toxicity, paradoxical effects, addiction, and withdrawal complications. Worst of all, it may also trigger adrenal crashes.

Chapter 2, *Hormone Basic, and the "Forgotten" Adrenals*, also described the function of some major hormones, along with their potential role in treatment. We revisit these hormones from a therapeutic perspective now in order to see the way we use them as part of a recovery program.

Pregnenolone

Some AFS sufferers report that pregnenolone replacement improves their energy, vision, memory, mental clarity, well-being, and often libido as well. In addition, some women report fewer hot flashes or symptoms of PMS while on pregnenolone. This is likely attributable to the relative rise of progesterone and thus, reduction in estrogen dominance. Remember that pregnenolone is converted in the body to progesterone and these two hormones have some overlapping similarities.

The clinical picture isn't completely clear, however, because other women report that pregnenolone worsens existing fatigue and may even trigger adrenal crashes. Such paradoxical reactions are common, especially as adrenal weakness advances.

In addition, many can take what appears to be a normal dose, but they don't benefit if the body is shunting it towards cortisol production, a phenomenon known as *pregnenolone steal*. On the other hand, overdose is possible if too much is taken over time.

Pregnenolone is the chemical mother of DHEA, which in turn may convert into androstenedione, testosterone, and estrogen. Pregnenolone supplementation may increase other hormones in the body, particularly testosterone.

That said, the following guidelines are important:

- Typical starting dose is 15 mg, increasing up to 50 mg for men or women.

- Use pregnenolone derived from a pharmacologically pure product and not a yam-derived "precursor."

- Oral pregnenolone pills work well for most.

- Sublingual administration is a good option; it bypasses initial liver metabolism that occurs after swallowing an oral pill. Because of its fast delivery to the bloodstream it tends to be spiky and not well tolerated by those who are sensitive or in advanced stages of Adrenal Fatigue Syndrome.

- Low doses can promote a relaxed feeling, while higher amounts may lead to irritability. The exact reason for this is unknown.

- Acne and hair loss can occur, probably because pregnenolone is likely converted into androgens.

- Headaches are possible with high dosages.

- Irregular heart rhythm and heart palpitations can occur even when the dose is low. These side effects are potentially serious in the elderly or in those with heart rhythm disturbances.

Given these side effects, you can see why a healthcare professional should guide you and oversee the results. Do not rely solely on blood or saliva tests to determine how much pregnenolone you should take.

Note: Pregnenolone therapy may be contraindicated in some people with a history of seizures, because it may interfere with the action of medications used to treat epilepsy and depression.

Pregnenolone and DHEA (discussed below) can be taken together for Adrenal Fatigue Syndrome. Since some pregnenolone is converted into DHEA, the intake amount of DHEA can be lowered if both are taken together.

Dosage Consideration: 10-50 mg daily in divided doses.

DHEA

The actions of DHEA tend to mimic pregnenolone, but are amplified, both in terms of desired results and side effects. Different doses appear to do different things, so we use DHEA judiciously.

DHEA converts into estrogen and testosterone. High dosages (100 to 200 mg or more) can lead to a redistribution of body mass as a result of the conversion of the DHEA into more androgenic steroid hormones. Significant side effects are similar to those of pregnenolone, only more severe. Hair loss and acne are particularly common.

For men, direct testosterone precursors such as androstenedione (and its metabolite androstenediol) may be more effective if anabolic results are desired. This, however, only applies to healthy individuals and not to those who are afflicted with Adrenal Fatigue Syndrome.

Even low dose DHEA can be problematic, because it tends to be quite stimulatory for those people with advanced adrenal weakness. In particular, those in Stage 3C and beyond (Adrenal Exhaustion) tend to react strongly even at minute dosages. Additional side effects are common and include: severe anxiety, feeling jittery, and increased PMS symptoms. These appear to be more prevalent in women.

Other important factors to consider include:

- DHEA is a slight mood elevator; it can potentially clash with antidepressants. Theoretically, antidepressant dosages can be lowered when the person is taking DHEA.

- DHEA has both a cholesterol lowering and blood thinning effect. Therefore, those taking cholesterol lowering drugs and blood thinning medications such as Coumadin® may need to have dosages lowered.

- DHEA is not regulated by a negative feedback loop in the body. In other words, taking DHEA supplements will not suppress the body's production of DHEA or cause the adrenals to rest and result in atrophy from disuse. Therefore, theoretically, patients do not need a resting period from DHEA, although it's probably good practice to have a resting cycle of a few weeks for each period of therapy lasting several months.

- Commercial DHEA products are made from *diosgenin*, an extract from the Mexican wild yam of the Dioscorea family. Biochemists can convert diosgenin to DHEA, but this happens only in the lab and not in the human body. Therefore, taking Dioscorea plant extracts does not lead to DHEA formation in the body.

Depending on the stage of AFS and individual constitution, both blood or saliva DHEA levels vary greatly as AFS progresses. Because of inconsistent clinical correlation, blood levels generally are not particularly helpful.

> *Dosage Consideration:* **10-50 mg in divided doses. Use DHEA for Adrenal Fatigue Syndrome only under professional guidance. Determining the right dosage is not straightforward and can be tricky. The many possible side effects are similar to those of pregnenolone.**

Cortisol

Cortisol, by far the most important anti-stress hormone in the body, is produced in the adrenal cortex. It has a critical role in helping the body handle stress, including normalizing blood sugar levels and making sure the body has adequate energy to deal with the demands of stress. Cortisol also is a player in the body's powerful anti-inflammatory response, and it is a strong anti-inflammatory agent itself. (See Chapter 2, *Stress, Hormonal Basics and the "Forgotten" Adrenals,* for a detailed discussion of cortisol.)

Conventional physicians have been using cortisol, also known as *hydrocortisone*, to combat Addison's disease for decades. The drug is widely available under the trade name Cortef®. Some clinicians have advocated using cortisol to treat Adrenal Fatigue Syndrome as well. However, advances in nutritional therapeutics over the years have greatly reduced the need to use this medication in all but the most serious cases of AFS. We believe overuse of cortisol as an Adrenal Fatigue Syndrome recovery tool is a serious concern. On the other hand, cortisol can be a lifesaver for someone with severe adrenal weakness.

Prescribe with Care

Symptoms of intolerance are common in the more advanced cases of Adrenal Fatigue Syndrome. In other words, a good portion of people suffering from advanced Adrenal Fatigue Syndrome can't tolerate corticosteroid such as hydrocortisone. Their condition often becomes worse, even at low dosages. The exact pathophysiology is not known. Those who are severely decompensated are particularly vulnerable.

Adrenal crashes may be triggered. Some patients require a few weeks to get used to the medication, and the beneficial effects may not be immediately evident. Still worse, we might have to deal with addiction and withdrawal symptoms. Anyone who has gone through that problem will tell you that most of the time the road is anything but smooth.

Fortunately, in most AFS cases, cortisol is unnecessary and is best considered a last resort. One of the key goals in AFS recovery is letting the body heal itself naturally. For those who have been on cortisol a long time, we support weaning off from it very slowly to break the dependency.

When cortisol is used, most patients find the following dosages effective:

- 5 to 10 mg in the morning
- Zero to 7 1/2 mg at noon
- Zero to 2 1/2 mg at 4 PM

This is a sample, and the actual dosage used by an individual must be adjusted to match the body's need. Some individuals do well on a morning dosage only, while others require an additional one to two doses each day. This should not be a long term recovery tool. If possible, those on cortisol should slowly decrease their dosage after a few months and eventually discontinue the treatment entirely. To avoid withdrawal side effects and adrenal crashes, we recommend first rebuilding adrenal reserves with natural compounds before titrating down cortisol dosage.

Many side effects of cortisol are possible and measures can be taken to counter them. For example:

- Shakiness can occur if the dose is too high, so lowering the dose is the solution.

- If patients experience an upset stomach, then they should take this steroid with meals. They can also lower the dose.

- If taken too late in the day, it can disrupt sleep.

- At a dose of over 20-30 mg a day, more toxic side effects of cortisol may start to appear. We don't recommend higher doses unless the benefits do clearly outweigh the risks.

For some, even proper cortisol replacement is inadequate or does not work. Remember that cortisol breaks the positive feedback loop between norepinephrine and CRH in the brain. If too little cortisol replacement is used, this effect will not be seen. On the other extreme, excessive cortisol can blunt adrenal cortex activity, leading to a reduced output of pregnenolone, DHEA, progesterone, testosterone, estrogen, and aldosterone. If this loss is large enough, calming signals from these hormones may be compromised. Norepinephrine and other anti-inflammatory responses may be dulled as well, leading to the opposite intended effect of cortisol treatment. This may explain why acceptance to cortisol therapy is not universally positive. In fact, some individuals feel worse while on the medication, reporting such things as increased brain fog, anxiety, and fatigue. At the same time, the autonomic nervous system (ANS) may put out more norepinephrine and epinephrine as a last ditch compensatory response, which contributes to a state of feeling wired-and-tired.

Cortisol mono-therapy (using cortisol alone) also does not work when AFS is accompanied by low blood pressure and electrolyte imbalance.

When Cortisol and Aldosterone Are Both Low

Cortisol and aldosterone can both become low, which usually happens in those who are already in Stage 3C and well on the way to Stage 3D, if not already there. Recall that aldosterone regulation is part of the renin-aldosterone hormonal axis system (RAS). In advanced AFS, low aldosterone can be the result of renin dysregulation, secondary to ANS imbalances, or as an independent event. Needless to say, the situation is dire. Extreme fatigue, low blood pressure, inability to stand for prolonged periods, orthostatic hypotension, and orthostatic tachycardia are the main clinical signs. In such cases, we consider the adrenal hormone, *fludrocortisones* (sold under the brand name Florinef® and available by prescription). This can be lifesaving because of its crucial salt regulation properties.

Florinef, also called 9α-fluorocortisol, is a synthetic corticosteroid with moderate glucocorticoid potency and much greater mineralocorticoid potency. It has been used in the treatment of cerebral salt wasting (extreme dehydration and low salt levels in the blood), where aldosterone levels need improvement. It is therefore commonly used in Addison's disease, the classic salt wasting (21-hydroxylase deficiency, an inherited disorder that affects the adrenal glands) form of congenital adrenal hyperplasia (a congenital condition in which the adrenals lack a necessary enzyme), and orthostatic intolerance. Side effects of this drug are extensive. They include edema, hypertension, headache, anxiety, hypokalemia (low potassium levels in the blood), worsening fatigue (especially at the start), increased sweating, hirsutism, peptic ulcer, insomnia, dyspepsia (generalized digestive problems), depression, and many more. Despite all the negatives, this is an important drug for those who have nowhere else to turn. This is truly a drug of last resort.

Unfortunately, many cannot tolerate Florinef, and a very slow and gradual build up is needed in the beginning. This is especially true for those who are very sensitive and constitutionally weak. The temptation is to rush into this drug too quickly, especially for those who are impatient and desperate to get well. While we do see good results with some, we must be reminded that some get worse because this drug can trigger further adrenal crashes. Close medical supervision is mandatory.

If blood pressure is pathologically low, we can consider adding anti-hypotensive agents such as midodrine hydrocholoride (sold under brand names Proamantine® or Midodrine®). Side effects of Midodrine include high blood pressure, itching, numbness, and the feeling of writing on your skin or scalp. They tend to be transient. Both drugs are usually taken along with salt tablets or extra sea salt in the diet. Licorice also might help, but we use it with extreme caution for AFS because of its potential stimulating properties.

> **Dosage Considerations:** Florinef is available in 0.1 mg tablets. Typical daily doses for mineralocorticoid replacement are between 0.05 mg-0.2 mg. Start with half a pill in the morning for one week or two, and then go up to one pill in the morning if no side effects occur. Renin plasma, sodium, and potassium levels are checked through blood tests in order to verify that the correct dosage is reached. Midodrine comes in 5 mg pills. Starting dosage is one pill in the morning and one pill in the afternoon. Up to two pills three times a day may be needed.

Testosterone Replacement Therapy (TRT)

Testosterone is produced by both men and women, however, the amount women produce is much smaller and is produced in the adrenal glands. In both sexes, a decline in testosterone levels is associated with a decrease in sex drive and libido, symptoms many patients with AFS report.

In healthy people, testosterone replacement therapy (TRT) reenergizes the entire body, increases lean muscle mass, and reverses fat accumulation and muscular atrophy, which are normal manifestations of aging. Unfortunately, in AFS patients, TRT is not so simple. It does not work all the time, and aggressive use of testosterone can worsen AFS.

Testosterone helps to reduce norepinephrine and increase dopamine signaling in the brain. It also helps to reduce pro-inflammatory signaling. These are potentially good attributes. However, testosterone also suppresses ACTH and directly inhibits adrenal cortex activity. The net effect depends on the sum of all signaling interactions and that is hard to predict with any accuracy.

Low dose testosterone can be helpful in women. Men, on the other hand, require normal dose replacement if TRT is used at all. Low dose testosterone does not help men since it actually can suppress endogenous testosterone production, leading to increased fatigue. This is one reason why certain healthy men, even if hypogonadal (deficiencies in secondary sex characteristics) with low libido, cannot tolerate TRT. Those with advanced AFS are particularly susceptible to this type of unintended consequence. This is why we recommend optimizing the rest of the body's systems before considering TRT in AFS for both sexes. Pre-TRT workups should include a complete history and physical examination, together with a battery of blood tests including a male hormonal profile. In addition, we recommend cancer screening tests such as prostate specific antigen (PSA). These tests are necessary to rule out contraindications to TRT.

Testosterone replacement can have undesirable side effects, including frequent or persistent erections, nausea, vomiting, jaundice, and ankle swelling. Men may also develop breast enlargement because testosterone can be converted to estrogen by way of an enzyme known as aromatase. More serious complications include water retention, liver toxicity, cardiovascular disease, sleep apnea, and prostate enlargement.

Alternatives to testosterone include testosterone precursors, androstenedione and androstenediol. These are available in oral capsules or sublingual sprays.

Dosage Considerations: While testosterone replacement is one of the most effective ways to boost energy, this hormone should not be used in people with normal testosterone levels. In addition, testosterone replacement is seldom necessary in the treatment of Adrenal Fatigue Syndrome; many more gentle nutrients are available that do not expose the body to this strong androgen.

Estrogen and Progesterone

Reducing estrogen overload is an important clinical goal in recovering from advanced Adrenal Fatigue Syndrome. Direct application of natural progesterone is one way we can balance estrogen and progesterone. This also indirectly supports the adrenals by making more progesterone available as the precursor of cortisol production. Both go hand in hand. In addition, natural progesterone itself has a relaxing, calming, and sleep supporting effect which will further help to restore the stressed adrenals.

Conventional physicians sometimes prescribe *synthetic* progesterone (progestin) to combat estrogen dominance. This form is not the same as natural progesterone.

Progestin is chemically *similar* to natural progesterone, but because it is molecularly different, its physiological actions are very different. Our bodies cannot convert progestin into cortisol to help the adrenals, or convert it to other hormonal compounds. However, *bio-identical* progesterone has this capability. In those suffering from advanced AFS, progestin can be highly toxic and hard to break down, which leads to a buildup of unwanted metabolites in the body. Therefore, the easiest way to restore balance to estrogen dominance is with *natural* progesterone.

Many delivery systems are available, but for most women, the low dose topical form is the most inexpensive and works well. The right time and dosage are keys to successful use, especially in the presence of AFS. Wrong dosage or timing can worsen AFS and could trigger adrenal crashes. Those in a low clearance state, characteristic of Adrenal Exhaustion, must be especially careful to correctly use progesterone, and in these cases even normal physiological doses may be too much for the body to handle.

There is great temptation to overcome estrogen dominance prematurely, especially if the clinical symptoms are severe. However, we believe it's best to any extent possible to heal the adrenals first and delay using natural progesterone until the body becomes ready. Many women can't tolerate progesterone if their adrenals are weak, because it taxes the liver, which metabolizes progesterone. As the body becomes stronger it is better able to tolerate natural progesterone.

Some controversy exists about the best delivery form of progesterone. Most physicians tend to favor the oral form (Prometrium), which is a prescription medication. A higher dose of the oral form is required, as compared to the cream form. This is the case because the oral form is assimilated in the gut and passes through the liver prior to being distributed to the rest of the body. This places an extra burden on the liver because it is the clearance center for this hormone. Since most with AFS are stressed and in a low clearance state to begin with, an overload of oral progesterone may trigger adrenal crashes because the liver is overwhelmed. However, this occurs subclinically, and liver function test results are usually normal.

Blood levels of progesterone tend to be short-lived, so women might need to split the total daily dose into two doses to achieve a more even or stable blood level throughout the twenty-four hour day. In short, we do not recommend the oral form of progesterone for those suffering from Adrenal Fatigue Syndrome.

Topical progesterone cream, which comes in a variety of concentrations, is the most common delivery form. For AFS patients the best option is the low dose over-the-counter (OTC) form. You simply need to apply 20mg of topical progesterone cream per day. Progesterone is lipophilic (dissolves in fatty substances) and it likes to stay in a fatty environment, allowing us to modulate the rate of release as follows:

- Application to an area such as the abdomen, which has a thick fatty layer, slows release.

- Application to an area such as the wrist, which has only a thin fatty layer leads to faster release.

Cream tends to be a bit messy, but for most in AFS, it is the best alternative overall, plus it's the least expensive. It's best to rotate the application site to allow the skin to refresh itself. Many OTC brands are available, but they vary greatly in quality.

Topical progesterone cream tends to release slowly over hours, days, or weeks from fatty tissue deposits. If used correctly, you can achieve a steadier blood level of progesterone with the cream than through any other practical method. Women suffering from AFS should be especially careful of compounded high potency progesterone cream, because it can trigger adrenal crashes. Even normal potency cream may sometimes be too much for those suffering from advanced Adrenal Fatigue Syndrome.

Side Effects of Natural Progesterone

Like most hormones, too much progesterone can cause problems. In the case of AFS, in addition to intolerance and sensitivity, too much progesterone is actually counterproductive. Consistently high doses of progesterone over many months eventually cause progesterone receptors to turn off, reducing its effectiveness. Furthermore, high doses may lead to toxic side effects, which can include:

- *An anesthetic effect such as slight sleepiness:* Excess progesterone down-regulates estrogen receptors, and the brain's responses to estrogen are needed for serotonin production. When this happens, simply reduce the dose until the sleepiness goes away.

- *Paradoxical estrogen dominance symptoms:* Some women report these for the first week or two after starting progesterone. After the initial application of progesterone, women who have been deficient in it for a period of years may experience some water retention, headaches, and swollen breasts. These are symptoms of estrogen dominance, but paradoxically they are exhibited in the initial stages of progesterone application as the estrogen receptors are being resensitized by the progesterone and waking up. This usually goes away by itself and is not a sign of toxicity.

- *Edema (water retention):* This is likely to be caused by excess conversion to deoxycortisol, a mineralocorticoid made in the adrenal glands that causes water retention.

- *Candida:* Specifically, *Candida albicans* is a naturally occurring yeast that lives in moist areas of the body, i.e., the intestines and genitourinary tract. It's troublesome when it is out of balance with the other flora and immune system cells in the body. This imbalance can occur for many reasons. Oral contraceptives and antibiotics are often pointed to as culprits. Excess progesterone can inhibit anti-Candida white blood cells, which can lead to bloating and gas.

- *Lowered libido:* Excess progesterone blocks the conversion of testosterone to DHT. This primarily occurs in men.

Applying Progesterone Cream

The best low dose progesterone cream should contain 1.7 percent of progesterone and yield 20 mg of progesterone per application. The simplest application method is a metered pump that measures the exact daily physiological amount (20 mg) each time the pump is pressed. Progesterone is best absorbed where the skin is relatively thin and well supplied with capillary blood flow, such as the face, neck, upper chest, and inner arms.

For maximum absorption, spread on as big an area as possible and allow as much time as possible for absorption. If you're applying it once a day, bedtime application is likely the most convenient. Twice a day application is actually best, but it may prove troublesome for some. In addition, for either once- or twice-daily application, rotate to different areas of the body to avoid saturation in any one particular site.

Here is a sample rotational application protocol for twice a day application:

- Day 1 morning: Apply to the right side of the back of the neck.
- Day 1 before bed: Apply to the left side of the back of the neck.
- Day 2 morning: Apply to the right wrist area, with palm facing up.
- Day 2 before bed: Apply to the left wrist area, with palm facing up.

- Day 3 morning: Apply to the underside of the right upper arm.
- Day 3 before bed: Apply to the underside of the left upper arm.

Repeat this cycle from day 4 onwards. In other words, day 4 will be the same as day 1, and day 5 will be the same as day 2, and so forth.

Practically speaking, the best gauge for the ideal dose should not be determined by laboratory tests alone. When figuring out the ideal dose, symptom relief is the best gauge. In other words, *the right dose is the dose that works.* This is especially critical in Adrenal Fatigue Syndrome.

Always start progesterone only after the adrenal functional reserve is well established. When in doubt, start with a small dose, only under professional guidance, and slowly scale up if deemed beneficial.

The following are *general recommendations* for a topical progesterone cream application schedule based on a normal physiological dose:

- **Women in pre-menopause, still ovulating:**
  Those taking no hormonal supplementation: Count the day the period begins as the first day. Apply 20mg of natural progesterone every day from day 12 to day 26. Those with longer cycles may wish to start from day 10 to day 28. Begin the cream after ovulation, usually occurring 10 to 12 days after your period begins. If bleeding starts before day 26, stop applying the progesterone cream and start counting up to day 12, and start again.

- **Women in perimenopause (still menstruating with menopausal symptoms and/or PMS but not ovulating):**
  Count the day the period begins as the first day. Apply 20 mg of natural progesterone from day 7 to day 27. If your period begins early, stop using progesterone cream while you are bleeding.

- **Women in menopause (not menstruating):**
  For those not on estrogen replacement therapy: Choose a calendar day, such as the first day of the month. Apply 20 mg of natural progesterone daily from day 1 to day 25. Let the body rest for the remainder of the month.

If a woman has not been taking progesterone for a number of years, body fat progesterone is probably low. In this case, double up on the application for the first two months, and return to a normal physiological dose thereafter. Those who are already on hormonal replacement therapy with estrogen should also be on natural progesterone. Dosage varies depending on the given individual.

Using Estrogen for AFS: A Complex Issue

Some physicians advocate using estrogen (synthetic or bio-identical) for AFS. However, they might be misled into thinking estrogen replacement is needed, along with testosterone, because they see an initial increase in energy when hormone replacement drugs are prescribed. Estrogen helps generate energy, motivation, drive, competitiveness, and libido; it is also important for neuron growth and enhances memory. Because of its ability to improve testosterone sensitivity, it is not unusual for physicians to prescribe estrogen and testosterone together.

Estrogen has monoamine oxidase inhibitor (MAO) type properties, meaning it potentially has antidepressant effects. It also enhances serotonin receptivity in the female brain. The result is an increase in the neurotransmitters, serotonin, norepinephrine, and to a smaller extend, dopamine. When serotonin levels are adequate, we see that release of norepinephrine, an excitatory neurotransmitter, is inhibited in the brain. The results: estrogen helps control norepinephrine.

When serotonin cannot be taken up by the receptor site, because the site is deficient in estrogen, one can become irritable, fatigued, and anxious. However, excess estrogen can be pro-inflammatory, which reduces free thyroid hormone. This in turn can lead to a compensatory response of increasing norepinephrine with simultaneous activation of adrenal cortex signals through the HPA axis.

Excessive estrogen can have a destabilizing effect.

Because of this, prolonged estrogen replacement may lead to HPA axis dysregulation. As far as fatigue is concerned, it is not unusual to see those on estrogen replacement (with or without testosterone) do well at first, only to get worse as time goes on. Those with advanced AFS are particularly at risk for this outcome. Estrogen replacement therapy is therefore a complex endeavor with many risks that can lead to bad outcomes.

Fortunately, we find that estrogen replacement is seldom needed for those with AFS. Most are in the opposite state of excessive estrogen, or estrogen dominance, making the primary goal to reduce estrogen, not increase it. We do find, however, that small amounts of estrogen may be needed in those who have clear signs of estrogen deficiency, even though they have symptoms of estrogen dominance. Generally, these are underweight women whose fatigue is worse from day 4-14 of their menstrual cycles. These women should be on the alert for estrogen deficiency.

We aren't sure why this occurs, but it may involve dysfunction in estrogen transport or receptor sites.

Most of the time, normalizing estrogen in AFS means reducing estrogen dominance through the use of natural progesterone. Proper timing is the key. Because estrogen is metabolized by the liver, the majority of those with advanced AFS will concurrently have weak liver function and slow clearance. Aggressively using estrogen before the liver and adrenals are normalized can worsen the condition and trigger adrenal crashes. Once a woman's adrenal function is stabilized, estrogen replacement can be of great relief if it's needed. Like testosterone replacement therapy, prior optimization of the rest of the system is the key to success.

Note: Because estrogen deficiency or dominance can produce similar symptoms, estrogen replacement, whether it is natural or synthetic, needs to proceed with care. For a detailed discussion on the proper use of estrogen, we suggest you read our mini-book *Estrogen Dominance* available separately as part of the Dr.Lam's Adrenal Recovery Series on our website.

Key Points to Remember

- Hormones commonly used for Adrenal Fatigue Syndrome include pregnenolone, DHEA, cortisol, progesterone, and testosterone.

- Premature use of steroidal hormones is a common recovery mistake and can worsen Adrenal Fatigue Syndrome.

- Compared to cortisol, pregnenolone and DHEA are both gentle hormones, but expect side effects in high doses or among those who are sensitive.

- Hydrocortisone is the most common steroid hormone prescribed. It should be considered as a last resort and for a limited amount of time, with an exit strategy well in place. We see potential addiction and withdrawal problems in addition to the many well known side effects at high doses or with prolong use.

- Estrogen and testosterone are normally not needed and have a limited place in AFS recovery.

- Estrogen and progesterone are important tools to balance female hormones, but to avoid taxing the liver and potentially worsening Adrenal Fatigue Syndrome, their use should be delayed until the adrenals are well healed.

Chapter 23

A Healing Diet for Adrenal Fatigue Syndrome

A poor diet, or one that is incompatible with individual needs, is a key and leading cause of Adrenal Fatigue Syndrome. Without a diet that is biochemically and metabolically compatible with the needs of a damaged adrenal gland, it's simply not possible to achieve complete recovery.

> **Note: The dietary guidelines mentioned in this chapter are designed for those in Stage 3 of Adrenal Fatigue Syndrome, a point at which adopting a diet that promotes healing is especially important. However, many of these guidelines would benefit others in earlier stages of AFS, along with individuals who would like to build their health and *prevent* AFS.**

Glucose/Sugar

Glucose is a simple sugar found in food. It is an essential nutrient that provides energy for the proper functioning of the body's cells. After meals, food is digested in the stomach and is broken down into glucose and other nutrients. The glucose is absorbed by the intestinal cells and carried by the bloodstream to cells throughout the body. However, glucose cannot enter the cells alone. It needs assistance from insulin in order to penetrate the cell walls. Insulin therefore acts as a regulator of glucose transport and metabolism in the body.

The Hunger Hormone

Insulin is also referred to as the *hunger hormone*. As the blood sugar level increases after a meal, the corresponding insulin level rises. For energy, glucose is transported from the blood into the cell. As energy is produced by the cell, the blood glucose level is slowly lowered, and the insulin released from the pancreas is turned off. As energy continues to be generated, the blood sugar level continues to drop. When blood sugar drops below a certain level, we feel hunger, which often develops a few hours after a meal. This drop in blood sugar triggers the adrenals to make more cortisol. The cortisol increases the blood sugar by converting protein and fat into its component parts. With this, the blood sugar rises to provide a continuous supply of energy to use between meals. Cortisol, therefore, works hand-in-hand with insulin to provide a steady blood sugar level twenty-four hours a day and keeps blood glucose levels in a tightly controlled range.

Carbohydrates, Proteins, and Fats

For Adrenal Fatigue Syndrome sufferers, it's especially important to balance the macronutrients: protein, fat, and carbohydrates. Those with AFS have an immediate need for sugar (glucose) when hunger strikes. However, to have sustained energy until the next mealtime they also need good protein as well as good fat. Therefore, the snack choice should resemble the components of regular meals.

Eating Schedule

It's important for those with AFS to commit to a program of regular meals. Hunger is a complicated issue, and no two people have the same sensations that signal when it's the right time to eat or abstain. For example, some of us have no appetite when our cortisol levels peak from 6:00-8:00 AM, and we may skip breakfast because we're not hungry. However, our bodies need fuel (glucose) to run on, the body's energy requirements don't change during this period of early morning. Even a small snack is better than nothing at all and will provide needed energy, even if you have no urge to eat.

If your blood sugar is low, the body instructs the adrenals to secrete cortisol because it activates *gluconeogenesis* (the synthesis of glucose from non-carbohydrate molecules, i.e., amino acids or fatty acids) to increase blood sugar levels, thereby allowing the body to function. This is why it's important to eat a healthy breakfast soon after waking and not later than 10:00 AM. An adequate breakfast prevents the body from having to play catch-up for the rest of the day.

> Ideally, you'll eat lunch between 12:15 and 12:45 PM. Sometimes we need a nutritious snack between 2:30 and 3:00 PM in order to sustain our bodies through the dip in cortisol levels that occurs between 3:00 and 4:00 PM. Then, the evening meal follows, ideally between 6:00 and 7:00 PM. In other words, every 3-4 hours, you should eat something healthy that includes some fat and protein.

All meals, which needn't be large, are best planned using low-glycemic index foods. (See Appendix B for a complete list.) It is important to avoid consuming high-glycemic index foods such as refined flour and high-sugar baked goods, fruit, and other desserts, especially by themselves. These sugary, high-carbohydrate snacks cause the blood sugar to rise, triggering a corresponding increase in insulin output. Then, over time, insulin secretion becomes dysfunctional, resulting in a hypo-glycemic state during the day and in the middle of the night, which manifests in symptoms such as anxiety, jitteriness, dizziness, nightmares, and night sweats. When this occurs, the body must activate the adrenals to put out more cortisol in order to raise the blood sugar back to its normal level. If this situation continues year after year, we eventually put an excessive burden onto the already fatigued adrenal gland.

The Primary Adrenal Fatigue Syndrome Diet

The primary diet for AFS is designed for those in Stage 3. However, as you can see, some of the guidelines are beneficial for most people, including those with sensitive blood sugar issues, allergies, or those who would like to adopt an anti-aging diet.

For optimal AFS recovery, design your diet to be high in raw food and low on the glycemic index (GI). Consider the following guidelines:

- Start each morning with a full glass of water and half a teaspoon to one teaspoon of sea salt as tolerated.

- Provided blood pressure is normal, sprinkle sea salt liberally on food to taste. (Foods high in potassium, such as bananas and dried figs, raisins, and dates can make the adrenals worse, so those in Stage 3 should avoid them.)

- Eat frequently—five to six small meals instead of three large ones, which means eating every 3-4 hours.

- Avoid fruit juices of all kinds.

- Avoid eating whole fruits alone, especially melons, which are high on the glycemic index, because sugar spikes soon after ingestion. It is best to eat fruits before a meal or that contain some protein.

- *Include in moderation:* organically grown fruits such as papayas, mangos, apples, grapes, berries, and cherries.

- Choose good quality protein from meat, fish, poultry, and eggs; these foods provide a steady source of energy between meals.

- Combine generous protein and fat at every meal and snack to maintain your energy supplies.

- If you have difficulty falling asleep, eat some protein and fat, such as nuts, turkey, chicken or eggs before retiring.

- If you tend to wake up in the middle of the night, eat a small healthy snack high in protein and fat, such as cottage cheese or nuts before going back to sleep.

- Avoid foods that stimulate the body, such as caffeinated coffee, caffeinated soft drinks, green tea and regular tea.

- Avoid foods that may increase inflammation in the body, such as wheat and dairy.

- If you have OAT axis imbalance, avoid foods that can cause hormonal imbalance such as unfermented soy like tofu and cruciferous vegetables.

- Avoid foods that stress the liver, such as alcohol.

- Avoid foods that cause more stress on the body, such as fried foods, refined foods, and highly processed foods.

- If you can find it, use raw (non-pasteurized) dairy. It's very nutritious. This is an exception to the guideline above that advises avoiding dairy. Further, goat milk is better than cow's milk for human consumption. Otherwise, avoid dairy as much as possible. The protein casein and the fats found in milk are chemically changed during the high heat of pasteurization, which creates more stress and promotes inflammation.

- Drink two cups of chicken broth (discussed next chapter) daily to help prevent the body from further breakdown of collagen and muscle—the body itself. Chicken broth provides gentle nutrients, easily absorbed by the catabolic body, thereby preventing further breakdown of collagen and muscle.

- To help the body clear the toxins, it is important to drink 8-10 cups of water daily. Add lemon slices or a splash of lemon juice to drinking water to gently improve liver function.

- Avoid fruits in the morning to prevent overloading the body with potassium and sugar.

If You Have Digestive Concerns

Those with digestive issues should take digestive enzymes and probiotics before each meal. In addition, it's also important to select the proper food combination at each meal to prevent bloating and gas. Correct food combinations help to improve digestion, meaning the use and assimilation of the nutrients in the diet. Here are some guidelines:

- Avoid eating fruits and vegetables in the same meal.

- Avoid eating starch and protein in the same meal.

- Vegetables and meat, or, vegetables and starch, can be eaten in the same meal.

- Many AFS sufferers have a lower level of hydrochloric acid (HCI), which is necessary to break down proteins. Symptoms of low-HCI include gas, bloating, and heaviness in the stomach after eating a meal containing protein. In such case, it's beneficial to take digestive enzymes, probiotics (acidophilus and other intestinal flora), as well as taking HCl replacements.

- If you feel worse after consuming certain foods, realize that this is the body's way of telling you that you are on the wrong track.

If You Have Acid Reflux

- Do not drink liquid during your meal. It's best to drink liquid between meals.

- Eat small meals—this guideline is especially important for those with acid reflux.

- Take digestive enzymes and hydrochloric acid before meals.

- Do not lay flat immediately after a meal.

- Take probiotics.

If You Have Food Sensitivities

Keeping a food journal is an effective and important way to identify foods that you are sensitive to. Once you have identified the food, avoid it. As your adrenals become stronger, you likely will find your food sensitivities decreasing. It is best to eat these foods only once every 7 days. For example, if you eat an allergenic food today, then don't eat the same food again for 4-5 days. It takes a food 4-5 days to clear out of your system; some foods take up to 7 days to clear.

A Word to Vegetarians

Vegetarians with AFS face a bigger challenge than others because of the nature of protein. Animal proteins contain complete proteins, meaning they provide *essential amino acids*. To clarify, 20 amino acids form the building blocks of the body's proteins, including muscles, tendons, organs, glands, nails, and hair. Our cells depend on proteins for growth, repair, and maintenance. *Essential* amino acids are so named because they must be obtained from the diet in the form of complete proteins, whereas the body manufactures nonessential amino acids from other sources that provide some but not all amino acids.

The body can produce 10 of the 20 amino acids, and we must supply the others through the food we eat. If we're missing the amino acids we can't produce, the body's proteins, such as muscle, begins to degrade. The body stores fat and starch, but it doesn't store excess amino acids, which is why the body demands protein every day.

Vegetarians have a challenge to obtain the *complete* proteins (containing all the essential fatty acids). The first step involves becoming educated about *food combining*. Animal protein, i.e., meat, dairy, eggs, poultry, and fish are complete proteins because they contain sufficient levels of all essential amino acids. Very few plant sources, one being soybeans, contain all the essential amino acids, which is why vegetarians need to be especially careful to ingest proteins that when combined form a complete protein. Lacto-ovo vegetarians are those who include dairy foods and eggs in their diet, and these foods provide complete proteins. Vegans eat plant foods only.

What is a Complementary Protein?

We derive plant proteins, which provide one or more essential amino acids, from foods such as beans, nuts, seeds, legumes, and soy products. For example, rice contains lysine, but beans tend to be low in that amino acid. However, when ingested together, these two foods make up a complete protein with adequate levels of the essential amino acids. In other words, these proteins complement each other. Vegetarians must plan their meals to make sure that the missing amino acids in one food are provided by another food eaten during the rest of the day.

We do not recommend relying solely on dairy products and eggs for complete proteins. Vegetarians and others should eat whole grains on a 4-5 day rotational basis. In other words, avoid eating the same grains day after day, but instead, vary them through rotation.

You will find complementary proteins in ethnic cuisines—and in some "humble" everyday foods that are staples in the west, including the Southern hemisphere. Traditional Middle Eastern and Asian cuisine also contain complementary proteins. However, few cultures across the globe rely 100 percent on plant foods to meet protein needs. Here are some dishes that contain complementary proteins:

- Beans with corn tortillas
- Tofu* with rice
- Almond butter on wheat/rye bread*
- Hummus with pita bread
- Chickpeas and other beans combined with rice

*Wheat and many soy foods are not recommended for the AFS diet. However, you can add miso or tempeh to your diet. (See Chapter 25, *Food and Chemical Sensitivities*, for more about wheat.)

Soy and OAT Axis Imbalance

If you are a woman with advanced Adrenal Fatigue Syndrome, it's likely you have developed some OAT axis imbalance. Soy acts like estrogen in your body, which adds to issues of estrogen dominance. Soy also affects the *goitrogens* (substances that suppress thyroid function) in the thyroid glands.

> **Ample evidence exists that the isoflavones found in soy products, including genistein, are toxic to the body. For example, isoflavones inhibit thyroid peroxidase, which makes T3 and T4. In other words, these elements of soy products interfere with the production of vital components of the thyroid hormone.**

Unfermented soy products, such as tofu and infant soy formula, contain:

- Allergens
- Enzyme inhibitors
- Hormone modifiers
- Mineral blockers
- Iodine blockers that interfere with thyroid function

Since the late 1950s, researchers have identified soy as a *phytoestrogen*, meaning a plant-based element with an estrogenic effect of about 1/500 the potency of the body's naturally circulating estrogen. Soy acts as a competitive inhibitor of estrogen at the cellular estrogen receptor site, reducing the effect of estrogen in your body. At the same time, over consuming soy can overwhelm many of the body's cells and may overload them.

How much is too much? This varies depending on age. For adults, just 30 mg of soy isoflavones per day is the amount found to have a negative impact on thyroid function. We can easily get 30 mg of soy from just 5-8 ounces of soy milk or 1.5 ounces of miso. Interestingly, while miso has a phytoestrogenic effect, it does not have the enzyme inhibitory effect because it is fermented. Other fermented soy products include soy sauce and tempeh.

What the AFS Diet Looks Like

As a general guideline, your daily diet should include:

- 30-40 percent above-the-ground vegetables (i.e., green leafy vegetables, winter and summer squash, tomatoes, green beans, celery, salad greens, and so forth). Broccoli, cauliflower, and cabbages are included, but we recommend reducing the amounts of these vegetables to no more than twice a week due to their estrogenic properties. About 50 percent of the daily vegetables should be consumed raw if possible provided they are tolerated.

> **Note: Vegetables such as carrots and turnips are root vegetables and grow below the ground. Consuming root vegetables raw is okay, because you can't consume too much of them. It is okay to eat cooked sweet potatoes, turnips, carrots, and beets in smaller quantities, i.e., half a cup a day.**

- 10-20 percent grains

- 10-20 percent beans and legumes.

- 20-30 percent animal foods, i.e., *organic* hormone- and antibiotic-free meats and poultry, such as turkey and chicken, as long as these products. Deep sea, mercury free fish (i.e., wild caught salmon and shrimp and some tuna caught in Canadian and U.S. waters) are allowed, too. Seafood must be purchased carefully because of the continuing issue of mercury and other substances polluting oceans and fresh water and adversely affecting living organisms.

- 20-30 percent good fats, i.e. nuts and seeds, extra virgin olive oil, coconut oil, grape seed oil, rice bran oil, avocado, flax seed, walnut oil. Purchase high quality, cold pressed oils.

- 10-15 percent whole fruits (except banana, fruits in the melon family, and dried fruits) taken with some protein.

> **Note:** You'll notice that the minimum percentages add up to 100 percent. The ranges however, are approximations and will vary day-to-day. Perhaps one day will include slightly more fat than fruit, for example. We recognize that the exact plan varies from person-to-person, and no one-size-fits-all approach exists. We customize dietary plans for those who seek our help in order to match the body's caloric and nutritional requirements according to the body's ability to assimilate. Those who are in advanced AFS, especially those in Stage 3C and 3D, often have poor assimilation and cannot tolerate most of the above general recommendations.

Tilting Toward Raw Foods

About 50-60 percent of the diet should consist of raw food, which means it's important to include 6-8 servings of a wide variety of vegetables each day. Vegetables high in sodium, and therefore recommended for AFS sufferers, include kelp, black olives, red hot peppers, spinach, zucchini, celery, and Swiss chard.

The easiest way to consume these vegetables involves introducing at least three types of different colored vegetables at your meals. For example, toss a salad of green and red leaf lettuce, spinach, red or yellow bell peppers, and celery. Use broccoli, carrot, cauliflower, zucchini, and red and green cabbages and/or bell peppers in other salads or in a vegetable stir fry. Add nutrients to meals with steamed or sautéed kale, Swiss chard, and other green leafy vegetables. You can add extra flavor to salads by adding a variety of chopped herbs such as basil, mint, parsley, cilantro, and green onions.

Multicolored vegetables, including many vegetables listed above, provide antioxidants (which help clear toxins and protect the cell) and phytonutrients (plant-derived nutrients) that benefit the body. These vegetables can be used both cooked and raw, because some phytonutrients deliver health benefits when heated. Still, a spinach salad, for example, has health benefits, too. As good as raw food is, not everyone finds it tolerable. The more advanced the AFS, the less tolerant of raw food one can be.

Seeds and Nuts

These are critical components of the diet and are sources of some amino acids and fatty acids, which the adrenal glands need to manufacture cholesterol, a precursor to all adrenal steroid hormones. Choose fresh raw nuts and seeds that are free of rancid (spoiled) oils.

Note: Rancid oils create and/or worsen symptoms of AFS, so avoid at all cost. Rancid oils, rancid nuts and seeds smell "off." We recommend storing nuts and seeds in the refrigerator or freezer.

> With the exception of peanuts, liberally include raw nuts in your diet. Excellent choices include: almonds, cashews, Brazil nuts, pecans, walnuts, hazel nuts, macadamia, chestnuts, pumpkin seeds, pine nuts, and so forth. Soak brown colored nuts at least 12 hours before eating; soak brown colored seeds 2-4 hours before eating. Soaking helps improve absorption by removing an enzyme inhibitor in the brown coating. Avoid peanuts because of the potential for allergic reaction among some people; in addition, peanuts may be contaminated with the mold aflatoxin.

Everyday Fats and Oils

The following tips are useful as you plan your meals:

- Use olive, avocado, flax seed, or walnut oil—cold pressed—for salad dressings, but not for high heat cooking. When heated, the chemical structure of beneficial oils changes and at higher temperatures will transform into trans-fats, which cause oxidative stress in the body.

- When cooking with these oils, in a stir fry, for example, use enough water to stir fry and steam the vegetables. Then add one of the above oils and seasoning after the vegetables are done cooking and you've turned off the stove burner. If you want to sauté or stir fry with oil, use grape seed or rice bran oil, which have higher boiling points.

- Butter improves the flavor of some foods—don't be afraid to use it.

- Use coconut oil and olive oil in protein smoothies to improve the number on the GI (glycemic index).

Sugar

We recommend avoiding foods high in sugar in order to avoid imbalances in blood sugar, which can lead to hypoglycemic reactions, discussed earlier in this book. Avoiding high sugar content foods also gives you evenly balanced energy levels throughout the day. Sugar is both an *overt* and *hidden* food. Avoid fruit juices, soda, and alcoholic drinks. Also, avoid ice cream and pastries, candy and cake—and on and on—foods that are obvious sources of sugar. These sweet foods are also called empty calories because they are high in calories, but low in nutrients. Hidden sources of sugar include many commercial salad dressings and sauces, including popular pasta and tomato sauces.

Decreasing sugar intake helps to improve the immune system, which in turn, helps the adrenal recovery, and reducing or eliminating the empty calories of sugar will help weight loss efforts.

Breakfast Ideas

It's true! Breakfast really is the most important meal of the day. It provides the necessary nutrients to start the day after the body has been in a fast during the night. This first meal of the day should include some protein and fats, along with some carbohydrates. Here are some suggestions:

- We agree with the old adage, *an apple a day keeps the doctor away*, so spread some almond or cashew butter (but not peanut butter) on apple slices. Or, eat an apple with a handful of nuts. Cut up fruits or berries into a bowl of wheat-free or gluten-free granola or wheat-free, whole-grain cereal, and then add whole milk yogurt.

- Be creative and make a delicious protein shake with protein powder (rice or whey, but not soy), raw hormone-free organic eggs, avocado, coconut oil, berries, and other fruits.

- Many individuals believe that consuming raw eggs is dangerous because of potential contamination with salmonella, a serious food borne bacterium. However, raw eggs are safe because salmonella exists in the eggshell, not inside the egg. If you carefully wash eggs before storing them, they are safe to use raw. Raw egg contains the best source of protein as well as un-oxidized cholesterol. It is truly one of nature's best gifts to AFS sufferers.

- You can also include soft boiled eggs and add a steamed or baked sweet potato.
- Cooked oatmeal with added ground nuts, berries or other fresh fruit, and coconut flakes is a good breakfast on a cold day.

Sample Food Plan, based on 2000 calories a day

Whole grains 10% = 200 calories = 1 slice of Ezekiel Sprouted Wheat bread, 1/2 cup of brown rice, and 1/4 cup of oatmeal, for example.

Vegetables 10% = 200 calories = 3 cups salad, 2 cups green leafy vegetables, and 2 cups mixed vegetables.

Root vegetables or starchy vegetables 10% = 200 calories = 1 cup winter squash, 1 sweet potato, 1 carrot, and potatoes in *small* quantities, such as homemade hash-brown potatoes, fingerling, or purple potatoes. Do not eat deep fried commercial and restaurant french fries or hash browns. The fats in these foods are unhealthy.

Beans or legumes 10% = 200 calories = half to one cup beans and legumes, such as black beans or lentils.

Nuts, seeds 15% = 300 calories = 1 oz nuts and seeds and 1 tbsp nut butter, for example.

Fat 15% = 300 calories = 1 tablespoon of olive oil, 0.5 tablespoon of coconut oil, and 0.5 tablespoon of butter.

Animal proteins 20% = 400 calories = 5 oz meat, chicken, fish, or eggs.

Whole fruits 10% = 200 calories = 2.5 medium whole fruits such as apple.

Adrenal Diet Do's and Don'ts

The following table summarizes and clarifies the dietary guidelines and the reasons for them.

Adrenal Fatigue Syndrome Diet
by Michael Lam, MD, MPH, and Dorine Lam, RD, MS, MPH

Goals

1) Eat before 10:00 AM.

2) Eat frequent, small meals: breakfast 6-8 AM, lunch 12-1 PM, dinner 6-7 PM, snacks 10 AM, 3 PM, and bedtime.

3) Eat 10-20% whole grains, 30-40% vegetables (50% should be raw), 10-20% beans and legumes, 20-30% animal foods, 10-15% fruit, 20-30% good fats, nuts and seeds.

Avoid

Banana, dried figs, raisins, dates, oranges, grapefruit	High in potassium - makes Adrenal Fatigue Syndrome worse
Fruit and juice in the morning	Raise and drop blood sugar fast
Refined flour products: pasta, white rice, bread, pastry, baked goods	Drops blood sugar fast, robbed of nutrients; wheat may cause inflammation in the body
Honey, sugar, syrups, soft drinks	Drops blood sugar too fast within one hour
Coffee, tea, black tea, hot chocolate, alcohol, colas, chocolates	Caffeine stimulates the body; alcohol causes liver congestion
Avoid foods you are addicted to or allergic or sensitive to	Cause additional stress on your body

Avoid rushed and hectic meals	Creates more stress for your body
Avoid deep-frying and browning; hydrogenated oils	Trans fats increase inflammation in the body
Most Beneficial	
Eat before 10 AM.	Replenishes waning glycogen supply
Eat frequent small meals Keep blood sugar and insulin balanced	Coast through low energy periods
Bedtime snack (use soaked raw nuts)	Helps to have more peaceful sleep
Combine fat, protein, and whole grains at every meal and snack	Provides a steady source of energy over a longer period of time
Mix 1-2 Tbsp. essential oils into grains, vegetables, and meats daily	Essential oils help reduce inflammation and help maintain satiety
Good quality protein (meat, fish, fowl, eggs, dairy, and legumes)	Provides good protein and fats
Take digestive enzymes and HCL with meals	Helps to properly break down protein and high fiber foods in the stomach
Eat 6-8 servings of a wide variety of brightly colored vegetables	Vegetables are low in calories; you will not gain weight; provides vitamins, minerals, phytochemicals, antioxidants which are crucial for optimal health

Sprouts	High quality concentrated nutrients
Sea vegetables	Rich in trace minerals, good quality vegetable protein, easily digested
Monounsaturated fats	Used for low heat cooking; put a little water in the pan before the oil to keep the oil from getting too hot
Fresh and raw nuts and seeds (soaked in water) - store in freezer	Good source of essential fatty acids
Acceptable - Use in Moderation	
Whole unrefined grains (exclude wheat)	Provides sustained energy and nutrients Caution: Take it easy as a breakfast food. Some people may need to avoid grains for breakfast.
Limited intake of fruits	Maintain blood sugar and insulin balance
Polyunsaturated fats (corn, safflower, sunflower, peanut oil)	Never cook with these oils, add after the food is cooked. Provides essential fatty acids

Plan Meals Using the Glycemic Index

The glycemic index (GI) provides a measure of the blood-sugar stress individual foods create. Controlling blood sugar is one key pillar in creating a successful diet for Adrenal Fatigue Syndrome, diabetes, hypoglycemia, and anti-aging. Elevated blood sugar is a direct reflection of high-sugar intake, so the ability of identifying low-sugar foods is important.

Eating low GI foods promotes an even flow of glucose into the blood. If you happen to eat a high GI food, such as puffed rice, we recommend adding a low glycemic index food such as nuts or whole milk yogurt. Doing so produces a balance between the high and low GI foods.

In Appendix B, you'll see a table of the glycemic index number for some common foods. These numbers use glucose as a baseline, using 100 as the value; all other values are relative to glucose.

To reduce blood sugar stress, focus on foods with *an index at or below 70.* Those with hypoglycemia type symptoms should focus on food with an index at or below 60. As indicated, always balance a higher GI food with a lower GI value food. You'll notice that meats, poultry, fish, eggs, seeds, and nuts are protein- and fat-containing foods and are automatically low GI foods.

Table Salt vs. Sea Salt

We recommend using sea salt because it contains additional trace minerals. Iodized table salt contains many additives that tax the body. Vegetable juice diluted with water and sprinkled with sea salt and kelp powder is a good fluid cocktail for AFS sufferers. Kelp contains about 90 mg of potassium and over 200 mg of sodium per serving and is easily absorbed.

Key Points to Remember

- A poor diet is a key leading cause of Adrenal Fatigue Syndrome and a trigger of adrenal crashes.

- Those in Stage 3 AFS must follow strict dietary guidelines; however, those with milder forms or those wishing to prevent Adrenal Fatigue Syndrome will do well by following the same dietary plan.

- All meals should be moderate in size and best planned using low-glycemic index foods.

- Frequent meals are needed for those prone to hypoglycemia.

- Simple sugar should be avoided, and moderate carbohydrates should be part of the meal plan that is balanced to offer quick energy.

- Avoid food high in caffeine and potassium.

- Soy should be consumed in moderation at best, due to its effect on the thyroid and ovaries.

- Adequate protein and good fats are necessary. Daily diet should include 30-40 percent above-the-ground vegetables, 10-20 percent whole grains, 10-15 percent whole fruits, 10-20 percent beans and legumes, 20-30 percent good fats, nuts, and seeds, and 20-30 percent animal foods.

  Again, the minimum numbers add up to 100 percent, but the range represents varying diets day-to-day.

Chapter 24

Soups and Juicing for Health

Your mother is right. Soups are an excellent source of nutrients when you come down with flu or a cold. Chicken soup, for example, has been used for centuries to deliver nutrients during illnesses, and for good reasons. During flu and other illnesses, the body automatically slows down the digestion process in order to conserve energy to fight unwanted bacteria. Those with advanced Adrenal Fatigue Syndrome face similar problems—and worse. Instead of lasting a few days as a normal flu would, poor assimilation can go on for years and decades. This is compounded if you have food allergies and sensitivities. Soups offer a gentle and nurturing way to restore adrenal health, especially when other modes may not be well tolerated. Those with Stage 3C and beyond may find soups lifesaving, sparing the AFS sufferer an admission to the hospital for TPN (total parenteral nutrition).

We also offer guidelines for vegetable juicing, which is beneficial for many patients. However, the benefits of both the easy-to-make soups and juicing are not limited to those with AFS, but are part of any sound prevention program and anti-aging effort. In other words, these soups and juicing are good for the whole family.

Chicken Broth Recipes

Homemade chicken broth provides vital basic and foundational macronutrients sorely needed in advanced AFS recovery. We consider it an important part of our complete program that includes diet and lifestyle changes, along with carefully selected micronutrients, such as vitamins. Chicken bone and its marrow provide key nutrients, easily assimilated by the GI tract, and thus made bioavailable to the cells when delivered in a liquid form like broth. We recommend making the chicken broth fresh every morning so it's ready to be consumed from mid-day onwards for the rest of the day.

Below are three recipes that are easy to follow and produce excellent broth.

> **Note: Do not substitute these ingredients with commercial off-the-shelf products, because many contain MSG and are too diluted to have any significant clinical impact.**

Each cup (8 fl oz) of our homemade chicken broth provides:
- 20 calories;
- 1 gram carbohydrates;
- 3 grams protein;
- 0.5 grams of fat; 0 grams of saturated fat; 0 grams of cholesterol.

The nutritional value goes far beyond what meets the eye; it rests with the bone marrow. Bone marrow is the essence of all mammals and contains all of the necessary nutrients for the human body, such as proteins, vitamins, B complex, and minerals (calcium, magnesium, zinc). Bone marrow also contains *lecithin* (a fatty substance occurring widely in animal and plant foods and a building block for other chemicals in the body) and *methionine* (an essential amino acid). It has been used as a whole food source since early civilization. Studies show it helps maintain healthy cholesterol levels, reduces inflammation, and promotes a strong immune system that is tied to the adrenal glands.

As we've said, most individuals suffering from Adrenal Fatigue Syndrome have salt cravings as well as fluid depletion. Drinking chicken broth helps restore fluid volume, and adding salt to chicken broth is an excellent way to replenish sodium in the body. We place no restriction on the amount of added salt, provided no signs of edema or high blood pressure are present and if your private physician approves.

Those who have a tendency to urinate in the middle of the night should restrict fluid intake in the evening to avoid excessive fluid buildup and urine retention in the bladder, which then leads to nighttime urination.

Our recommendation is to drink one cup (8 oz.) chicken broth twice a day, preferably midmorning and mid-afternoon, times that the body often runs out of steam. At these times, chicken broth can recharge the body. If you can only drink the broth once a day, then have it at the time of your worst low-point of energy. Three common lowest energy times are midmorning, mid afternoon, or immediately after work. You can also add a cup of chicken broth after exercising.

For those recovering from AFS, we recommend doing adrenal exercises (See Chapter 27, *Adrenal Fatigue Syndrome and Healing Exercise*) midmorning followed by a cup of chicken broth and a small healthy snack.

Some individuals with severe AFS need a more aggressive nourishment protocol. These individuals should have a cup of chicken broth five times a day, preferably:

- in the morning right after waking up (using the leftover broth from the previous day is acceptable as a matter of practicality)

- freshly prepared chicken broth at midmorning

- with lunch

- early afternoon (two hours after lunch)

- late afternoon (4-5 PM)

Again, for maximum effectiveness, before you drink the broth do short sessions of Adrenal Breathing Exercises (8-24 breaths lasting 1-3 minutes), designed to help stimulate the parasympathetic nervous system and thus prepare the GI track for optimum assimilation of nutrients into the bloodstream.

If desired, you can add some raw nuts along with the broth as a snack. The protein and fat from the nuts enhance sustained energy release; the salted broth will generate an immediate energy boost. In addition, you can take your adrenal supplements at the same time as the broth.

For maximum benefit, follow these guidelines:

- Make the broth fresh daily in the morning, rotating the three recipes, thus making a different recipe each day.

- Drink the broth warm to hot as tolerated, one cup each time.

- Reheat on your stove top, not in a microwave.

- Each recipe makes 3-5 cups, but the longer you boil it, the less liquid remains.

- You can have 2-6 ounces of the chicken meat before bedtime, along with some nuts, to combat sleep onset or sleep maintenance insomnia. (See Chapter 26, *Adrenal Fatigue Syndrome and Healing Sleep.*)

Remove the skin and fat from the chicken before making the broth; if some oil remains after boiling, skim it off with a spoon or a shredded paper towel.

Note: As you will see, the recipes and instructions are essentially identical except for the vegetable choices in each.

Chicken Broth Recipe 1

1/2 chicken, skin and fat removed. Use all the bone. The breast meat can be saved for other uses, but use the bones for the broth.

1 medium onion, chopped

2-3 stalks of celery cut in 3-inch segments

1 medium carrot chopped

Add enough water to cover the chicken and vegetables, plus three more inches. Bring to a boil, and then decrease heat to medium and cook for 30 minutes. Then reduce heat to medium-low for another 90 minutes.

Carefully remove the chicken to remove the meat from the bones, and then drain the vegetables to make a broth.

Salt to taste before serving.

Chicken Broth Recipe 2

Instead of carrots, use:

1 medium beet root, peeled and chopped

Chicken Broth Recipe 3

Instead of carrots, use:

One 6-10 inch lotus root peeled and chopped

Juicing

Juicing tends to be one of those health recommendations that many people are attracted to, but it seems both expensive and a lot of work. However, we recommend reviving your interest in juicing because of the many benefits listed below.

Three general categories of juices exist: green juices, vegetable juices, and fruit juices. We emphasize green and vegetable juices for those in advanced AFS, and recommend limiting fruit juices to those who are in mild stages of AFS only.

Benefits of Vegetable Juicing

The benefits to vegetable juicing are many if the body can tolerate it. They include:

- Easy to digest and absorb.

- Enzymes, vitamins, minerals, and phytochemicals remain intact and active and in much larger quantities than if the piece of vegetable is eaten whole.

- Flushes out acid wastes and detoxifies the liver to improve clearance of byproducts.
- Improves the immune system.
- Rich in chlorophyll.
- Cleansing, rejuvenating, and energizing.

Note: Do not start juicing on your own without professional supervision if you have advanced AFS. Improper juicing can worsen AFS and trigger adrenal crashes.

Buying and Preparation Tips for Vegetable Juicing:

- Don't buy more than a week's worth of fresh fruits and vegetables, for they may spoil before you use them.
- Buy organic produce if possible.
- Thoroughly wash the produce before juicing. Use a vegetable brush to remove any residue and waxes. (You may also want to use vegetable washes that are found in health food stores.). Let the produce sit in a tub of clean water filled with activated charcoals for 20 minutes. Store the cleaned vegetables in containers to keep the freshness.
- When using potatoes for juicing, avoid those with a green tint. The green coloring is caused by a chemical called solanine. It can cause diarrhea, vomiting, and abdominal pain. Also, remove any sprouts or eyes on them.
- Stems and leaves of most vegetables can be left intact when juicing, except for carrot and rhubarb greens which must be removed.
- To make leafy green vegetable juices (spinach, lettuce, greens, etc.) more palatable, mix them with ½ carrot, 1 slice apple, or ¼ beet root.
- As a general rule, don't mix vegetables and fruits together when juicing.
- Strong tasting vegetables such as broccoli, onions, and rutabaga should be used sparingly.
- Garlic is a wonderful, immune building addition to your juices. Before juicing your garlic, it must be immersed in vinegar for one minute to destroy any bacteria and mold on the surface. Those with a sensitive stomach may need to avoid this.
- Stop the vegetable juicing if you feel more wired or tired.

Juicing Machines

The best juicing machine is the cold press. Reputable brands include Green Machine, Omega, or Champion. But for the adrenal recovery process, if budget is a concern, a regular centrifuge type of juicer will serve the purpose.

Quantity

Not everyone can tolerate juicing. We recommend starting slow, with two ounces in the morning on an empty stomach every other day, or as directed. Increase the frequency to daily slowly as tolerated over a few weeks. Increase by one ounce per week until you reach 8 ounces daily. Excessive juicing is not recommended in advanced AFS because of the risk of developing re-toxification or die-off reaction as toxins tend to recirculate in the body.

Good Vegetables for Juicing

Base vegetables for juicing –1 celery stalk, ¼ carrot, 4 lettuce leaves

Add two of the following for variety:

- alfalfa sprouts
- cucumber
- beet greens
- dandelion greens
- parsley
- endive
- spinach
- lettuce (romaine, red leaf, green leaf, etc.)
- cilantro
- wheatgrass
- barley greens
- pumpkin
- sweet potato, potatoes
- bitter melon / bitter gourd
- summer squash

Cruciferous vegetables such as:
- bok choy
- mustard greens

- kale
- cabbage (red, green, napa, etc.)
- watercress
- collard greens
- turnip root and greens
- arugula
- radish, daikon
- broccoli, cauliflower
- kohlrabi
- Brussels sprouts

Note: Those who have estrogen dominance and thyroid issues should avoid cruciferous vegetables.

Preparation Tips for Fruit Juicing

While we generally do not recommend fruit juicing for those with advanced AFS, juicing can be part of a recovery program when AFS is mild or if there are no hypo-glycemic issues. Proper preparation is the key to an effective juicing program. Here are some tips:

- Wash and prepare the fruits as you did the vegetables.

- Fruit juicing should be done in a blender so you also get the benefit of the fibers.

- Remove the skin before juicing apricots, grapefruits, kiwis, oranges, papaya, peaches, and pineapples.

- As a rule, leave small seeds in the fruits, except apple seeds, which contain cyanides. Therefore, remove all apple seeds before juicing.

- Always add a serving of whey protein and a few soaked raw nuts (you don't need to soak cashews or macadamia nuts) to fruit juice. This modulates the effect of the sugar content.

- Add 1-2 cups of water to dilute the thickness of the fruit juice so you can drink it.

- Rotate the fruits used daily—always have 1 berry, and 2 other fruits.

- The best time to have fruit juice is around 3-4 PM when your blood sugar is the lowest.

Whether they are from fruit or vegetables, fresh juices you make in your own kitchen are the best quality and are our first choice for juicing. However, we realize that juicing is time consuming and difficult for some. Fortunately, fresh organic juice blends are available in refrigerated cases in many supermarkets today. Those with AFS can fill in with these commercial blends if home juicing is not an option. Because nutrients are lost if they sit around too long, it's best to drink the juice immediately after making it.

Key Points to Remember

- Soups are an important way to deliver macronutrients to those with advanced AFS, as their gastric assimilation system is invariably compromised.

- Chicken broth is particularly nutritious and is easily absorbed, making it ideal for those in a weakened state.

- Juicing vegetables can be detoxifying, but aggressive use can lead to excessive re-toxification or die-off reactions. In those who are compromised, this can precipitate adrenal crashes.

- Fruit juices should be avoided except when AFS is mild.

Chapter 25

Food and Chemical Sensitivities

Sensitivities, sometimes loosely referred to as allergies, are a worldwide phenomenon. For example, allergies to peanuts, dairy, and wheat are very common and often show up in allergy testing. However, we can't rely on testing alone to establish such sensitivities. As in other situations discussed throughout this book, laboratory testing often shows a normal result, but the medical history and observations point to an abnormality or dysfunction. Sensitivity to wheat is often subtle—hidden—and a negative result on an allergy test isn't determinative. We discuss wheat sensitivity in detail because it's so widespread in Adrenal Fatigue Syndrome.

We also offer guidelines for vegetable juicing, which is beneficial for many patients. However, the benefits of both the easy-to-make soups and juicing are not limited to those with AFS, but are part of any sound prevention program and anti-aging effort. In other words, these soups and juicing are good for the whole family.

Wheat in the Modern Era

After maize and rice, wheat is the third most produced cereal. Wheat has been around a long time, too. Domestically cultivated since 9,000 B.C., the human civilization would look drastically different had it not been for wheat, an inexpensive staple food much of the world relies on for energy. Wheat products include flour used for many thousands of varieties of breads, breakfast cereals, pasta/noodles, plus many kinds of cookies and cakes. Fermented wheat is used to make beer and other alcoholic drinks, and it's the base of some biofuels. It's no exaggeration to say that in many parts of the world, wheat, in all its forms, is a sunrise to sundown food and more recently, a fuel.

Unfortunately, the wheat of today differs from wheat of ancient times. Over the past several decades, the drive to increase production has ushered in an era in which food scientists have developed technological advances designed to lower cost, extend shelf life, and increase variety, while also increasing production. Wheat producers and processors have achieved their goals through hybridization. Wheat has been selectively bred to produce larger quantities of lectin protein, a type of wheat germ agglutinin (WGA), and glycoprotein.

This manipulation of the wheat plant is not without negative consequences. For example, hybridization has greatly increased the amount of gluten protein now found in wheat. It is estimated that lectins are present in about 30 percent of the western diet. Today's pure wheat flour is processed into refined white flour. The principal parts of wheat and white flour are gluten and starch. The problem begins when lectins bind to the sugar in cells in the gut and blood, initiating a cascade of inflammatory responses. Scientific literature shows that dietary lectins can drastically reduce natural killer (NK) cell activity directly and through disruption of intestinal flora. Natural killer cells are one of the body's most vital defenses against unwelcomed bacteria and virus.

Lectins in the human body appear on the vascular endothelial lining in order for blood cells to escape into the tissue. (Lectins should not be confused with leptin, an endocrine hormone.) They are also present in the liver to help capture microorganisms. Finally, lectins act as a defense system by coating foreign antigens, making them more susceptible to destruction by the body's immune driven cells. Lectins, however, have a dark side. We now understand that lectin proteins found in wheat are often the primary cause of many of today's illnesses and allergies. WGA lectin has the potential to:

- damage major tissues of the body
- promote inflammation
- impede digestion and absorption
- disrupt bacteria balance
- disturb endocrine function

WGA lectin proteins are also capable of circulating in the blood and crossing the blood-brain barrier. Lectin itself also acts to defend the wheat plant from its natural enemies, such as fungi and insects, which is why lectin has been bred into the plant in modern times. Ever increasing production is the goal, and the hardier the plant, the greater the production.

Lectins are also called agglutinins because of their ability to bind to many cell surfaces, causing agglutination (cell clumping) reactions. Lectins bind to sugar on the cell membrane, proteins, and fat.

Because this protein lectin is very small and difficult to break down and is virtually resistant to digestion, it hampers normal biological processes and is stored in important tissues, thereby acting as an *anti-nutrient.*

Usually, sprouting and fermenting, or the process of digesting grains, can work against some anti-nutrient effects. However, lectins are resilient proteins and resist these processes; lectins may even subsist in sprouted breads, which are purported to be a healthier form of wheat.

WGA lectin is very hard to break down because it is formed by the same chemical bonds that produce vulcanized rubber and human hair, both of which are tough, flexible, and durable. WGA lectin has unique properties in that it has the potential to directly harm most of the body's tissues even in a body that has no evidence of genetic or immune system susceptibilities. This might be one reason why chronic inflammatory and degenerative conditions are endemic to wheat consuming populations. What is surprising is that WGA is found in its highest concentration in "whole wheat." The push toward more whole grain bread may actually promote the onslaught of lectin-driven illnesses. While most healthy people are not affected, those with AFS are particularly vulnerable.

Foods with the highest concentrations of lectin include all dried beans (especially soy), grains of all kinds (especially wheat), seeds and nuts, dairy, and plants in the nightshade family (i.e., white potatoes and tomatoes). The large concentrations of lectin in plant seeds decreases with growth, so sprouting the grains and seeds before eating reduces the lectin concentration. However, avoiding soy, wheat, and dairy is the best action. Soaking nuts for at least twenty-four hours improves their digestibility.

Threats of Wheat Lectin

Exactly how does lectin harm your health? Lectin:

- **Promotes inflammation:** Even at minor concentrations, WGA lectins stimulate the production of pro-inflammatory chemical messengers.

- **Is toxic to the immune system:** WGA lectin may fasten to and stimulate white blood cells.

- **Is toxic to the nervous system:** WGA lectin easily passes through the blood-brain barrier and binds to the myelin sheath that protects the nerve. It can also inhibit the nerve growth factor, which is important for growth, maintenance, and survival of certain target neurons.

- **Is toxic to the cells:** WGA lectin has the capacity to induce programmed cell death.

WGA lectin enters the body through the intestinal membranes, which then allows it to circulate in your body.

Almost everyone has antibodies to some dietary lectins in the body. Many food allergies and delayed food sensitivities are actually immune system reactions to lectin. Ultimately, our intrinsic constitution will determine to a large degree how we respond. The weaker the body, the more problematic this becomes. It should come as no surprise that those with advanced AFS are particularly vulnerable to lectin sensitivity due to their low gastric assimilation and clearance capability.

Looking at Wheat Gluten

Gluten originates from the Latin word for glue, implying the bonding properties that bind or hold together wheat products, such as cake and bread. These qualities might be advantageous to cooks and bakers, but they are also responsible for standing in the way of effective breakdown and absorption of nutrients. Eating gluten results in a constipated lump in the gut rather than a nutritious, easily digested meal. This lump of undigested gluten then provokes the immune system to launch an attack on the lining of the small intestine, leading to symptoms such as diarrhea or constipation, nausea, and stomach aches. As time passes, the small intestine becomes more injured, making it harder to absorb certain nutrients such as calcium and iron. This in turn leads to osteoporosis, anemia, and other problems.

Two Types of Allergies

You might be aware that two kinds of food allergies exist. At times, individuals are severely allergic and have serious immediate anaphylactic reactions (a reaction commonly associated with peanuts and shellfish, for example) characterized by respiratory symptoms. This is a "true allergy." When most people hear the words "food allergy," they associate them with the severe and sudden anaphylactic response.

The second type of food allergy is much more common and far less understood by the general public. It is referred to as an IgG food intolerance, food sensitivity, or delayed food allergy, better known as delayed food sensitivity. IgG is the type of allergy to wheat, dairy, and soy we see at work in AFS. Delayed food sensitivity brings many different types of reactions, which may take place hours or even days after you've eaten the offending foods.

You may be unaware that some of our physical problems are related to foods you consume, much less foods you ate three days ago. If you do associate a physical response with something you ate, you usually try to think of an unusual food. But you're most likely reacting to a food (or foods) you eat regularly. Allergies to wheat, dairy, and soy are among the most common culprits within the universe of delayed food allergy, largely because they comprise so much of the average diet. At times, you can be sensitive to a specific combination of foods that you don't react to individually, or a certain food was okay, but overnight you become sensitive to the same food.

Conditions and Symptoms Associated with Delayed Food Sensitivity

Aside from the obvious gastric symptoms (indigestion, diarrhea, constipation, and so forth), delayed food allergies can also manifest themselves in ways most people would never think to connect. Examples include: rheumatoid arthritis, migraine headaches, asthma, attention deficit disorder (ADD), autism, fibromyalgia, and other autoimmune syndromes. All these and many other conditions have food sensitivity triggers, and those who have identified their food sensitivities and eliminated them from their diets see dramatic improvements in their health.

Day to day complaints can also be caused by delayed food allergies. Consider this list of seemingly ordinary symptoms:

- cloudy thinking/inability to concentrate
- lethargy/fatigue
- headaches, including migraines
- joint pain
- muscle weakness
- depression
- chronic sinus issues/plugged ears or chronic ear infections
- weight gain
- dark circles under the eyes, red/ruddy cheeks/acne
- cravings for the allergenic foods
- itchy mouth and ears, or feeling itchy all over the body

Wheat and Adrenal Fatigue Syndrome

Because of the high frequency of wheat allergy or intolerance, it plays an especially important role in Adrenal Fatigue Syndrome. Among those with AFS, the slow onset food intolerance is the most common type of allergy. It is characterized by delayed subclinical allergic reactions that can take hours or days to manifest symptoms. However, at times we might not even recognize a reaction, or we attribute it to another cause.

Such delayed reactions include:

- low energy
- dry skin, itchiness
- heart palpitations
- blurry vision
- irritability/anxiety
- irritable bowel syndrome (IBS)

Normally, we don't see hives and respiratory difficulties typical of *acute* allergic responses.

As you can see, these delayed symptoms are rather general, which is why their potential link to wheat is overlooked, even though wheat is omnipresent in everyday diets of many millions of individuals. Unlike acute responses, these general symptoms typically develop in a stealth manner and gradually worsen over years. This is one reason conventional doctors fail to connect these symptoms to wheat. Unfortunately, this kind of allergy does not show up during allergy testing and remains subclinical. In other words, as an allergy, wheat can elude detection while it causes havoc in an already weak adrenal system.

As with other allergic responses, cortisol is the key hormone regulating the response. In Adrenal Fatigue Syndrome, cortisol output first rises in the early stages, but eventually falls, a progression that usually takes place over years of chronic stress. As Adrenal Fatigue Syndrome progresses, cortisol output reduces and allergic responses become more symptomatic.

As discussed earlier, lectin sensitivity is a major contributor to this problem. It is often accompanied by sensitivity to other foods, such as soy and dairy. As the adrenals weaken, multiple food sensitivities become prevalent. In addition to food allergies, we also see multiple chemical sensitivities.

Food intolerance weakens the body, especially the lining of the stomach and intestines, which means that the body expends more energy than normal to assimilate and metabolize foods. Then, the already stressed adrenals are unable to maintain the energy supply to the body. As this downhill process continues, the GI tract typically becomes irritated and inflamed, and over time, the continuous irritation leads to stomach pain, heartburn, gas, and/or other uncomfortable digestive symptoms. In addition, it's possible to develop leaky gut syndrome, which occurs with increased permeability of the intestinal walls. This means that undigested proteins and fats leak out of the intestine and into the bloodstream, where they set off an autoimmune reaction. This irritation triggers a further increase in demand for the adrenals to produce more cortisol to calm the inflammation. However, this occurs at a time when the adrenals are already stressed.

What You Can Do

Fortunately, you can prevent or reverse delayed food allergy or intolerance. The best way is to eliminate the offending food from your diet while you also normalize adrenal function. Then, as adrenal function improves, the body's ability to combat food intolerance also improves, and these allergens cause fewer symptoms. As time passes, many people are able to tolerate the allergenic foods, and provided the adrenal functions are normalized, these individuals no longer have problems with the foods that once caused so much trouble.

Gluten Free or Wheat Free

As a larger issue, however, most people would live healthier lives if they stopped eating wheat, and perhaps other refined grains. Even those without gluten intolerance tend to feel better when they eliminate wheat and other grains. The reason is that grains break down into sugar in the body and elevate insulin levels, which are linked to many other health problems, including obesity, high cholesterol, high blood pressure, type 2 diabetes and cancer. In other words, with or without obvious reasons and consequences, wheat-free diets have health benefits.

AFS and Gluten

As a preventive measure, everyone with Adrenal Fatigue Syndrome should eliminate wheat from their diet (along with dairy). This sounds easy enough, but wheat now hides in many foods including soy sauce, soups, cold cuts (processed deli meats), candies, and certain low-fat or nonfat products. Read labels carefully and avoid other starches and additives, some of which may be derived from wheat. These include:

- malt
- hydrolyzed vegetable protein (HVP)
- texturized vegetable protein (TVP)

- natural flavorings
- some pharmaceuticals
- alcohol

The following is a (long!) list of common products that may contain wheat, essentially any products that contain flour, bran, wheat germ, wheat starch, or gluten, including:

- baked goods, including bagels, biscuits and rolls, doughnuts, cakes and pies of all types, cookies, and muffins
- bread and bread crumbs, crackers and cracker meal, packaged stuffing
- pancakes and waffles (homemade or packaged mixes), breakfast cereals
- pasta (macaroni, spaghetti, lasagna, and egg noodles)
- breaded meat, fish, and poultry, plus deep fried foods (chicken, fish, vegetables, cheese sticks, and so forth)
- ice cream cones and ice cream sandwiches
- hot dogs, luncheon meats, and pizza
- products containing malt
- coffee substitutes
- bottled salad dressing (unless labeled gluten free)
- gravy, sauces that have been thickened but are opaque (e.g. cream sauces)
- most prepared cream soups
- soy sauce

The Practical Approach

At least at first, it can be difficult to cut out all wheat products in your diet, although today, many alternatives and substitutes exist. First, avoid the most obvious foods, such as bread and pasta, for a couple of weeks. Then eliminate crackers, cakes, cookies, pies, and other desserts. It may take you up to six months to get over your cravings for wheat products. That is normal. However, as your body detoxifies and gains strength because you have avoided wheat, you will notice ill effects if you reintroduce wheat into your diet.

Good alternatives: Today, an increasing number of wheat-free/gluten-free foods, from bread to salad dressing, are available in health food stores and regular supermarkets. In addition, brown rice products, such as rice flour bread and other products are appropriate for both vegetarians and non-vegetarians. You also can use sprouted breads (Ezekiel bread) or gluten-free bread for toast or sandwiches. Rice flour wraps are also good substitutes for bread. You can also use other rice and rice flour products, oat flour, kamut, and quinoa. Those who have cravings for carbohydrates will not necessarily see any difference by using gluten-free products.

If you begin eating some of these wheat containing foods again, you may note that your body isn't reacting well to them, which provides additional incentive to stay away from wheat.

Multiple Chemical Sensitivities

Many individuals develop sensitivities to substances other than food. We see this developing frequently among those with Adrenal Fatigue Syndrome. For example, along with being environmentally unfriendly, commercial household cleaning products are also highly toxic to many people. In order to avoid these products, we've listed some common, safe, and environmentally friendly cleaners to use around the house.

- Baking soda—can clean, scour, and deodorize, and it can even soften water.

- Borax—also known as sodium borate, works like baking soda and can even clean wallpaper and painted walls.

- White vinegar—especially good for removing grease, mildew, odors, stains, and wax build up.

- Citrus solvent—good for removing oil and grease, and can clean paint brushes as well.

- Lemon oil—effective against many bacteria found in homes.

- Isopropyl alcohol—an excellent disinfectant.

- Cornstarch—use to shampoo carpets and rugs, and also to polish furniture.

Your home floors are often in direct contact with the soles of your feet; use these floor cleaners and polishes to keep your body safe:

- **Wood**: Use a one-to-one ratio of vinegar and vegetable oil. Apply a thin coat on the floor and rub in well.

- **Painted wood:** Mix 1 teaspoon of washing soda with 1 gallon of hot water and clean.

- **Brick and stone tiles:** Mix 1 cup of white vinegar with 1 gallon water and clean, then rinse with clear water.

- **Varnished wood:** Add a couple drops of lemon oil into a half cup of warm water. Pour into a spray bottle and shake well. Spray onto cloth and wipe. Finish by wiping furniture again with a dry soft cotton cloth.

- **Unvarnished wood:** Mix 2 teaspoons of olive oil and 2 teaspoons of lemon juice and apply using wide strokes.

Keeping so many products can be a handful, so try out these all-purpose cleaner formulas you can make yourself:

- **For all purpose general cleaning:** Mix a quarter cup of baking soda with a half cup of vinegar into a half gallon of water. This mixture can be stored for a while. It is useful for bathroom cleaning such as the removal of water deposit stains on and around shower stalls, windows, mirrors, and chrome fixtures.

- **For laundry:** Mix 1 cup of Ivory® soap or Fels Naptha® soap with ½ cup of washing soda and ½ cup of borax. Use 1 tablespoon for lighter loads and 2 tablespoons for heavier loads.

- **For bathroom mold:** 1 part 3 percent hydrogen peroxide with 2 parts water in a spray bottle. Spray on affected areas and wait for 1 hour before rinsing.

- **For carpet stains:** Use equal parts white vinegar and water and mix in a spray bottle. Apply directly on the stain and let sit for several minutes before cleaning with a brush and warm soapy water.

- **For really tough carpet stains:** Mix a quarter cup each of salt, borax, and vinegar to form a paste. Rub the paste into the carpet and leave for a couple of hours before vacuuming.

These household remedies have the advantage of being simple and eco-friendly. Most people find that once they begin using these safe products, they have no desire to return to the harsh cleaning products that will one day fade into the past.

In the next chapter, we address another key component of recovery, which is how to get a good night's sleep. Sleep disturbances plague so many with AFS.

Key Points to Remember

- Food and chemical sensitivity is very common in those with AFS, especially those in advanced stages.

- Wheat and dairy products are the main culprits of delayed food sensitivity. Everyone with AFS should try to reduce or eliminate wheat from their diet.

- WGA lectin found within wheat is linked to a variety of inflammatory reactions within the body.

- Gluten, found in most grains, triggers sensitivities to the digestive system.

- We are exposed to many chemicals that are toxic to the adrenal glands. Commercial cleaning products are especially common. Fortunately, there are many natural alternatives to these chemicals, including the use of vinegar and baking soda.

Chapter 26

Adrenal Fatigue Syndrome, Insomnia and Healing Sleep

Insomnia is a classic sign of Adrenal Fatigue Syndrome, and is usually a result of the malfunction of the hypothalamic-pituitary-adrenal (HPA) hormonal axis, over-activation of central nervous system neurotransmitters such as norepinephrine, and imbalances with the sympathetic nervous system and adrenal medullary hormonal system (AHS) discussed in Chapter 2, *Stress, Hormone Basics and the "Forgotten" Adrenals.* Rather than being a single, discrete condition, insomnia in AFS more closely resembles a complex condition, because it is quite different from regular insomnia experienced by healthy individuals. The main complaints include part or, frequently, all of the following:

- difficulty falling asleep (sleep onset insomnia, or SOI)
- disturbed sleep and being easily awakened at night
- difficulty falling back to sleep (sleep maintenance insomnia, or SMI)
- seldom or never feeling rested, leading to morning fatigue, a slower morning start, and feeling fatigued during the day

Sleep Onset Insomnia (SOI)

Most people think of SOI, a situation in which it's difficult to fall asleep, as what insomnia is all about. In fact, it is only one manifestation of insomnia. For normal sleep to occur, and to awaken refreshed and energized, it's important that cortisol be at its highest level in the morning and at its lowest level at night. When the cortisol balance is off, sleep patterns can be affected. High cortisol levels are typical of people suffering from mild Adrenal Fatigue Syndrome. This happens when the adrenals are on overdrive, putting out excessive cortisol throughout the day in order to deal with constant stress. Some of the excess cortisol carries into the night and affects the ability to fall asleep, thus contributing to SOI. Lack of sleep is also a trigger that further increases cortisol output, which in turn worsens insomnia. This forms a vicious cycle.

At the same time, stress and insomnia trigger the AHS. The adrenal medulla is activated to produce adrenaline, which is, as you recall, a hormone responsible for the fight-or-flight response. A high adrenaline level can independently disturb sleep patterns by putting the body on full alert, commonly referred to as being wired. Besides, when the body is on full alert, as is expected and advantageous during threats of danger and other emergencies, sleep is the last thing the body needs. The problem arises when adrenaline is high when no immediate danger is at hand. High cortisol and high adrenaline can occur simultaneously, a common situation among those who suffer from Adrenal Fatigue Syndrome. On top of this, the brain usually is already on overdrive with norepinephrine overload, leading to a concurrent state of constant arousal. This situation is made worse if stimulatory natural compounds are used such as certain vitamins, herbs, and glandulars. It comes as no surprise that advancing AFS often equates to worsening insomnia.

Below are some general tips to help you fall asleep more easily:

- *Sleep in a cool and completely quiet and dark room.* A dark room enhances the production of *melatonin*, an important sleep regulating hormone. Draw and close all the window coverings; even a small amount of light in the environment can reduce melatonin output from the brain.

- *Go to bed and get up at about the same time every day, even on weekends.* Sticking to a schedule helps reinforce your body's sleep-wake cycle, and doing the same things each night tells your body that its time to wind down. This may include taking a warm bath or shower, reading a book, or listening to soothing music. Relaxing activities done with lowered lights can help ease the transition between wakefulness and sleepiness.

- *Remove all electrical appliances, such as nightlights and alarm clocks.* Put them at least ten feet away from the bed to reduce EMF (electromagnetic field) emission, which can alter sleep patterns.

- *Do not do strenuous aerobic exercise or power yoga after dinner.* You want to avoid over stimulating the SNS (sympathetic nervous system), which is frequently on overdrive in people who already suffer from Adrenal Fatigue Syndrome.

- *Turn off your computer, TV, loud music, and hyper-stimulating video games.* After 6:00 PM, these and similar devices can trigger an adrenaline rush. Try reading books in a quiet environment during the evening; if you do watch TV, then avoid channel surfing and don't watch violent action shows.

- *Avoid adrenal stimulators.* It's important to avoid certain foods and chemicals in order to avoid excessive stress on the adrenal glands. Stay away from sugary foods and both caffeinated and decaffeinated drinks of all kinds, along with other common offenders including nicotine, alcohol, allergic foods (histamine is an adrenal stimulant), green tea, and chocolate. In addition, you should avoid herbs and glandular products, unless approved by your healthcare professional. We also recommend avoiding partially hydrogenated fats, such as those used in deep fried foods and shortenings, which inhibit steroid hormone synthesis. Artificial sweeteners should be eliminated as well—they block the conversion of phenylalanine to tyrosine, which is needed to synthesize catecholamines (particular types of substances that function like hormones or neurotransmitters) in the adrenal medulla. Non-stimulating herbal teas, such as chamomile, are permitted.

- *Perform gentle Adrenal Restorative Exercises in the late afternoon* (*discussed in the next chapter*). This helps the body transition from (presumably) the end of a work day to the evening. However, do not perform them in the evening. Low intensity aerobics, such as long, slow walks should be done in the morning or late in the afternoon. Taking a short walk after dinner is an exception, provided that the body does not feel drained immediately afterwards.

- *Always go to sleep before 10 PM at the latest.* If you are tired, go to sleep earlier. Do the Adrenal Breathing Exercises (addressed in the next chapter) just before bedtime and not at any other time in the evening. This will help with the transition to sleep. Adrenal Breathing should always be part of your relaxing bedtime routine.

- *A small snack of protein and fat (a handful of nuts or cottage cheese) before sleep is beneficial.* A light snack before bed can help promote sleep, and pairing tryptophan-containing foods (such as turkey and certain dairy products) with carbohydrates, helps to calm the brain, which allows the body to sleep better.

- *If you don't fall asleep, get up and do something like Adrenal Restorative Exercises or Adrenal Breathing Exercises.* Go back to bed when you're tired, but don't agonize about falling asleep. The stress will only prevent sleep. It is common for many people with advanced AFS to feel wired and tired at the same time, so if your mind is racing and can't stop, use the energy to think positive thoughts. Try to set aside worries and negative thoughts and form the habit of engaging in positive thinking at bedtime. To the extent you can, occupy your mind with images of relaxing places or happy events.

- *A good bed is subjective and different for each person.* Make sure you have a comfortable bed that offers orthopedic comfort. If you share your bed, make sure there's enough room for two. Children and pets often disrupt sleep, so you may need to set limits on how often they can sleep in your bed with you.

- *Take a natural sleep aid as directed by your healthcare professional.* Many are available, and each has individual characteristics. Finding the right one or combination might require trial and error. We discuss this later on in this chapter.

Sleep Maintenance Insomnia (SMI)

Sleep maintenance insomnia involves the tendency to wake up in the middle of the night but be unable to go back to sleep. Usually, a number of factors trigger SMI. Metabolic imbalances, such as problems with blood sugar and insulin regulation, may occur during sleep and cause wakefulness. When the body must deal with excessive daytime stress, the body can sometimes fall asleep simply because the magnitude of the physical fatigue overwhelms high adrenaline and cortisol levels. The wired and tired body needs a break, so it crashes, allowing for a few hours of sleep. However, cortisol and adrenaline levels remain high during this time, and these sustained high levels in the middle of the night eventually awaken the body. The physical tiredness is reduced by a few hours of rest, leading to sleep maintenance insomnia. Once awakened, it is hard to fall back to sleep.

Those who suffer from advanced AFS often have concurrent metabolic imbalances, such as insulin dysregulation and subclinical hypoglycemia. When the body's glucose supplies (from food) are inadequate, the blood sugar level drops below a certain threshold level during sleep; this can activate the SNS and AHS, which leads to norepinephrine and adrenaline release, both of which can contribute to wakefulness.

By conventional laboratory standards the blood sugar level may be normal, but individuals may be extremely sensitive to the rollercoaster ride of the blood sugar level; even a small drop within normal ranges during the night can trigger awakening. These wakeful periods are often accompanied by symptoms such as heart palpitations and cold sweats. So, to avoid SMI we need to practice the aforementioned good sleep habits and follow the protocol for *SOI*, along with ensuring the stability of the blood glucose level throughout the evening. When your blood sugar level falls, healthy adrenals restore it back to normal. If the blood sugar levels are not stabilized, then we don't see optimal results when attempting to correct the adrenal status.

Below are dietary guidelines which are beneficial to both prevent and treat AFS, but also help stabilize both daytime and nighttime blood glucose levels. As you can see, they are much like the dietary guidelines listed in the previous chapter:

- *Do not skip breakfast.* In fact, it should be the biggest meal.

- *Follow the mealtime guidelines for AFS*, being sure to eat every 2-3 hours during the day.

- *Snack only on low glycemic foods*, such as nuts, seeds, hard-boiled eggs, and so forth. For sustained energy release, add a small amount of carbohydrate, such as a few raw carrot sticks to supply instant energy to the body.

- *Avoid all fruit and vegetable juices.* Whole fruit, such as apples, are acceptable.

- *Never consume high glycemic fruits (or other foods) without a source of protein and fat to balance them.* For example, a whole fruit along with some almond butter balances the carbohydrate of the fruit with protein and fat supplied by the almond butter spread.

- *Take the prescribed natural compounds designed to stabilize blood sugar and calm the autonomic nervous system.* Your healthcare professional will guide you on this.

- *A bedtime snack is especially important.* This snack may be a small portion of protein, carbohydrate, and fat, but for some, it may be nearly a full meal.

- *If you wake up in the middle of the night, have another light snack to normalize blood sugar, thereby allowing you to go back to sleep.*

Sleep issues may take time to resolve, so begin by being patient. Stick with your routine and slowly but surely you will begin to experience the benefits of a good night's sleep.

Natural Sleep Aids

A great variety of sleep aids are available, but we know which work or don't work only through trial and error. Each sleep aid nutrient has specific pathways and affects individuals in different ways. For example:

- GABA (gamma-amino butyric acid, an amino acid that helps to regulate sleep and anxiety) works best for those with Adrenal Fatigue Syndrome and who are adrenal dominant.

- 5-HTP is usually more effective for the thyroid dominant type.

Because of individual reactions to different types of sleep aid nutrients and the predominance of paradoxical reactions in Adrenal Fatigue Syndrome, experienced clinicians use different combinations of natural compounds.

Considering Melatonin

Melatonin is a hormone produced by the pineal gland, located deep in the brain. Many older individuals use melatonin as a supplement and sleep aid because this hormone declines with age, thereby causing sleep disturbances in many people.

Although sleep patterns are often disrupted as we age, this reduction of the nightly release of melatonin by the pineal gland also occurs among those with AFS. Many individuals have discovered that bedtime doses of melatonin will restore their ability to have a sound and peaceful night's sleep. Taking oral melatonin helps with both SOI and SMI.

Low doses of melatonin (0.5 to 3 mg) act as a natural sleeping pill, but the dosages are individualized, especially with Adrenal Fatigue Syndrome. Trial and error is almost inevitable. We recommend starting with 0.5 to 1 mg, gradually increasing if there are no adverse side effects. The upper limits of dosage vary from person to person, and some need as much as 30 mg. A higher dose isn't necessarily better, however, and some people feel better on smaller doses.

When you first begin taking melatonin, you may feel slightly disoriented or dizzy during your first few waking hours. This hangover sensation should subside after a few nights of use. If it persists, then reduce the dose.

Note: High doses of melatonin are contraindicated in children, pregnant or nursing women, women trying to conceive, people taking prescription steroids, or who have mental illness, severe allergies, or immune system cancers such as lymphoma.

To effectively use melatonin, always take the hormone supplement just before bedtime. If you take it earlier in the daylight hours, it may disrupt sleeping and waking cycles. If you have a hangover sensation, then try taking melatonin earlier in the evening instead of at bedtime (but not during daytime hours).

Other Sleep Aids

If sleep continues to be a problem, other supplements and compounds might be helpful. For example, consider: phosphaditylserine, glutamine, magnesium, calcium, fish oil, progesterone, glutamine, theanine, flower remedies, herbs such as valerian, GABA, inosital, and 5-HTP (hydroxytryptophan). Interestingly, the herb, ashawandgha, may enhance sleep in some people for reasons not well understood.

It is not unusual for natural sleep aids to be grouped into a cocktail to work best. Those who are sensitive may need to be on a special schedule to avoid toxic metabolite buildup. Sometimes sleep improves but is short-lived. Other times, things can actually get worse, and then all of a sudden get better. Even in the best of hands, some trial and error is required.

Prescription Sleep Medication

Those who have unrelenting insomnia may need prescription sleep medication for a short time. However, proceed with extreme care and consider this only under close medical supervision because of potential addiction problems and the liver clearance complications frequently seen in those with advanced AFS. Nevertheless, these prescription drugs are sometimes clinically necessary to help the body get much needed rest in order to reset itself during the recovery process. As much as we advise caution with these substances, their proper use can be of tremendous benefit.

Here, too, because each person reacts differently to prescription medications, expect a period of trial and error. Those with a weak constitution and high sensitivity must be on extra alert for paradoxical reactions, meaning that the action of the sleep medications leads to a state of hyperarousal.

We recommend starting at a very low dose. Those who are already on prescription sleep medication should not stop abruptly as sudden withdrawal can trigger adrenal crashes. The best time to reduce dependence on sleep medications is after adrenal reserves have been re-established. Many have reported a spontaneous reduction in insomnia as adrenal health returns. This is normal, and often reflects a reduction of the sympathetic overtone so common in adrenal exhaustion.

Sleep is so important for general health and for preventing and recovering from Adrenal Fatigue Syndrome that we recommend doing whatever you can to get a good night's sleep, both in duration and quality.

Key Points to Remember

- Most people with AFS complain of insomnia to some degree. The more advanced the AFS, the more serious this is.

- Sleep onset insomnia (SOI) is often due to an overflow of adrenaline or a cortisol imbalance in the body. A person usually feels wired-and-tired.

- Sleep maintenance insomnia (SMI) refers to the inability to fall back to sleep after waking up in the middle of the night. This can be due to a variety of metabolic and hormonal imbalances and this situation can be quite challenging.

- Most insomnia improves as Adrenal Fatigue Syndrome improves.

- Many sleep aids are available. Trial and error is required, and often a cocktail of natural sleep aids works the best.

- Melatonin is an excellent sleep aid. The dosage requirement varies greatly. Other important sleep aids include GABA, 5-HTP, magnesium, progesterone, and so forth.

- It is important to have good sleeping habits to facilitate restful sleep. The most important is to sleep in a completely quiet and dark room.

Chapter 27

Adrenal Fatigue Syndrome and Healing Exercise

Most people think of exercise in terms of *aerobic* activities, such as brisk walking, jogging, cycling, rowing, and other activities that elevate the heart rate and condition the cardiovascular system, or as *anaerobic*, such as strength training that builds and maintains muscles. These are beneficial to general good health, but for advanced Adrenal Fatigue Syndrome, they are not the best types of exercise. In fact, the wrong exercise program may make Adrenal Fatigue Syndrome worse and can easily trigger adrenal crashes. Let's look at the reasons for this dilemma.

One common misconception is that Adrenal Fatigue Syndrome equates to low energy only, which can be linked to the body's inability to overcome stress, whether it is physical, mental, or emotional. In addition, because all body functions require energy, low energy is the most prominent outcome in those with Adrenal Fatigue Syndrome. This sounds logical, but at the root level, however, AFS is much more complicated.

Think of a car running low on gas, plus it has a steering wheel problem, a gas pedal that continues to accelerate at will, and a brake pedal that malfunctions intermittently. In other words, many of the systems that ensure a smoothly running vehicle are broken. No longer under your control, the car is an accident waiting to happen—and it can't get you where you want to go. Translate these circumstances to your body and you are not far away from advanced Adrenal Fatigue Syndrome.

Like a car, the body needs to run smoothly for us to feel and perform well, which means we need perfect synchronization of numerous organs and systems. In AFS, the body is drained and low on energy, like a car running low on gas, and we see numerous concurrent imbalances. Since many hormones are dysregulated, low energy may exist with:

- hypoglycemia, low blood sugar, which we can liken to not enough gasoline in the gas tank

- feelings of being wired, like a sticky gas pedal that's stuck in acceleration

- foggy thinking, like a driver who texts while driving

- depression, which tells us the brake pedal has burned out

With the internal equilibrium of the body dysregulated, it is no wonder that the adrenals crash with each little stressor.

An Exercise Strategy

A successful Adrenal Recovery Exercise Program requires a strategy that helps you regain control of the core functions of the body. Returning to the analogy of the car, controlling the body involves more than adding gasoline to the tank. If the steering system is not functioning, you are still unable to get where you want to go, even with a full tank of gas. The goal is a complete rebalancing of the internal systems, so they can operate together smoothly and get you where you want to go. This involves a total mind-body approach incorporating lifestyle, exercise, diet, and nutrition, plus both mental and physical components. If done properly, exercise helps the adrenals boost their function, and thus, energy.

Energy and Exercise

Individuals in early AFS (Stages 1 and 2) may feel tired only intermittently and tend to quickly recover from any low energy state. As you recall from our discussion of the stages of AFS, those in advanced AFS (Stages 3 and 4) experience a constant low energy state and fatigue, which worsens over time. For those with advanced adrenal weakness, it is important to custom tailor an exercise program for the best use of limited energy.

Over-use of energy for exercise may trigger adrenal crashes. Therefore, it's of paramount importance to reach the right balance of intensity, length of exercise sessions, and frequency. Exercise makes many individuals in more advanced stages of AFS feel drained of energy, so they tend to avoid it. However, except during an adrenal crash, it's not beneficial to avoid exercise altogether. Other individuals treat their energy drain and fatigue by forcing themselves to do more and more. Both approaches can be wrong. This is why we recommend a personalized exercise program designed specifically for the level of adrenal function.

For vital organs to overcome a low energy state, we need to maintain a consistent energy stream, and any excess energy can be channeled into exercise. However, the amount of exercise must be adjusted to avoid over-stimulation of the fight-or-flight response mediated by epinephrine. The right exercise performed at the right time is tremendously beneficial, but the opposite is true as well. (See exercise graph in the next section.)

During the initial stages of healing advanced AFS, experienced clinicians want to conserve energy as much as possible, so the goal is *not to choose* exercises that are overly focused on increasing energy. A more gentle, nurturing approach starting from the core is more appropriate to increase internal reserves. After a comfortable level of reserve is accomplished and built up in the body, then over time, the body can go from a catabolic state into an anabolic state, in which muscles start to rebuild and strengthen. This level of healing must be accomplished gradually, step-by-step, which goes a long way in avoiding the common mistake in AFS recovery, over exercising.

A well designed Adrenal Recovery Exercise Program includes breathing, muscle toning, stretching, strength training, motion fluidity, control, and overall circulation. It considers the stage of AFS, the body's remaining reserve, the biological constitution, age, metabolic issues, past medical history, and injuries. (As with any exercise program, always consult and seek approval of your personal physician before beginning.)

The AFS Exercise Toolbox

Each tool has its place and must be deployed at the right time for maximum benefit. The proper program allows the body a total healing experience, starting at the cellular level in the core of the body. Remember, too, that the body has an internal repair system in place, and fortunately, the body is forgiving.

The tools are:

• Adrenal Breathing™ Exercises for basic harmony and ANS balance.

• Twelve Adrenal Restorative Exercises to enhance blood flow/oxygen delivery.

• Twenty-one Adrenal Yoga™ Exercise sessions, with three major components: the beginner phase, with a focus on breathing and stretching; the intermediate phase, with a focus on toning and strengthening; and the advanced phase, with a focus on fluidity and control.

In addition, we briefly describe *regular yoga, power yoga,* and *aerobics.* In this book, we're limiting our detailed discussion to the first two tools, but the graph below illustrates the way a comprehensive exercise program in stages can help restore the adrenal function and energy:

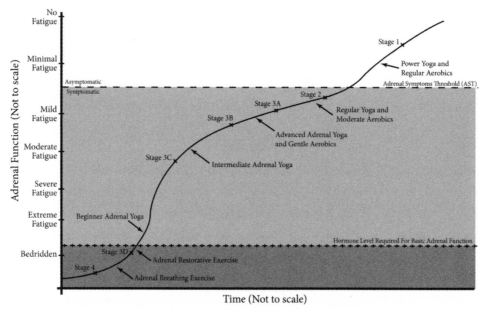

Figure 19. Adrenal Fatigue Syndrome Exercise Progression

Breathing as Therapy

Because breathing is an automatic function, the western medical world has not taken the time to understand its therapeutic significance. Only when breathing is compromised or obstructed is it considered and evaluated. Therefore, most people in the west are not taught the significance of proper breathing, let alone its healing power. As a result, the vast majority of people do not breathe properly, either while in a normal healthy state or when the body is weakened, as occurs with AFS.

Three main sets of muscles are active when you breathe normally: the intercostal muscles, the abdominal muscles, and the respiratory diaphragm. All muscular activity of the body is under the guidance of the nervous system, e.g., contraction of individual cells, isotonic (with normal contraction) or isometric (without normal contraction) exercise, agonist or antagonist activity, and concentric shortening or eccentric lengthening. Breathing is special in that it involves both the somatic nervous system and the autonomic nervous system, the ANS. In other words, you can voluntarily control breathing, or if you choose not to do so, the body automatically takes over. Both systems are connected. The ANS is self-regulating and usually not controlled by the somatic nervous system. For example, you cannot voluntarily decide to speed up or slow down your heart rate. This is normally regulated by the ANS and is beyond control of the somatic nervous system. However, you can influence the heart rate by consciously regulating the respiratory rate because breathing connects both nervous systems. *Long exhalations slow down the heart rate.*

So, by modulating our respiratory rate at will, we influence the ANS. Therefore, breathing offers an important gateway into the world of the ANS. This is important because in advanced Adrenal Fatigue Syndrome, the autonomic nervous system is invariably dysfunctional.

Remember from earlier discussions that the ANS is broadly divided:

1. Into the sympathetic nervous system (SNS), which is responsible for adrenaline release and the fight-or-flight response; and

2. The parasympathetic nervous system (PNS), which is responsible for rest and relaxation of the body's internal functions.

We need less air in quiet times, and the PNS mildly constricts the smooth muscle that surrounds the airways. However, in times of emergency or increased physical activity, the SNS opens the airways and allows air to flow more easily.

To modulate and maintain homeostasis in the body's inner world, the PNS, through release of its neurotransmitter, acetylcholine, works in a dynamic balance with the SNS, through release of its neurotransmitter, norepinephrine. Advanced Adrenal Fatigue Syndrome is invariably tied to over-stimulation of the SNS and the AHS. Extensive experiments have compared Type A (aggressive and high strung) with Type B (laid back and relaxed) personalities. They found that during exposure to various laboratory and clinical stressors, Type A individuals have about threefold larger plasma norepinephrine responses and fourfold larger adrenaline responses than Type B individuals. These chemical transmitters flood the body in Type A individuals, which puts the body on constant alert. This leads to a viscous downward spiral of compensatory response and ultimately adrenal burnout.

One key to adrenal recovery is to reduce SNS tone and enhance PNS tone. This is where Adrenal Breathing can help greatly, because it influences the autonomic circuits that slow the heartbeat and reduce blood pressure, producing calm and a sense of stability. Further, it calms the mind, and allows the body's internal homeostatic system to reset itself. Controlled respiration consciously gives us access to autonomic function that no other system of the body can boast.

Those with severe adrenal weakness often exhibit abnormal breathing patterns that can over-stimulate the SNS, which in turn can trigger panic attacks and contribute to adrenal crashes. We tend to breathe shallowly or even hold our breath when we are feeling anxious or under stress, and sometimes we're not aware of it. Shallow breathing also limits oxygen intake and adds further stress to the body, thus creating a vicious cycle. As we'll describe in the instructions for Adrenal Breathing, holding the breath at the end of inhalation or exhalation stimulates the SNS, thus aggravating adrenal weakness if the body is already in a state of low adrenal reserve.

Adrenal Breathing Exercises are so important because they can break this negative cycle by rebalancing the ANS, thereby gently delivering more oxygen to the body to naturally generate energy without over-stimulating the SNS. Proper Adrenal Breathing enhances the PNS, the parasympathetic nervous system's function, and shifts the body's basal resting mode from a sympathetic to a parasympathetic bias.

Bear in mind that in eastern cultures, breathing is also used to stimulate the SNS. We see this in certain types of yoga breathing. Various techniques involve holding the breath with increasing intensity and performing quick breathing exercises with high frequency (bellow breathing).

Another technique, called thoracic or paradoxical breathing, involves using only the chest wall to affect breathing. The chest wall expands while the abdominal wall is drawn inward toward the back during inhalation and outward during exhalation. While these breathing techniques are empowering and increase energy flow, they can drain the body of the already low energy state in Adrenal Fatigue Syndrome as the SNS is already fully activated.

In Adrenal Breathing, the goal is to *reduce* sympathetic tone. Therefore, we recommend restricting all sympathetically driven breathing techniques until the adrenals are healed or unless directed by your healthcare professional.

Other Benefits

After a few weeks of consistent practice, this abdominal breathing technique will automatically lead to stronger diaphragm muscles. You will notice an automatic increase in your inhalation and exhalation capacity with the same effort, often extending to 90 percent or even 95 percent of capacity. This is achieved effortlessly, calmly, being fully relaxed and with no need to force your breath.

Note, too, that the muscles that connect the ribs (intercostal muscles) are passive and not actively engaged during Adrenal Breathing. Therefore, your chest wall expands and contracts naturally as air flows in and out of the lungs, usually with minimal movement. Since no special effort is directed toward the chest wall to help the breathing process, you won't note any significant rise and fall during the Adrenal Breathing process.

When properly done, Adrenal Breathing Exercises use the diaphragm to help restore adrenal health by:

- enhancing parasympathetic tone
- improving lymphatic circulation, thus clearing toxic metabolites
- improving vital capacity
- supporting healthy ANS balance
- improving tissue oxygen saturation
- optimizing musculoskeletal tone
- effecting gentle rhythmic massage on the GI track and internal organs including the adrenals

This is one of the easiest and most effective exercises anyone with Adrenal Fatigue Syndrome can do at anytime and anyplace to support adrenal recovery.

Adrenal Breathing Exercise

Let's begin with the Adrenal Breathing Exercise. Here are step-by-step instructions:

1. Lie down on your back on a flat but comfortable surface, arms and palms facing up and slightly away from the body with legs uncrossed and apart at shoulder width. Loosen your clothes as needed. Make a conscious effort to relax and feel the weight of the body on the floor. You can also do this breathing in a sitting position with your spine straight (do not arch your back because the abdominal muscles wrap around to the rear). Those in advanced AFS and who are weak should begin practicing this exercise in the supine position. As the body strengthens, you can do this exercise in either a sitting or standing position. (If space does not permit the supine position during this breathing exercise, then a sitting or standing position is acceptable.)

2. Close your eyes. (If desired, you can cover your eyes with a small towel.) Drop your tongue to its natural relaxed resting position toward the back of the mouth without obstructing air flow. It is very important to keep your spine straight, drop your shoulders and let them relax. Check yourself for these items before going any further.

3. Exhale completely through your mouth, making a small whoosh sound. Now you are ready to start.

4. Close your mouth and inhale quietly through your nose. Start at 50 percent of capacity in a smooth and rhythmic fashion. (Working yourself up to 80-90 percent of capacity depends on how well you can perform this breathing.) From this point on, don't breathe through the mouth.

5. Imagine the air entering your body through your left nostril, which according to ancient tradition, is calming. Your belly should be expanding outward as you inhale comfortably. If you put your hands on your stomach, they will be pushed away from the back. This ensures that you are breathing properly.

   Imagine you are filling your body with air from the bottom up. Focus your attention on the flow of air in and out of the nasal passages, in through the left and out through the right nostril. Breathe evenly, and do not force the breath.

   During this breathing exercise, the chest wall does not move significantly, but the abdominal muscles must be completely free and relaxed. (If they are even mildly tensed you can't do the breathing correctly.) The rest of the body is stable except for a slight backward movement of the head during inhalation. Don't forget that eyes are closed, with shoulders dropped and relaxed throughout.

6. Do a mental count of four slowly and comfortably (about 1-2 seconds per count). At the end of the inhalation, spontaneously progress to exhale naturally and without effort. Inhalation can occur only as a result of muscular activity; however, exhalations are different, as the lungs have the capacity to get smaller because their elasticity keeps pulling them, along with the rib cage, to a smaller size.

Do not hold your breath intentionally at the end of inhalation or exhalation. What we want from relaxed, even breathing is a smooth rhythmic transition from inhalation to exhalation and from exhalation to inhalation—no jerky movements.

The actual pattern of breathing is elliptical rather than circular. Even though no air is moving in or out at the ends of inhalation and exhalation, you can smoothly merge inhalation with exhalation (and exhalation with inhalation) without effort if you focus on rhythmic movement along the ellipse.

7. Exhale completely through your nose, while imagining the air coming out of the right nostril, quietly and smoothly. There is no count required on exhalation. Feel your stomach contract slowly until most (but not all) of the air is out naturally. Exhalation is normally a little longer than inhalation. Do not force, overextend, or hold after the exhalation, because that will activate the SNS. Simply let the body control the exhalation time and intensity naturally.

This is one full breath. Now inhale again and repeat the cycle seven more times for a total of eight full breaths. A full set is eight complete breaths, which takes most people 1-2 minutes.

It's important to do at least one set of eight full breaths each time you start Adrenal Breathing. Let's examine why. When you first maintain a stationary position that is comfortable, especially in a flat position with face up (supine), most of the motor neurons that innervate the skeletal muscles are still firing nerve impulses automatically. With each breath, however, the number and frequency of nerve impulses transmitted to your muscles starts to decline. This is an automatic physiological response of Adrenal Breathing. With practice, within a minute or two (1-2 sets of 8 breaths each), the number of nerve impulses to the muscles of your hands and toes is drastically reduced and relaxation increases. Within five minutes (3-4 sets of breathing), the motor neuronal input to the muscles of your limbs diminishes and approaches zero if you are in a supine position. This effect, along with the rhythmical movement of the respiratory diaphragm, draws you into even deeper relaxation with full activation of the PNS. The mind and body is fully connected and engaged.

Immediately following the Adrenal Breathing Exercise, most individuals report a sense of calm, peace, reduced fatigue, and renewed sense of "being," a result of the mind-body connection. However, although it seems paradoxical, any *drastic* improvement in energy immediately after the exercise indicates over-exertion. Similarly, if you feel lightheaded or agitated when you first breathe this way, reduce frequency or intensity until you feel comfortable and relaxed during the entire exercise.

The key to success is persistency and consistency. Most people start reporting benefits within a few days, but it can take up to 20 or more days, depending on the degree of Adrenal Fatigue Syndrome and ANS dysfunction. Those who have a high sympathetic overtone bias or bad breathing habits will take longer to see results.

Adrenal Breathing uses basic techniques of abdominal breathing, or belly breathing, because this is where movement can be seen and felt. During inhalation, the belly expands and moves away from the back of the body toward the front (anterior). During exhalation, the opposite happens and the belly contracts and moves toward the back of the body (posterior). What makes Adrenal Breathing unique is the focus on intensity that is matched to the body's capacity.

Caution: Follow the above instructions; start slowly and work your way up. Start with 50 percent breath intensity and increase to 80 percent as tolerated.

These exercises are much more powerful than they appear, and if you're in advanced AFS (e.g., Stages 3C and 3D) you may not be able to tolerate them when you first try. Immediately reduce the intensity of each breath if you experience shortness of breath, increased pulse rate, strengthening heartbeat, or fatigue, and reduce the length of each session accordingly. Make sure you're not taking too many breaths per set, and do not hold your breath at the end of inhalation or exhalation. You should feel good after each session, not worse. Always listen to your body, and remember that overzealous breathing may trigger an adrenal crash.

Tip: Adrenal Breathing Exercises can help you relax before you go to sleep for the night, or fall back to sleep if you awaken in the middle of the night. If you cannot fall asleep, do not simply lie in bed and fret about not sleeping or passively feel the time go by. Instead, do a few sets of Adrenal Breathing Exercises.

Recommended Protocol

- **Day 1-3:** Start by doing one set (8 breaths) twice a day, once upon awakening and before breakfast and again at bedtime right before going to sleep. The sessions should take 1-2 minutes each.

- **Day 4-6:** Increase to one set five times a day: on awakening, midmorning (10-11AM), early afternoon (1-2 PM), late afternoon (4-5 PM), and at night before going to sleep.

- **Day 7-9:** Continue five times a day, but *increase from one set to two sets* each session (16 complete breaths). This should take 2-3 minutes per session.

- **Day 10-12:** Continue five times a day, but *increase from two sets to three sets* each session (24 complete breaths). This should take 3-4 minutes each session.

- **Day 13 onwards:** If you feel up to it, continue five sessions a day, but *increase from three sets to five sets* each time (40 complete breaths). This will take about 5-6 minutes per session. If you do not feel well with this intensity, decrease back down to three sets per session, but keep the five sessions a day unchanged.

Consider the protocol a general recommendation only. Those in severe Adrenal Fatigue Syndrome may not be able to progress as recommended and in fact, can get worse if they progress too quickly. Always seek professional guidance prior to beginning. A detailed audio CD on Adrenal Breathing is available from *DrLam.com*.

While you cannot overdo Adrenal Breathing, we recommend that you do not exceed five sets of breathing exercises each session and no more than five sessions a day without consulting your healthcare professional. Once you practice Adrenal Breathing, you could be ready to proceed to the more advanced adrenal stretches and restorative and rebuilding exercises to speed up your recovery process.

Advanced Adrenal Breathing Exercises

After mastering basic Adrenal Breathing, those wishing to expand the breathing capacity further may engage in mild contraction of the lower thoracic muscles during exhalation to further close the chest wall and expel the air. Mild backward contraction of the scapulas (flat bones in the back) during inhalation will also help to open the chest wall. The body remains relaxed during the entire process.

Advanced breathing using both abdominal and thoracic muscle will activate both the PNS and ANS. Because of the stimulatory component, advanced Adrenal Breathing is a good auxiliary form of strengthening the adrenal glands *only* if used at the right time. Overzealous self-navigation programs or inexperienced clinicians can use this breathing incorrectly and worsen AFS, triggering adrenal crashes.

Adrenal Restorative Exercise (ARE)

A complete Adrenal Fatigue Syndrome recovery program must incorporate techniques and exercises designed to restore the health and balance of the nervous system. Adrenal Restorative Exercise (ARE) is a set of specially designed exercises that promote deep and active relaxation. These exercises adapt established restorative yoga poses to enhance adrenal function; they focus on a key aspect of Adrenal Fatigue Syndrome, repairing the mind-body connection and restoring nervous system homeostasis.

ARE is unlike regular exercise, which directs you to focus on stretching and strengthening. For those in Adrenal Fatigue Syndrome, the regular approach leaves sufferers feeling physically strained and exhausted, and in some people this triggers adrenal crash. On the other hand, ARE is designed to help those people with Adrenal Fatigue Syndrome, for whom even gentle stretching is too active and for whom a priority is the need to restore their health and regain balance in their lives. Those with injuries, recent surgery, or prolonged and chronic physical conditions, such as high blood pressure, will find ARE a breakthrough experience.

Adrenal Restorative Exercise focuses on being—connecting the mind and body—thereby allowing signals from the mind and body to reconnect in a restorative and nurturing mode. These exercises rely on a customized sequence of specially designed postures in which your body is comfortably supported. This allows your joints to open and the muscles to relax and melt into place instead of stretching and straining into position. Blood flow to the adrenals is increased, and the nervous system switches to a calm state and a mode that promotes deep inner healing.

The Essence of Adrenal Restorative Exercise

- Promotes activation of the parasympathetic nervous system (PNS) without over-stimulating the sympathetic nervous system (SNS) or the adrenomedullary hormonal system (AHS).

- Promotes joint motility and range of motion to overcome the immobility that is common in Adrenal Fatigue Syndrome.

- Improves postures and biomechanics of the body function.

- Allows muscles to relax without worsening the catabolic (breakdown) state.

- Enhances blood flow to the adrenal glands to support recovery.

What you need and what to do:

Equipment: Soft support such as a towel, pillow, cushion, chair, or sofa. If a cushion is uncomfortable, then use a folded towel adjusted to a comfortable height. A yoga bolster is not required but is useful if your body is flexible.

Environment: A quiet room, free of distraction and noise. Clothing should be loose and not constrictive at the waist or over the rest of the body.

Breathing Technique: Use only Adrenal Breathing throughout the session. Take full breaths up to 80-90 percent of vital capacity, using the diaphragm only, with smooth, regular, rhythmic nasal breathing, imagining the air coming in through the left nostril and going out through the right nostril. Do not force any breath.

Duration: This program consists of 12 sequential positions or poses that you assume for one minute per pose for poses 1-11, and three minutes for pose number 12. The entire session takes about 15 minutes but can be as long as one hour simply by proportionately extending the amount of time spent in each pose. Beginners may start with as little as 20 seconds per pose and slowly increase the time.

Protocol: The protocol is divided into four parts, with three poses per part. It is best to perform the exercise in sequence, from 1-12.

Note: Adrenal Restorative Exercise can be too simulating for those with advanced Adrenal Fatigue Syndrome, especially during an adrenal crash. Do not start this protocol unless recommended by your healthcare professional. Stop at any point you have a sense of the body becoming overexcited, anxious, or jittery, and report the experience to your healthcare professional.

Part 1: Neck Restorative Sequence

We start ARE with relaxing the neck. The neck represents the anatomical area of the body that is critical in the overall nervous system, because this is where the major nerves and arteries branch off. Your neck muscles and your posture control the spine and set the muscular tone for the rest of your body to follow. You cannot have a relaxed body if your neck is tense. Conversely, the body cannot help but relax once the neck muscles are rested.

Pose 1: Half Lotus:
This pose focuses on neck relaxation, breathing, and calming of the body.

Sit on the floor comfortably, with your legs crossed in half lotus position (left foot touching the right inner thigh or vice versa, as you are able to perform). Beginners will find comfort by sitting on some

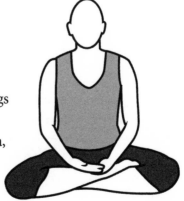

form of support (folded towel, pillow, or cushion) to prop up the hips just a bit.

Make sure the spine is straight.

Your hands are comfortably extended in front of you, with the elbows resting on the inner part of the hips or thighs. Palms are facing up.

To ensure that the neck muscles are not tense, relax and drop your shoulders. Head is straight, eyes closed. Tongue is dropped backwards.

Start Adrenal Breathing.

Tip: For maximum restorative effect, place extra support on the outside part of each knee.

Tip: If you find it difficult to sit on the floor with legs crossed, sit on a chair with your feet resting on a stool if possible. Do not cross your feet.

Pose 2: Half Lotus Variation:

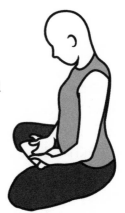

This pose focuses on neck and shoulder muscle relaxation.

While in half lotus position (pose 1), drop your head forward with eyes looking at the belly button. Now close your eyes. The back remains straight, shoulders are dropped.

Experience total relaxation of the neck as the head comfortably rests in its natural flexed position. Tongue is dropped backwards. Eyes remain closed.

Start Adrenal Breathing.

Tip: If you are doing this while sitting on a chair, place a cushion on a table and rest your forehead on the support

---

Pose 3: Child Pose:

This pose focuses on relaxation of
the neck, shoulder, and upper limbs.

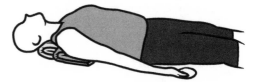

Remain on the floor (or in the chair).

Spread the knees as wide as is comfortable,
keeping the big toes touching, with knees flexed.
The back of your thigh is now resting on your calf muscles.

Bring the belly to rest between the thighs, with the forehead to the floor.

Bring the arms alongside the thighs with the palms facing upwards.
Experience the total relaxation of neck, shoulders, and upper limbs.
Shoulders are dropped. The back is still straight but not stiff.
Tongue is dropped backwards. Close your eyes.

Start Adrenal Breathing.

> **Tip:** For extra restorative effect, place support underneath your knees, between
> your thighs, and under your forehead.

Part 2: Spine Restorative Sequence

The next three poses are designed to open up the spine and properly realign
body posture. This is important because all key muscles in the body are connected
to the spine directly or indirectly. Proper spinal alignment controls muscles, and
therefore, the vessels and nerves that run through it.

Pose 4: Supported Fish Pose:

This pose focuses on expanding
the chest wall.

Fold a towel to a comfortable height and place on the floor. You can use a
thick cushion or bolster if you wish.

Lie down (supine), face up, with the upper back resting on the support.
Feet are at shoulder width, arms along the side of the body, palms up.

To support the neck, place a rolled up towel underneath the neck.

Tilt your head back, with the chin facing upwards toward the sky. The neck is hyper-extended but comfortable.

Feel how the chest wall opens up, and your lung capacity is increased.

The body is now totally relaxed. Shoulders are down. Tongue is back. Close your eyes.

Start Adrenal Breathing.

Tip: For extra restorative effect, place support beneath both knees and neck.

Pose 5: Supported Lumbar Expansion:

This pose focuses on expanding the lower back and the pelvis.

Move the support used in pose 4 to the lower back (lumbar) area. Head returns to normal position and resting comfortably on the floor, with a towel behind the neck for support as needed. Do not tilt the head.

Flex both knees, bringing the feet together, with the bottom of each foot touching the other if possible. Note how the pelvis is opening up. Tongue is back, shoulders are down, and all limbs are in a comfortable position. Close your eyes.

Start Adrenal Breathing.

Tip: For extra restorative effect, place support on the outside of each knee.

Pose 6: Supported Full Spine Expansion:

This pose focuses on the entire spine, with upper back and lower back simultaneously expanded.

Roll your towel(s) the long way, enough to reach from the shoulders to the tail bone. Lay your back over the towel, so the towel is under your entire spine. Support neck with a folded hand towel.

Open your legs to a position about shoulder width apart. Arms are extended to the side, horizontal to shoulder, with palms up. You look like a starfish. Experience the entire back curving around the raised towel from left to right. The chest wall and lumbar areas are expanded. Tongue is back, shoulders are down.

Start Adrenal Breathing.

Tip: Place your arms next to you if you find a horizontal position uncomfortable.

Part 3: Circulation Restorative Sequence

Now that the neck and shoulder muscles are relaxed (poses 1-3) and the spine is opened (poses 4-6), we are ready to restore the body's circulation to maximum flow, while removing any strain on tissues that may interfere with this process. We accomplish this by opening the two key outlets where circulation flows: the thoracic outlet and the femoral outlet.

Pose 7: Supported Bent Knee:
This pose focuses on increasing the circulation to the head.

Lie supine on the floor, with knees bent and feet resting comfortably on a sofa or chair. (A support for the lower back often helps.)

Place your arms alongside the body, palms up. The back lumbar area is resting on the floor and free of tension. Tongue is back, shoulders are down. Eyes are closed.

Start Adrenal Breathing.

Pose 8: Diagonal Thoracic and Femoral Outlet Expansion:
While in supine position with pose 7, lift and bend your left knee and place the left foot comfortably on the right thigh.

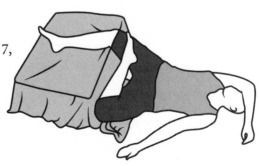

Let the left knee drop comfortably (as you can tolerate). Use extra support to prop up the bent knee. This relaxes any connective tissue impingement around the groin area (inguinal) and opens up the femoral artery, allowing maximum blood flow to the lower extremities.

Now raise your right arm, and place it over your face without impeding your breathing. The inside part of the elbow should be resting comfortably on the forehead, with palm facing down, and the forearm resting in a comfortable position. This opens up the thoracic outlet. You can actually feel the softness in the lower mid-clavicle space, that is, the area on either side of the neck. Use support to prop up any uncomfortable area(s). Tongue is back, shoulders are down. Eyes are closed.

Start Adrenal Breathing.

Pose 9: Reverse of Pose 8: Repeat the sequence using the right knee and arm.

Part 4: Mind-Body Restoration Sequence

With the neck and shoulders relaxed, the spine opened, and blood flow optimized, we come to the final sequence designed to connect the mind and body. All previous poses are designed to prepare the body for this mind-body reconnection.

Pose 10: Supported Fetal Left:
This pose focuses on the body's calm state of being. A calm mind helps us to direct our body energy toward healing to balance the nervous system and the adrenal glands.

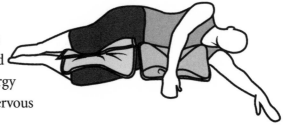

Place support on the floor and lie down on your left side in a fetal position, with the left side of the body on the support. The degree of support can vary depending on the person. Bolsters are excellent tools. Place additional support like a pillow between your knees.

Both arms are in a comfortable position. Head is supported. Abdominal wall is unimpeded. Tongue is back, shoulders are down. Eyes are closed.

Start Adrenal Breathing.

Pose 11: Supported Fetal Right: Repeat Pose 10 on your right side.

Pose 12: Deep Relaxation (In traditional yoga, this is also called Savasana or Corpse Pose): This is the last and most important of all 12 restorative exercises. It is also the most difficult pose to do well, but the most vital to perform correctly. This exercise promotes total body calm.

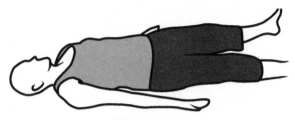

Lie down on the back, letting the feet fall out to either side. Bring the arms alongside, but slightly separated from the body, palms facing up. Relax the whole body, including the face. Let the body feel heavy.

The position of the head is crucial. Keep your chin even with the forehead or slightly lower, which is a relaxed position. (When the head is tilted back, the position is stimulating and, therefore, undesirable.) The tongue is back, shoulders are down, and the eyes are closed.

Start Adrenal Breathing.

To come out, first begin to deepen the breath, and then awaken the body by moving your fingers and toes.

Bring the knees into the chest. Turn to the right side and slowly sit up. (Do not abruptly rise from a supine to a standing position as this may lead to dizziness.)

Note: Stay in this position three times longer than all other poses. For example, if you stay one minute per pose from pose 1-11, then stay 3 minutes for pose 12.

Adrenal Yoga Exercise

Some individuals mistakenly believe that yoga is a religion, but though it developed centuries ago in India, it is not a form of Hinduism. Modern yoga dates back to the late nineteenth century, and today, Christians, Buddhists, Jews, Muslims, and many other groups, even agnostics and atheists, happily practice yoga. Certainly, a spiritual side to yoga exists, but we don't need to subscribe to any particular belief to benefit.

Those without a particular religious bent often speak of the inner or human spirit or the highest self, concepts that affirm the value of life.

We recommend yoga for AFS because it is a systematic technology to improve the body, understand the mind, and free the spirit. Overall, yoga practitioners tend to be more flexible, stronger, more energetic, thinner, and more youthful than others, and all these attributes are welcome and desirable in Adrenal Fatigue Syndrome recovery.

Yoga practice leads to strengthening and calming the nervous system, thereby balancing the dysfunctional stress-response system we see in AFS sufferers. Blood flow to internal organs is increased, and the body delivers more oxygen to the adrenal glands, which promotes healing. Equally important, yoga practice helps clear mental clutter—mind chatter—that interferes with finding clarity and even helps in listening to the voices of intuition and creativity.

Yoga practice cultivates spiritual and physical muscles, which over time, leads to greater happiness, less anxiety, and greater peace. Because yoga builds on itself, it becomes more effective over time. It is equivalent to learning how to play a musical instrument: The longer you stick with it and practice, the better you become and the more benefits you reap.

Adrenal Yoga takes the best of *traditional* yoga and modifies it to suit those with Adrenal Fatigue Syndrome. For example, certain stretching and strengthening exercises known as asanas are removed, because they can stimulate the SNS, along with certain breathing techniques known as pranayama that can trigger a release of adrenaline. On the other hand, posture and lung capacity are improved as are bowel function, lymphatic draining, and the function of the immune system.

Gradually, one feels more balanced and the body is better able to endure the inevitable stress of daily living. Therefore, Adrenal Yoga is about restoring internal balance, and with balance, internal control. It is not about physical flexibility. We see many individuals with Adrenal Fatigue Syndrome who are already quite flexible. It is not about increasing strength, as many men and women are strong and still suffer from Adrenal Fatigue Syndrome. Adrenal Yoga enables us to transform liabilities such as fear, inability to relax, low energy, anxiety, and depression into strength, giving the person more control and a more balanced feeling. Here are the levels of Adrenal Yoga:

- Beginning Adrenal Yoga focuses on breathing and stretching. This forms the foundation of internal control.

- Intermediate Adrenal Yoga focuses on strength and toning. This serves to reverse the catabolic state and stabilize metabolic function.

- Adrenal Yoga focuses on fluidity and control. This serves to fine tune internal body homeostasis.

Note: Adrenal Yoga consists of 21 sessions and is available on DVD at *www.DrLam.com.*

Regular Yoga

When you are ready to do yoga in a commercial yoga studio, health club, gym or local Y, or you choose to follow a DVD at home, remember that you are still recovering from AFS and, as such, building your reserves. We recommend choosing a level of yoga that challenges you and goes beyond what you have accomplished with Adrenal Yoga. However, we've observed a tendency to be overly aggressive, and even with yoga, this kind of pushing can trigger adrenal crash. Whether you are practicing yoga at home or in an outside setting, the following tips may help you avoid any backlash or injury:

- In your poses, find an edge for yourself where you are challenged but not overwhelmed. At this edge, practice maintaining a clear, open, and accepting mental state.

- Give yourself permission to rest when you feel overworked.

- Pay close attention to what you are saying to yourself as you practice, and make an intentional effort to appreciate your own efforts and innate goodness.

- Faithfully go to class or practice at home. If you practice outside your home, arrive at the class early to give yourself time to talk to others in the class.

- Realize that the development of qualities like patience, discipline, wisdom, right effort, kindness, gratitude, and many others will arise from your yoga practice. These qualities create a steady and soft mind.

- Find a teacher who offers a balance of gentleness and firmness and whose teaching inspires you to practice from your highest self.

Recognize that simply attending class is a major statement of courage, self-care, and positive momentum. Realize that you are inspiring others as you become truer to your deepest desires.

Power Yoga

Power yoga represents an advanced form of yoga that focuses on the core strength. Power yoga is a general term used in the West to describe a vigorous, fitness-based approach to yoga, generally modeled on the Ashtanga practice style. The term *power yoga* came into common usage in the mid 1990s, when several yoga teachers sought ways to make Ashtanga yoga more accessible to western students. However, unlike Ashtanga, power yoga does not follow a set series of poses. Therefore, power yoga classes can vary widely from one to the next, but what they share is their emphasis on strength and flexibility.

Power yoga heralded the current popularity of yoga in the U.S. and brought it to studios and gyms all over the country, especially because so many individuals began to see yoga as a way to work out. Back in the 1950s and '60s, gentler forms of yoga became popular in the U.S., which gradually led to its wide availability. Power yoga has its greatest appeal among those who are already quite fit and enjoy exercise. With consistent practice, muscle definition becomes prominent, toning is enhanced, and strength is improved.

Another Component: Aerobics

As you probably know, aerobic exercise includes long duration and slow paced activities such as walking, slow jogging, rowing, cycling (including slow cycling), and any other form of exercise that involves endurance. This type of exercise will help decrease cortisol levels and aid in burning body fat as well. Aerobic exercise benefits those who have stressed adrenal glands in the early stages, where cortisol output is high. However, keep in mind the following principles:

- Intense aerobic exercise can also worsen adrenal function. Those with advanced adrenal weakness should not consider any activities more strenuous than walking (or exercise recommended by their healthcare provider). Excessive aerobic activities drain the body of already low energy reserves.

- We recommend that those in advanced Adrenal Fatigue Syndrome avoid all aerobic activities other than walking. Frequency and duration varies from person to person. Some in advanced stages might be able to tolerate only five minutes of walking every other day.

- We generally introduce aerobic exercise carefully and slowly as recovery returns to Stage 3B. Then, as Adrenal Fatigue Syndrome improves to Stage 3A and later Stage 2, the frequency and intensity can be increased.

As you can see, we consider it a goal in AFS recovery to return to exercise and develop the mind and body from the core through a series of systematic gentle exercises. Those who take these exercises seriously will be happy to know that many have gone from a bedridden state to running long distance races within a short time after starting with us, and an important tool used in their recovery and training were the exercises we mention and describe here. Exercise is part of what we know as, and consider to be, "regular" life.

Relationships also are a component of normal life, but relationships can be stressful, too. In the next chapter, we talk about the way relationships can interfere with AFS recovery.

Key Points to Remember

- Exercise is an important tool for AFS recovery, but it has to be done right. Engaging in the wrong exercise regimen can often trigger adrenal crashes.

- Those with advanced AFS must be careful in exercise progression, starting with Adrenal Breathing Exercise, progressing to Adrenal Restorative Exercise, and then ending with Adrenal Yoga Exercise.

- When properly done, one should not feel drained after exercise.

- Most of us do not sufficiently appreciate the healing power of breathing. Adrenal breathing is the most important exercise for many in advanced stages. This is different from other types of exercise in that it helps to lower sympathetic tone while enhancing parasympathetic response.

- Aerobics and power yoga exercise can be added to the overall exercise program as AFS recovery proceeds.

Chapter 28

Your Relationships Influence Adrenal Fatigue Syndrome

Earlier, we discussed the mind-body connection, and now that you understand more about it, and about Adrenal Fatigue Syndrome, you likely can see how important the mind is in maintaining and enjoying good health. In the past, this has often been overlooked. Neuroscience research has now proven beyond a doubt that the mind and the body are connected. Nothing affects the mind more than our relationships, because unpleasant or dysfunctional relationships cause enormous emotional stress.

Chronic stress is the leading cause of Adrenal Fatigue Syndrome, and as you know, stressors come in all shapes and sizes, so to speak, including physical, emotional, or financial. Those who regularly physically over-exert, such as serious professional or even amateur athletes, are at high risk of developing AFS. However, as athletes learn through experience, the effects of physical stress can usually be reversed and the body nurtured back to health with rest and other measures. Other stressors, such as overwork, poor diet, and overexertion, usually act as underlying triggers of adrenal crashes. However, we've also noted that in and of itself, financial distress is seldom the root stressor cause of AFS.

Emotional and mental stress and distress represent the most common stressors that contribute to AFS. Issues related to unresolved toxic relationships usually cause such stress because they gradually wear our bodies down over time. We have found it truly amazing how much your emotional health can influence your physical health. As we've said, advanced AFS can be considered a mind-body disorder in its broadest sense. A strong mind-body connection is a powerful healing force we can harness to improve and maintain health. However, on the flipside, as in Adrenal Fatigue Syndrome, the mind-body connection can also have a devastating negative force that's capable of ruining your body.

Those who are in advanced AFS will tell you how easy it is to have an adrenal crash after a heated debate or an unpleasant encounter, especially if it is with someone close to you. Your adrenaline starts pumping, anxiety sets in, heart rate goes up, force of heart beat goes up, you become drained, and quickly become bedridden.

Clearly, maintaining a good relationship with those around you is conducive to the healing process.

Numerous studies support the belief that individuals with an upbeat and positive perspective tend to be healthier and enjoy longer lives than those who take a gloomy and cynical attitude about the future. We now see an emerging influence factor, *epigeneticism*, which contends that environmental factors such as diet and stress influence the expression of your genes.

> Remember that the *expression* of your genes, not the genes themselves, dictate whether you develop certain diseases. For example, if you have *constitutionally* weak adrenal glands, stress may cause this weakness to be expressed, which then leads to Adrenal Fatigue Syndrome. On the other hand, the absence of stress can delay the expression of this weakness for an indefinite period.

As you age, your genes do not change, but your epigenome changes dramatically. It is influenced by how you react to physical and emotional stresses. Virtually everything that happens in your environment, from something as amorphous as climate change to something as specific as marriage, ultimately affects your epigenome. Everyday issues such as the building up to taking final exams or the lingering effects of childhood abuse, also influence your epigenome.

Relationships and Well-being

Relationships also influence the expression of your genes and have a direct impact on your tendency to either avoid or develop unpleasant conditions, from heart palpitations to Adrenal Fatigue Syndrome to depression. For example, studies have shown:

- Heart surgery patients with strong spiritual and social support have a mortality rate 1/7th of those who do not have these advantages.

- Meditating for just 30 minutes a day can be as effective as the use of antidepressants.

- Elderly people with positive attitudes have an over 20 percent reduction in risk of death from cardiovascular disease and over 50 percent lower risk of death from all other causes.

We can clearly see that the ability to build positive mental attitudes greatly affects your physical health, and this applies to Adrenal Fatigue Syndrome. In fact, if emotional stressors are present but not resolved, they impede recovery.

It can be liberating to know that the ability to manifest positive emotions and happiness is perhaps one of our greatest human characteristics. You needn't feel bad because you're getting older or are tired much of the time, or because your life isn't going exactly as you had planned. Once you make your mind up to be happy, you really don't have to feel bad for any reason at all. In addition, if you view it from a positive perspective, AFS might turn out to be one of the best things that has happened to you.

A Wakeup Call

For many, AFS serves as a much needed wakeup call, signaling that one or more areas of life are out of balance or misaligned. Addressing Adrenal Fatigue Syndrome often becomes the starting point for an exploration of life at a deeper level. For some, this involves recognizing the role of toxic relationships.

Day to day, most of us tend to live superficially, and we may need a significant wakeup call, such as AFS, to nudge us to live at a much deeper level. This often involves understanding the body and mind from a spiritual perspective, perhaps relearning and focusing on what we once knew about the truly important things in life—inner peace, love, forgiveness, contentment, and so forth.

No matter how tempting to believe otherwise, Adrenal Fatigue Syndrome, or any serious condition, can't merely be dismissed or handled with a quick fix. If you try for a fast and easy path, you not only fail, you also likely miss the great blessings of self evaluation and the rewards waiting for you when you take the time to reorder your life. We always recommend using AFS as a tool to learn to really listen to and get to know your body, along with rediscovering the broader meaning of your life.

Gaining insight into ourselves and our healing process also means cultivating subtle changes in our thinking and attitudes. For example, we need to transform superficial concerns that focus on negative thinking and feeling like a victim to attitudes that value serenity and peace, no matter how painful the circumstances of the moment. Bear in mind that having a positive attitude is not about being happy all the time, and part of being happy involves accepting that you'll feel down at times.

Although we already have the full potential to be happy, and we control our capacity for happiness, most of us find it extremely difficult. At any given time, the majority of people are unhappy with one thing or another in their lives, from their homes to their jobs to their incomes. However, of all possible challenges and concerns, relationship difficulties remain the most difficult to overcome.

A Barrier to Healing

In the process of examining your life, it's also essential to develop the willingness and strength to let go of toxic and harmful relationships. Again and again, we've seen that AFS patients must heal the mind before the body can fully heal, because the mind controls the body. If we carry emotional baggage, we need to discard it and lighten our emotional load. Since much emotional baggage results from difficult relationships, we need to address them. If we don't, we won't see the mind-body healing we desire.

Of course, at some point, our important long-term relationships, including marriage, family, and close friendships, encounter rough patches involving disagreements and disappointments. Deepening relationship bonds during difficult times and growing through the experience is a hallmark of emotional maturity.

On the other hand, we must face that some relationships are just plain toxic. No matter how we try to work through troubles, conflict and friction poison the well and we and the other person continue to be hurt, and at least one person ends up in an emotional desert.

To be in a toxic relationship doesn't necessarily mean that the individuals involved are bad. Rather, it's more likely that the individuals are a bad fit, and goodness or badness isn't the issue. When personal styles clash, a toxic relationship often develops. Perhaps good chemistry existed at one point, but over time, and perhaps because important events intervened, the people involved changed, thus altering the relationship. This is all part of the human experience. Still, although no one is to blame, the relationship is toxic all the same.

Relationships you consider toxic put your emotional health at risk. Perhaps the other people involved have short tempers, mood swings, inconsistent behavior, or are impulsive and in denial about their behavior. Or, they might admit to behaving badly, but then never try to correct their ways. Sometimes, this kind of toxic relationship can be quite abusive, even if the bad behavior is limited to thoughtless or hostile words. At times, one partner may show only shallow feelings for the other person, or they refuse to engage in meaningful discussion, but instead, threaten to break off the relationship. Some individuals withdraw and withhold their concern and love, leaving the others feeling left out in the cold.

Overall, a person who is toxic to you no longer cares about the marriage, partnership, or friendship and for various reasons remains self-centered. Typically, toxic individuals manipulate their companions and situations to keep a one-up-one-down, dependent relationship and use shame, insult, and sarcasm as weapons against others. Then they look down on the very people they're abusing; this kind of treatment of other people is emotionally abusive and far more common than we may realize.

If you're in the midst of a toxic relationship, isn't it true that you have found yourself chronically tired and angry, and perhaps even frightened? You might constantly be nervous about finding a safe or unsafe time to talk to your partner, or you may question your right to express yourself.

All abusive relationships are by definition toxic. Unfortunately, many individuals stay in these relationships because they have forgotten their rights and options. This kind of low self-esteem can come from depression, fear of loneliness, or harmful threats from an abusive partner. Some probably no longer believe that their lives could improve if they left the toxic relationship behind.

Sadly, marriages and long term partnerships can become abusive over time. It seems that suddenly, the relationship has deteriorated. Some individuals become subtly conditioned to being badly treated, and may forget that the behavior going on in their relationships and home is truly abusive. However, danger signs invariably appear. Here are some important signs to watch for and consider.

Your partner:

- separates you from your family, friends, and children;
- keeps watch over you;
- publically or privately verbally abuses you;
- dominates you and the entire household, not leaving space for your desires and preferences;
- blames you for ruining the relationship and tries to make you change to make things work; and/or
- controls you by being overly possessive and overpowering.

Meanwhile, you:

- begin to believe your own thoughts, words, opinions, and accomplishments have little or no value anymore;
- lose your individual self identity as you depend more on your partner, and you may no longer have confidence that you can survive without him/her;

- become afraid to tell the truth for fear of upsetting your partner; and/or

- find your self esteem has plummeted to a low level as you absorb your partner's abusive remarks meant to make you feel worthless and unattractive.

Emotions and Toxic Relationships

Some specific emotions help people evaluate their relationships. In addition, these feelings may sneak up, so to speak, and only when they see a list or someone asks pointed questions do they suddenly say, "Hey, that's me. That's how I feel much of the time." Like AFS itself, this realization is its own wakeup call. Consider if any of the following currently relate to you:

- Unsupported
- Dissatisfied
- Fearful
- Exasperated
- Depleted/Drained
- Unaccepted/Unrewarded
- Judged
- Guilty
- Tired
- Angry
- Untrusting
- Unequal
- Stifled
- Shamed
- Stressed

Recognizing a Toxic Relationship Cycle

Most of us want to find love and intimacy, but we're also afraid of being hurt; we worry about making a commitment, but we dread abandonment. The feelings around commitment and fear of abandonment are also known as anxiety. The relationship comfort zone is flanked by highly individual behavior patterns, which are not close enough to trigger *fusion anxiety*, nor too distant to trigger separation *anxiety*. We formed these boundaries in our childhood and unless we bring them into the realm of our conscious awareness we seldom change. Our boundaries are capable of creating positive patterns, of course, but they also create patterns that can lead to a toxic relationship cycle.

In a toxic relationship cycle, power struggles arise again and again, but no solutions are found. Intimacy turns into conflict, which then leads to anxiety, often triggering fear of loss. These anxieties and fears trigger arguments that end with hurt feelings and withdrawal. Though withdrawal might bring temporary relief, it ultimately turns into feelings of isolation and loneliness, thus setting off anxieties about abandonment. We often see this separation anxiety leading to new declarations and proposals, which renew intimacy; the couple (even couples involved in truly abusive relationships) goes through a *honeymoon* period. However, this closeness soon triggers fusion anxiety and trouble starts all over again, thus initiating another repetition of cyclical behavior.

In terms of AFS, each time the cycle occurs, the adrenals take another beating. With each stress, the adrenal glands increase their demand for cortisol. With time, this output eventually declines, and symptoms of Adrenal Fatigue Syndrome surface.

When couples fail to understand the cycles they go through, they often forget the positive elements in their relationship. Many relationship problems are the product of varying comfort zone settings. When one person hits one side of the comfort zone boundary and is already experiencing fusion anxiety, the other person might just be following his/her desirable depth of intimacy. As the first person reverses direction and comes back into the comfort zone, the partner might feel abandoned; their mutual anxiety explodes and accusations are thrown back and forth.

If we don't understand the role of anxiety in relationships, we're likely condemning ourselves to constant hurt. However, if we try to face our anxiety, we can alter the comfort zone boundaries and transform our relationship into a healthy, mutually reinforcing growth process. In such a relationship not only does our sense of self grow, but also the couple-bond tends to deepen.

In order to change a static comfort zone relationship into an actively growing relationship, we must train ourselves to stop in the middle of a conflict and engage in self awareness. We can ask questions like:

- How did this fight start?
- What am I anxious about?
- What about this situation feels so threatening?

Using these questions allows us to forge a path to self-knowledge and deeper peace in our relationships. Intimate relationships awaken our deepest anxieties, and therefore, if we use them intelligently, relationships have the capacity to help us grow as individuals.

When Removing Yourself Is Needed

The positive possibilities notwithstanding, it is also true that some relationships do not have the potential for growth, at least not without significant commitment to change. As we all know, we can't change other people, so one-sided commitment is not necessarily enough. In fact, being around a toxic person for a long time might greatly decrease self-worth, along with capability and competence. For this reason, you must stop the harm caused by another person (or more than one person); only then can you determine if a relationship can be maintained or must be ended.

First, recognize that if your life is distressing, only you can change the situation. Here are some tips on how to live a better life by nullifying the negative influence of toxic relationships:

- **Take Responsibility:** Understand that some part of you is contributing to the negative—toxic—behaviors. Then, ask yourself why you're willing to allow the behaviors to continue. What can you learn from your own behavior?

- **Set Boundaries:** Let your partner know that you won't be bullied or ignored. Describe what changes you want and tell your partner your expectations for the future.

- **Forgive:** Remember that individuals generally are not born toxic. Our environment and circumstances over time mold us into who we are. Regain your sense of the good in the person beneath the surface toxicity. Regardless of the ultimate outcome, learn to forgive and return love; we believe this is our primary purpose on earth. When possible, use love to heal one another.

- **List the positive characteristics of the person:** If you focus only on negative characteristics, the person will be negative whenever he/she is around you. By altering your focus, you influence the other person's behavior for the better.

- **See a new perspective from a neutral party:** Counselors, coaches, neighbors, or co-workers are individuals who likely have no bias for or against your relationship, whereas relatives and close friends may well have strong opinions one way or another. The key is to avoid creating a situation that triggers pity. You want another person to help you focus on the situation, examine the part you have played, and determine what you are willing to do to move forward.

- **End the relationship:** If nothing changes after you have tried all other constructive steps, you can walk away from your relationship with your head held high. You know you have tried to change the relationship but have also protected yourself from further harm.

Unless you transform or remove the negative toxic relationships from your life, you will generate the constant negative energy flow needed to sustain the toxicity. Clearly, this situation prevents healing Adrenal Fatigue Syndrome. The key to healing is first to recognize that the toxic negative energy must be transformed and rechanneled into the constructive energy needed to heal, and in the long run that will change your life for the better.

Key Points to Remember

- Relationships and well-being go hand in hand.

- Stressors come in all kinds. Emotional and mental stress tops the list, with toxic relationships being one of the most common contributors.

- Recognizing a toxic relationship is an important step to finding love and intimacy.

- In a toxic relationship, power struggles arise again and again, but no solutions are found.

- If a toxic relationship cannot be resolved, you must remove yourself by setting boundaries and taking responsibility for yourself. Terminate the relationship if needed.

Chapter 29

Managing Adrenal Crashes
and Recovery

Because adrenal crashes are invariably part of the recovery process, it is imperative that we have a comprehensive plan in place specifically to handle crashes and subsequent recovery. This chapter focuses on special tools and other considerations we use to minimize crashes and maximize the recovery potential.

The key to successfully managing an adrenal crash entails efforts to reduce the velocity and intensity of the crash, and to administer the right nutrients at the right time in order to propel the system into stabilization and follow up recovery as soon as possible. *Minor* adrenal crashes in Stages 1 and 2 usually go unnoticed, but all crashes are noticeable in Stages 3 and 4 of Adrenal Fatigue Syndrome. Crashes involving a loss of 30 percent (level 3 or higher) or more of pre-crash energy are considered major events and can be devastating at any stage.

As AFS advances, the body has less reserve, and the crashes are faster in onset and intensity, if all else is equal. The same stressor that takes a few days to trigger a crash in those with Stages 1 and 2 may take only a few hours or minutes to cause the same damage in those with Stage 3 and 4 Adrenal Exhaustion. In the later stages, symptoms become greatly magnified as well. Effective crash management requires individualized attention. What might be right for one person might actually make another person worse.

We must address the following key areas during crash management:

- *Physical Activity:* Usually, sufferers immediately reduce unnecessary physical activity and increase rest. It is important to adjust activity levels to match the energy state of the body during the crash. Those in early AFS may actually find exercising invigorating because exercise increases adrenaline release and improves blood circulation. Those with more advanced AFS, on the other hand, may find any attempt to exercise draining, to say the least. Some can still walk and perform household chores, while others need to take time off and rest. For those with the most severe AFS, bed rest is the only option. In general, all exercise should be reduced and followed by adequate post-exercise rest. Over exercise can drain the body, leading to delayed recovery. While we caution against over-exercise, complete bed rest is not necessarily the best path either.

It's helpful to begin a personalized program of Adrenal Restorative Exercises and Adrenal Breathing Exercises (described earlier in Chapter 27, *Adrenal Fatigue Syndrome and Healing Exercise*). Because the body is sensitive to even the slightest stress, to avoid triggering further crashes, sufferers must be careful to adjust the intensity and frequency of these exercises to match the body's state. Improper breathing techniques, such as holding the breath for prolonged periods or breathing too deeply, can also increase sympathetic tone and worsen existing crashes.

• *Dietary Adjustments:* Hypoglycemia and metabolic imbalances are common during an adrenal crash (Stages 3+), so sufferers must focus their diet on stabilizing blood sugar by balancing the amount of macronutrients (carbohydrate, protein, and fat). In addition, gastric assimilation is often compromised during a crash, so it is important to consider the best way to deliver the macronutrients for maximize absorption. For example, raw milk (where permitted) may be superior to regular milk, and raw egg is better than cooked egg in such cases.

Those who have had severe crashes might not be able to tolerate regular food; these individuals often need to be on a diet of soups (Chapter 24, *Soups and Juicing for Health*) for foundational nutritional support. Those who are in late, severe AFS stages might actually need to be hospitalized and given total parenteral nutrition, where nutrients are delivered directly into the bloodstream.

• *Electrolyte Adjustments:* Salt craving is a common symptom of AFS and can be caused by the sodium imbalance that results from hormonal dysfunction. This imbalance is usually worse during a crash, so to avoid exacerbating the situation, rebalancing must be carefully controlled. Too much sodium relative to water may lead to hypertension and too little water may lead to dehydration, thereby compounding the crash. Too much water relative to sodium may lead to inadequate sodium in the blood. All are undesirable and may be problematic. Unfortunately, laboratory values may be normal during the crash and may or may not be abnormal until the crash is well advanced or much later.

Those on diuretics or other medications and who also have a history of high blood pressure need to be especially careful. Symptoms such as nausea, vomiting, headache, malaise, and foggy thinking are common. Severe cases may need hospital admission.

• *Nutritional Supplement Adjustments:* Taking nutrients during an adrenal crash requires great care, because AFS can worsen if patients blindly take the same dosage of supplements *during* a crash as they took *before* the crash. The body is in a very different state during a crash. For example, animals under stress need up to ten times more vitamin C than they normally do.

Various factors determine the amount of key nutrients needed during a crash, including: biological constitution, clearance state, history of paradoxical reactions, and autonomic nervous system sensitivity. There is no one-size-fits-all recommendation, because none exists. For this reason, we recommend you consult your health practitioner for supplementation recommendation when you are experiencing a crash.

Trial and Error

During a crash, the body first goes through a series of adaptations in order to return to homeostasis. When this fails, various internal emergency systems are automatically activated. The more intense the crash, the more such response becomes evident and exaggerated. As the crash progresses, unpleasant and paradoxical symptoms worsen as fatigue accelerates. At the peak of the crash, one may become bedridden for days or even weeks.

Except for those who have very weak constitutions or unresolved stressors, usually the body is eventually able to regain some level of internal control with time. It then enters a stabilization period, followed by a preparation period before the body starts its honeymoon period of recovery.

During the crash, the body is actually hungry for more nutrients to overcome stress, and in its effort to soften the crash, much internal reserve is used and metabolized. Once used, nutrients need to be replenished as quickly as possible, and we may need to consider additional nutrients to support the body during this time. Unfortunately, during AFS, the body is usually also in a low clearance state. In an effort to conserve remaining energy, many organ systems enter a slow down mode. The result is that there is further weakness in gastric absorption and reduced rate of liver detoxification. As excretory capacity is compromised, breakdown byproducts accumulate within the body and can turn toxic. Symptoms such as brain fog, joint pain, muscle ache, and so forth, are more common and intense.

This forms a vicious cycle. If not properly managed, things can get worse quickly. In particular, if extra nutrients are administered during a time of stress and low clearance, a variety of toxic and paradoxical reactions may arise. In other words, instead of getting better, the crash worsens.

Because crashes are inherently complex, expect some trial and error even in the best of hands, because the underlying physiology is still poorly understood. On the other hand, although an adrenal crash is one of the most difficult events to manage in AFS, we often see a silver lining.

Recovery Management

The adrenal crash phase usually takes a few hours to a few days to complete its course. It is one of the most dreaded experiences. The ensuing recovery phase, however, usually takes much longer—often weeks and sometimes months. Those with weak constitutions are especially vulnerable to an overall delayed recovery phase. This is why it is critically important during any recovery program to avoid crashes at all times. There are no good crashes, as every crash is damaging to the body. We are proactive in our program to prevent crashes rather than reactive and play catch-up afterwards. The absence of crashes is, therefore, a sign of good recovery.

The main focus of adrenal crash management involves reducing crash intensity and duration, analogous to quickly assembling a safety net to soften the harsh landing of a person falling. On the other hand, in recovery management our focus involves providing the body with enough tools for it to heal itself.

> Adrenal recovery management is analogous to leading a blind man across a stream, wisely moving slowly and gently. One foot is always ahead trying to feel where and how secure the next rock is before actually putting body weight on it. That is how one avoids falling into the water, or in the case of adrenal recovery, crashing again. There is nothing worse than rolling crashes, where one crash is followed by another one. In such cases, the body hardly gets a chance to recover properly.

For sure, the recovery process is a long distance run, not a sprint. It requires systematic planning, training, testing, and allowing for setbacks. Imagine training for a marathon. At first you may simply walk to the finish line to gauge your energy reserve when you have completed the course. If that is successful, you then slowly work to higher speeds. Most successful marathon training programs stress a gradual approach, with intermittent challenge runs along the way to gauge your body's reserve and energy level. The recovery plan from adrenal crashes is similar.

The body is not a light switch that can be turned on and off at will. AFS often takes years to develop, so it may need ample time to heal itself. Some mistakenly focus on a speedy recovery, usually through the use of stimulatory compounds or medications. That ignores the more important goal and concept of rebuilding the underlying reserve. Pushing the body ahead of its readiness is a recipe for future crashes and recovery failure.

A successful recovery management program incorporates the following factors:

Stabilization immediately after an adrenal crash: After a severe crash has occurred, the body goes into a period of stabilization. It is important to manage the body well at this time. Emergency systems triggered during the crash need to be deactivated by reducing the frequency of alarm signal activation. This is best accomplished by properly adjusting diet, lifestyle, and nutritional supplementation to match the functional level of the adrenal system. Although this varies from person to person, we may need more nutrients at certain times and fewer at others. As the body stabilizes, paradoxical reactions gradually resolve and the low clearance state improves. As a result, follow up crashes are less easily triggered.

Prepare the body for the honeymoon period: After stabilization, we evaluate and examine various dysfunctional systems, starting with the most prominent dysregulation. For example, those who have ovarian-adrenal-thyroid (OAT) axis imbalance may be thyroid dominant, meaning their primary symptoms are more related to thyroid dysfunction than ovarian or adrenal irregularity. Similarly, some may have dominant adrenals, prominent sympathetic symptoms, and adrenaline rushes. These individuals are wired-and-tired, a symptom of ANS imbalance.

As much as possible, the priority is to help the body heal the most damaged system. The total recovery process is only as strong as the weakest link. Identifying the most damaged system and prioritizing treatment is, therefore, important.

At times, fatigue can be so overwhelming that sufferers and doctors tend to focus only on regaining energy instead of fixing the underlying dominant dysfunction. It's tempting to fix the worse symptom, usually fatigue, but short term improvement doesn't help identify the weakest link. In fact, it is often masked. For example, low energy could result from low blood sugar or electrolyte imbalance, but these can have different root causes. Low blood sugar can point to metabolic dysregulation;

electrolyte imbalance could point to aldosterone insufficiency. So, boosting energy alone is not going to help the adrenal recover over time.

Most people present multiple symptoms that require careful analysis. If energy is good in the morning, but fatigue sets in late in the afternoon, then modulating the blood sugar level is a priority. This is in contrast to taking steroids or other stimulants to prop up energy levels. Without proper normalization, the body struggles every day to maintain homeostasis, and lacks reserves to rebuild itself. As a result, it is unable to enter the honeymoon phase with vigor, and recovery will invariably be delayed or fail over time. Those who fail to prepare and plan for a sustained recovery are in effect preparing themselves to fail.

Take properly dosed nutrients to match adrenal function for recovery: In addition to identifying the most prominent dysfunction for action, it is important to note that such dominance can change along the recovery path. A good clinician is always on the lookout for this. For example, we may see a prolonged period of stabilization without significant improvement and then suddenly the person improves. The body may also go through sudden turbulent periods for no apparent reasons, reacting erratically and negatively to a once helpful supplement. Astute clinicians need to be on special alert to quickly adjust nutrients to match the body's specific needs each step along the way. Identifying and titrating nutrient dosages is more of an art than a science, and requires extensive clinical experience.

Prevent follow up crashes that can set back the internal homeostasis: One of the hallmarks of successful recovery is the absence of follow up crashes. Those with advanced AFS or weak constitutions simply cannot afford any crashes at all. The worst recovery pattern possible is the fast recovery followed by many rolling crashes. Therefore, the primary goal is to avoid crashes by giving the body extra supports so that its marginal reserve is increased. The speed of recovery takes a back seat in favor of steady recovery. Nutrient doses that are too large increase the energy, but carry a higher risk of adrenal crash. Multiple crashes over time are a sign of poor recovery, so we make every effort to avoid them.

Prepare a set of tools to prevent, abort, or soften future crashes: Not all nutrients are treated the same way by the body. The adrenal recovery nutritional toolbox should have a good mix of all. The strong ones need to be identified, and used sparingly, while gentle nutrients can be used more frequently. Those particularly well suited for emergency situations are identified and set aside. They form an emergency nutritional kit that the sufferer can reach out to in case of crashes. Having such a kit handy has helped many avoid and better manage their crashes.

A Closer Look at the Recovery

During the *stabilization/plateau period* many patients become discouraged and impatient when their energy levels are not immediately restored. This can go on for months. They believe they are merely treading water. This is perhaps one of the most frustrating times. Many give up on their doctor because they do not feel any improvement.

> It must be remembered that the adrenals secrete over 50 different hormones; some act quickly, while others take time. Energy is not the only parameter of recovery, and patience is required. Quick fix stimulants and aggressive use of nutrients put patients at risk of crashes. Driving up energy without proper counterbalances will eventually lead to an overall weaker state of adrenal function.

After each mini-recovery cycle up, we like to see a plateau period, similar to the stabilization period, but it happens only after the honeymoon period and not after an adrenal crash. It is prudent to allow the body to rest during the plateau. After rest and consolidation of energy at this level, the body will be ready for the preparation period, that is, a time to get ready for the next honeymoon period of adrenal recovery. If we don't allow the body this plateau phase, we increase the risk of subsequent crashes.

Resetting State

Oftentimes during the recovery phase, the body may go through a period where it tries to reset and kick start itself for reasons we don't completely understand. Perhaps it is nature's last resort to try to help itself when all else fails. During a crash, the body often goes into an emergency mode. This resetting may be part of the delayed survival mechanism that activates automatically. If resetting occurs, the timing varies from person to person. As we've said, during the resetting, the body suddenly behaves differently for no apparent reason.

This is a turbulent time for the body and is discouraging for patients who may not know what to do next. The resetting state usually occurs sometime during the late initial stabilization period, late in the plateau period, or sometime during the preparation periods of subsequent mini-recovery cycles.

Duration of Adrenal Recovery Phase and Recovery Factor (RF)

So, how long does recovery take?

No single answer exists, but we can say that the length of the recovery phase varies because it is dependent on the stage of AFS. The more advanced the AFS, the longer the recovery phase.

Recovery factor (RF) is a quantitative measurement of the length of the recovery phase relative to the duration of the crash phase. RF is a numerical number derived by dividing the recovery time by the crash time.

If the crash duration is one day and the subsequent recovery time to return to the immediate pre-crash baseline is four days, then RF = 4/1 = 4. In other words, it takes the body four times longer to recover relative to the length of the crash. The more severe the crash and the more advanced the AFS, the larger the number. Those in Stage 3C or higher frequently have a recovery factor of 10 or more. In other words, it takes more than 10 days to recover from one day of crash. You can see why we are so vigilant in preventing crashes.

When Good News Turns Bad

Unfortunately, programs using stimulatory compounds (natural or prescription) may appear to bring about improvement for a short time, and sufferers are misled into believing they've found the right path. Invariably, symptoms return and are worse, and a more severe second crash occurs, which continues the downward cascade of symptoms. The body weakens as additional crashes occur. These crashes propel the body into advanced stages of Adrenal Fatigue Syndrome that could have been avoided if a good recovery program had been followed early on.

Those who do not pay attention to the lessons learned from the recovery phase invariably will miss important clinical perils and thus lack a plan to handle future crashes. The result is a body that is subjected to repeated crashes over time.

Understanding the crash and recovery cycle in detail and their characteristics will help the clinician and sufferer better manage the crash as it happens, prepare a soft landing, set a realistic recovery time, and select the proper tools to effect maximum adrenal healing in the shortest time with minimum risk of triggering a subsequent crash. It also helps the sufferer to understand the natural progression of Adrenal Fatigue Syndrome and to have realistic expectations of the road ahead.

Crash Prevention Tips

We can't always prevent adrenal crashes, but you can use these tips to slow down crashes that may be coming your way:

- Increase Adrenal Breathing Exercises to 5 times a day or more.
- Increase Adrenal Restorative Exercises to 3 times a day.
- Cancel all nonessential activities outside the house.
- Delay dealing with stressors.
- Stay away from refined sugar and watch your diet.
- Maintain your body's hydration by drinking water.
- Increase salt intake to as much as you can tolerate.
- Have a snack every two hours and eat more food if you have signs of hypoglycemia.
- No watching TV, computer surfing.
- Minimize negative thoughts and avoid arguments.
- Avoid alcohol or caffeinated beverages.
- Avoid direct sunlight or prolonged indirect sunlight.
- Take nutritional supplements specific for crashes.
- Avoid over-exercise.
- Avoid any form of massage, sauna, colonics, enemas, cleanses, and detoxification programs.
- No sex.
- Reread Chapter 12, The Adrenal Crash and Recovery Cycle.

Overall, stay alert and tune in to your body's needs, signs, and symptoms so you can record any changes that happen and report them to your doctor. This is best done systematically with an adrenal journal which we present in the next chapter.

Key Points to Remember

- A key to success in your adrenal recovery program is to prevent crashes while building adrenal reserve gently. Since some crashes are inevitable, especially if external factors are involved, learning how to manage adrenal crashes and recoveries is critical for all because all adrenal crashes worsen the condition.

- Effective crash management requires individualized attention. The key is to avoid physical activity and allow the body to rest. Proper dietary and nutritional supplement adjustments are usually required. Whether to increase or reduce supplements depends on the kind of crash, the individual constitution, and the stage of AFS. Incorrect applications can worsen the crash.

- Recovery management is much more difficult compared to crash management. The more advanced the AFS, the more complicated this is.

- If done properly, recovery management can be an important stepping stone to help the body prepare and enter the next phase of improvement.

- Duration of the recovery phase as measured by the recovery factor is an important clinical indicator of adrenal function.

Chapter 30

Your Adrenal Recovery Journal

As you recover from Adrenal Fatigue Syndrome, we recommend keeping a journal, which encourages you to keep good notes about your symptoms and progress. Keeping a journal promotes a state of mind that focuses on details and keeps your memory fresh so that you don't forget recommendations.

Journaling also allows you to reflect on what you're doing right and perhaps figure out how to improve when you believe you are falling short on carrying out your plan. This allows you to track any immediate adjustments before too much time has lapsed and the damage is done. We also recommend recording questions you may have for your doctor or recovery coach.

Over time, your journal will serve as an authentic self-navigational tool that will help you to recover from Adrenal Fatigue Syndrome. The only equipment you need is a notebook and a pen. Include the following things in your journal:

Your Supplement Instructions: Record the times you are advised to take your supplements each day and the quantity.

Fatigue Scores: Fatigue scores record two important parameters of your energy state each day. It is comprised of two components. First, the amount of resting time you need each day in order to have the energy to perform your regular chores. Second, the percent of normal daily activities you can do.

For example, if you *needed* a 30 minute nap to get through the day smoothly (whether or not you were actually able to take a nap), your score is 0.5. If you were capable of doing or did 70 percent of your normal daily activities, such as performing your job or business, or carrying out a normal load of errands, your score is 70. Similarly, if you were capable of or performed 90 percent of your normal household chores without feeling tired, your score is 90. Your entries for these categories would look like 0.5/90. Tracking this fatigue score over time will give you an objective measurement of your progress.

Optional Categories

- *Food intake*, as well as restrictions and adjustments.

- *Exercise regimen*, paying special attention to how you feel before and after exercise, specifically, how much energy you have after exercising.

- *Sexual activities*, and if you feel drained afterwards.

- *Hypoglycemic episodes*, frequency, intensity, and the time between episodes.

- *Bowel movements*, the patterns, especially if there is constipation, loose stool, or diarrhea.

- *Sleep patterns*, describing the problem, as in going to sleep (sleep onset insomnia or SOI) or waking up and being unable to go back to sleep (sleep maintenance insomnia or SMI). The sleep aids you took and your use of other sleep supports. Write down your sleeping and waking times. Since sleep often is especially challenging, consistent recording will help you spot a trend.

- *Emotional states* such as anxiety, depression, jittery, anger, or irritability.

- *Menstrual cycle*, tracking the dates and duration of your cycles along with symptoms. This is particularly important for those who tend to crash during their menses.

If any one of these areas is of particular concern, begin tracking it on a scale of 1-10, with 10 as the worst, 5 being average, and 1 being the best. For example, if you have had no hypoglycemic episodes today, the score is 1. The importance of these numerical parameters will be evident to you over time. However, do not track more than 3-5 categories at any one time. Trying to assess too many issues all at once can be stressful and overwhelming. You can always add categories to track later.

To begin, we recommend focusing on the key category of fatigue. Energy levels reflect most other underlying root issues in Adrenal Fatigue Syndrome. When the fatigue and energy levels improve, many of the underlying symptoms, such as sleep and anxiety, will have automatically improved as well.

It's a good idea to do all the scoring and recording at the end of the day, putting the relevant scores on the bottom of each day's entry. Briefly note what transpired that day, and if you experienced any changes.

Avoid Over-Journaling

If you don't have anything special to put in your journal and you have no overall change, skip that day and wait for the next. The key is to record significant events that alter the scores, most commonly, an adrenal crash—or the lack of a crash. Also note other negative life events, i.e., loss of a loved one, an infection, troubles on the job or in your business, problems arising with family, and so forth. The presence or absence of a crash or symptoms provides information on your adrenal reserve and the body's ability to withstand stress.

When there is significant change in any of the scores, take some time to reflect on the reasons and write them down. Your journal should be informative and act as a memory trigger. However, we don't want journaling to become a stressful activity. Most of the time, it takes no more than 5-10 minutes a day. Remember, too, that the information is for your personal use only.

Key Points to Remember

- Keeping a simple personal journal is an important recovery tool.

- It serves as an authentic self-navigation tool in the future.

- Important entries include supplement schedule, the fatigue score, and overall well-being.

- Do not over-journal, as it can drain you of precious energy.

Chapter 31

Tips for Special Occasions and Travel

As you now understand, recovering from Adrenal Fatigue Syndrome requires self care and vigilance. Recovery (and crash prevention) also requires adjusting your daily lifestyle to minimize stress and allow for adequate rest. However, you may need or want to travel and enjoy special occasions, too. We included this chapter to help you manage a variety of events and offer pre-crash management tips.

Special Events

Weddings, holidays, birthday parties, commemorations, and gatherings of all kinds are stressful for many people, regardless of their health status. Family conflicts and other personal issues tend to surface, schedules become crammed with events, and for some, travel looms. We've all seen pictures of travelers stranded in airports because of delays. Seldom do holiday seasons progress smoothly and without stress.

Obviously, for those with Adrenal Fatigue Syndrome special occasions and holidays can be an ordeal beyond the typical hustle and bustle of that time of year. For many, Christmas/Hanukkah shopping or days of wedding planning, for example, are presented as fun and rewarding, but they can be extremely stressful activities. Without realizing it, we change our breathing patterns during stressful times and events, causing the body to go into a sympathetic overtone. If you have AFS, it is imperative that you do your Adrenal Breathing Exercises at various times during your daily activities:

- Before you leave the house.
- During the car/bus/train ride to the store.
- While walking through the aisles.
- During snack/meal breaks.
- After you have returned home.

Other Tips for Special Occasions

- If possible, celebrate holidays (any of the major holidays in your country) or other special events away from home. This avoids the additional stress of concerning yourself with all that goes into getting ready for company. If you feel up to it, bring a dish along for the holiday meal. However, listen to your body. If you don't feel up to cooking, don't push yourself—you have alternatives and choices. Plan to go out for a birthday dinner or if possible have food for a wedding or baby shower catered. Overwork can trigger an unwanted adrenal crash.

- Plan in advance. Rushing around at the last minute causes adrenaline to start flowing, which in turn can increase your anxiety level, which is certainly not conducive to enjoying yourself.

- If you are traveling any distance and might be away more than a day, bring sufficient supplements to cover last minute delays and change of plans.

- Everything is ramped up during busy holiday and common vacation weeks: airports are not only busy, but chaotic; parking lots are packed; and all kinds of transactions, from airport check-in to finding restaurants on the road seem to take longer than expected. That's why we recommend that you travel with snacks in your glove box, handbag, or briefcase, so you can keep your energy level up no matter what life throws your way.

- Snack regularly and bring snack foods with you, even when you're headed to a meal at someone else's house or are heading to a restaurant. Your meals are often delayed, and if you encounter crowded restaurants, everything slows down from ordering to delivery.

- Care should be taken to avoid any formula that contains alcohol as a preservative, due to its potential negative effects on the liver.

- Strictly watch your sugar intake! With Adrenal Fatigue Syndrome, the body is highly sensitive to sugar, and unfortunately, sugary foods are extra plentiful during parties and holiday celebrations of all kinds.

- Try to maintain a normal sleep schedule and do your best to avoid staying up too late. If you're tired, find a way to take a short nap to recover the energy spent.

Air Travel Tips

At one time, most people considered air travel quite manageable. In recent years, however, even the hardy among us have had to adjust to changing conditions, including increased security, frequently cancelled flights/fewer flights, and increased costs and decreased services. While most people adjust, those with Adrenal Fatigue Syndrome dread the grueling experience of air travel. The weaker the adrenals, the higher the chance that air travel can trigger an adrenal crash. The following tips serve to prepare you for departure and ensure you arrive in the best shape possible:

Pre-Travel Tips:

- If possible, plan to travel with a companion, a person willing to be the runner, so to speak, able to take care of your needs during the trip and handle most of the check-in process and the baggage.

- Try to schedule your travel during your best and freshest time of the day. Avoid red-eye flights because they disrupt your circadian cycle.

- To the extent possible, avoid layovers, but if you must stop, try to schedule a long layover of 48 to 72 hours, thereby allowing the body time to adjust.

- If there is a weight limit imposed by the airline, weigh your luggage at home to avoid last minute surprises.

- To conserve energy, do not engage in strenuous exercise on the day before and the day of departure.

- Take an additional recommended booster dose of your supplement prior to departure.

- Print out the boarding pass ahead of time with the seat assignment on it.

- Choose a rolling carryon bag and keep it as light as possible—avoid a backpack as a carryon bag—but do take a neck pillow or regular pillow, as well as lumbar support for the plane ride.

- Pre-pack at a leisurely pace, starting a few days prior to your departure date, and remember to include prepackaged snacks in your carryon baggage. Check your travel documents and store them in your carryon baggage.

- To minimize stress, arrive at the airport well ahead of schedule. Have your travel companion or cab driver drop you off at the terminal doors.

- If possible, confirm your seat assignment to avoid being bumped. For convenient access to restrooms and to minimize walking, ask for an aisle seat toward the front of the plane.

- Many international airports provide short term beds and showers at reasonable prices within the terminal. If necessary, take advantage of these services.

At the Check-in Counter:

- Luggage is best checked at curbside; if that's impossible, seek help from a porter to get to the check-in counter or wait for your companion. Do not lift any heavy baggage by yourself.

- Once inside the terminal, find a place to sit down, using your upright luggage if necessary. Do not stand in line unless no alternative exists. Again, wait for your travel companion to handle the check-in for you. Try to stand as little as possible.

- Ask for the "meet and assist" wheelchair/cart service (usually provided free of charge) from the check-in counter to the gate, especially if the walk to and from the gate is long.

- Carry an empty water bottle with you to bring past the security checkpoint, unopened snacks, and extra supplements accessible at any time, along with your books and music devices and headphones. The idea is to go through security with ease.

From Security Check Point to Gate:

- This is often the most chaotic area within the airport and has the most potential to drain your energy. We often forget that the brain is bombarded by the noise and x-ray emissions. It's also stressful to follow the many instructions for passing through security, i.e., taking off your shoes, belts, jewelry, hats, and so forth.

- If you can, preserve your energy by sitting on your carryon baggage if the line is long. Lean against your companion as needed, but don't force yourself to stand for long periods. Do your Adrenal Breathing Exercises whenever possible.

- Once you've passed through security, sit down if you are tired and do the Adrenal Breathing Exercises. Go to the restroom where you can sit and do these exercises.

- Ask your travel companion to fill your water bottle, and as a precautionary measure, drink some water and eat a snack—even if you don't feel like you need it.

- Take your time and rest for a few minutes before continuing to the gate.

- Unless you're traveling alone, ask your companion to guide you to the correct gate, so that you don't need to look up and search for it. Do not stop to window shop along the way.

- Walk slowly—you've allowed extra time, so you aren't pressured to rush. Use the escalators or moving sidewalks, terminal trains or busses, or golf cart service to conserve energy. Sit when you can and ask for help with your carryon bag.

At the Departure Gate:

- Sit in the least congested place in the departure lounge. Ideally, stay as far away as possible from computer monitors, TV screens, and loud music, and as close as you can to a water fountain and restroom.

- Stay relaxed with quiet reading or listening to personal music. Don't chitchat unless you have to—unnecessary talking will drain your energy.

- Purchase a meal to bring with you on the plane so your scheduled mealtimes are disrupted as little as possible.

- Go to the bathroom immediately before the boarding phase.

- Do Adrenal Breathing Exercises as often as needed.

- If you are not using a wheelchair service, be the last to board, so you don't have to stand in a long line. By the time you board, others will have cleared the aisles.

On the Plane:

- If you have luggage for the overhead compartment, ask your companion to stow it for you, and if you're traveling alone, ask the flight attendants for help.

- Avoid watching action oriented TV or any videos. Enjoy music instead.

- Put down the window shade to avoid bright sunlight and/or use eye shades to block light and visual stimulation.

- Stand up, stretch, and walk to the restroom as needed, but avoid standing in the restroom line for a prolonged period of time.

- Drink fluids frequently—the air is very dry inside the plane. Ask for water as needed.

- If your current seat is noisy because of passenger conversation and activity, ask if a seat change is possible.

- If meal service is included, ask the flight attendants not to wake you if you are sleeping, but do ask that your meal be saved for a later time; however, don't depend on the airline for the proper food. Always bring your own.

- If you have a tendency to be hypoglycemic, it's especially important to have plenty of snacks with you, so you can eat according to your body's schedule, not the airline's.

- If you anticipate being tired upon arrival, ask the cabin crew to prearrange wheelchair/ cart service on arrival.

- Fill in arrival forms ahead of landing.

- Do Adrenal Breathing Exercises frequently.

On Arrival:

- Unless you are seated in the front of the plane, let others exit first and take your time.

- Ask for help retrieving your overhead baggage.

- If it's a long walk to the baggage claim, drink water and eat a snack, even if you don't feel as if you need it.

- Don't stop to shop.

- It is normal to be excited when you arrive at your destination, but try to remain calm and serene throughout this last leg of your trip.

- At the baggage claim, let your travel companion take over. If you're traveling alone, always ask for help.

- Once you've arrived, take a nap—consider it mandatory. Then you will feel up to other activities.

We wish you safe and healthy travels!

Key Points to Remember

- Special events are an unavoidable part of balanced living.

- Learning to plan ahead will greatly reduce any chances of crashing and help you enjoy the occasion.

- Air travel is one the most common triggers of adrenal crashes. Fortunately, this too can be managed calmly and systematically.

Chapter 32

A Return to Simplicity: The Ultimate Solution

We need a new approach to life that matches our particular moment in history. Until roughly the last century, human civilization lived in a community-based and relatively simple environment. Research studies of centenarians repeatedly show the link between a simple life and a long life. Those who live a long life tend to live in simple dwellings, eat simple foods that are locally grown and prepared simply, and they do simple exercises such as walking. In addition, these individuals have simple loving relationships.

While some may argue that the body has proven its ability to adapt and survive over time, we must not forget this applies only to a select few with the strongest genes. All of us are born with multiple defects within, though they may not be evident for decades. Those who are constitutionally weaker are at a disadvantage relative to those who are strong and have ample internal reserve. Designed as it is, the body can't sustain the kind of persistent complexity modern society places on it, not without regular rest and replenishment, both physically and emotionally.

When the body's ability to overcome complexity is overwhelmed, the body then slows down, which is its way of returning to simplicity. This is a survival mechanism and reflects the body's knowhow or wisdom. AFS is the body's way of awakening us to this wisdom. If we can only embrace it, we see that the return to simplicity is a good thing.

Until recent years, simple goals were the norm in human civilization. However, today, many are taught that the human spirit can conquer and control all things. This belief in our supremacy intensifies the shock when an earthquake or tornado rips through our communities and destroys almost everything in its wake. Suddenly, we realize that much of life is out of our direct control.

Yes, the human spirit is strong, but it does have limitations. Sad to say, few take the time to fully evaluate this aspect of their lives. Have we forgotten that we are biological creatures, not machines? Adrenal Fatigue Syndrome is nature's way of asking us to pause and ask ourselves if the life we are living is worth the price we are paying. It is a simple yet profound question that is easy to ask but difficult to answer.

AFS forces us to reckon with this question and come to terms with our answer. It forces the best of us to face the consequences of the decisions we make as we journey through life.

For many, the same effort that makes us successful in our career and life goals turns into a runaway train, and those with Adrenal Fatigue Syndrome are in a slow motion train wreck. The problem is that the train wreck process is so slow that few of us notice until too late. Yet, in retrospect, it is clear that we'd built a house of cards that inevitably would fall.

Instead of welcoming fatigue as a warning sign and slowing down accordingly, most people march into their physician's office in denial, demanding a cure so life can go on as usual. Clinicians are often pushed into the common strategy of prescribing stimulating compounds such as hormones, herbs, and glandulars to achieve this goal. When these compounds are used correctly, they can be *temporarily* beneficial, but this is seldom a long term solution and in fact may backfire. At the root level, this strategy involves suppressing symptoms, and is exactly the opposite of what the body needs and wants: *proper nutrition and rest.*

A New Approach to Daily Life

To truly heal or avoid Adrenal Fatigue Syndrome, we must consider a new approach to life. Instead of continuing to lead a highly complex life in a complex world, our goal should be greater balance. The body is designed to take in fresh air and sunshine, along with whole fruits, nuts, and vegetables as the primary source of nutrition. Energy derived from these elements focuses on driving the daily energy expenditure of living a simple life, allowing the nutritional reserve drawdown at any point to be well within acceptable limits. The adequate rest we need at the end of each day then replenishes the energy store.

For proper healing, a continued and conscious effort to gently replenish the nutritional reserve is the key. It is important not to further stimulate the body unless absolutely necessary. We should reach equilibrium by striving for complexity only to the degree that the marginal return justifies the effort, and our primary focus should be a general default balance toward simplicity.

Contrary to popular belief, a simple life is one rich in quality. Bringing simplicity into our lives can bring many gains in areas we may have forgotten about. This is not easy, because the trend toward complexity is a social phenomenon, and in the developed world, striving toward a simple life means going against the tide. Yet, this is the path you must choose if you have Adrenal Fatigue Syndrome or wish to avoid developing it. When we peel back the veneer of complexity, we allow the simplicity beneath to triumph again.

Return to Simplicity

Unfortunately, most people do not make significant changes until they feel pain, and for many, AFS is this pain. Those who ignore AFS as a warning sign are setting themselves up for more pain and ultimately, extinction. Fortunately, when we see the light, so to speak, the body is forgiving; the body has great self-healing abilities if the damage is not too severe.

At some point in our lives, most of us face a choice: either we listen to what our body is trying to tell us and slow down, or the body will force us to do so by down regulating its function. Remember that the body is designed to perform with fundamental efficiency. Adrenal Fatigue Syndrome returns us to that simpler form of function. For example, in certain circumstances, the body shuts down the menstrual cycle and will not allow reproduction to begin until the healing process is complete. Or, those who over-exercise will feel drained and need extended rest. The body needs quality nutrients, and, therefore, consuming unhealthy food, such as sugar, increases fatigue.

To many, the return to simplicity also is psychologically unwelcome. We are used to our old habits of doing what we want and being *productive*. Little did we know that this productivity is actually destructive to the body. The energy needed to generate this output requires a higher level and quality of energy input. Regardless of how noble our life goals may be, the body knows we cannot help others until we first help ourselves to good health. For our own survival, charity does indeed begin at home. Dipping into our energy and nutritional reserves can only last so long. Just like our bank accounts deplete when we withdraw money, our energy depletes when we withdraw energy without depositing more nutrients and rest to restore the reserves.

The call to live simply again within our emotional and physical capacity is a gift, not a curse. Those who deny this may brilliantly succeed in life's endeavors, but from the perspective of their health, they are not so wise. However, the call to return to simplicity is nature's way of saving us from further self-guided destruction—it is practical wisdom.

When the body is forced to rest, we could liken it to a teacher sending a student to the detention room. The signals telling us the body is breaking down are the body's way of sending us to the detention room to do some self reflection. In the body's infinite wisdom, it forces us to do what our conscious minds can't do well, that is, take care of ourselves. As elemental as it seems, it is truly amazing how many of us have ignored the body's wisdom for long periods of time. If we respect the body, we have no problem accepting this thesis, and we know this is the best conclusion possible after we consider all scientific facts and logical reality. Many connected physical derangements and emotional disconnects exist, but these represent symptoms of a body in a state of complexity well beyond its ability to handle. The good news is that symptoms tend to resolve once we embark on the right course of healing.

> To be clear, the simple life is by no means boring or mundane and can include a variety of creative tasks, including computer work, intellectual debates, and heavy exercise from time to time, with reserve left to handle emotional and psychological issues, unexpected stress, and so forth. Life is a celebration when our body is finally in harmony with its environment the way nature intended it. We may need to admit that the complexity of modern society has failed, and our refusal to go along with the expected complexity deserves celebration, too. Overall, it's a process of returning to what really counts in life in a balanced way in accordance with the makeup of our body.

Generally, the simple life doesn't include intense, on-the-go lifestyles as typified by Type A personalities, which usually include subclinical obsessive-compulsive traits. These characteristics are made worse if superimposed on a dysfunctional environment that induces excessive physical and or emotional stress.

Simplicity Framework

Adrenal Fatigue Syndrome is ultimately the body's strategy to return to simplicity from a complex state, but we often feel punished when AFS occurs. But let's remember, the body is a complex closed system, which is self-maintaining and self-healing. Given that, it is also most content in a simple mode of operation, which modern civilization challenges every day. Adrenal Fatigue Syndrome is one way the body reminds us that it is always right.

It's not wise to argue with your body. On the contrary, if you listen, AFS is the best thing that can happen. It is the way of crying out for a return to basics—love, prayer, and nutrition.

The basic premise of healing Adrenal Fatigue Syndrome is to return to a more simple way of life, one that matches the body's capability. Ultimately, this is the long term solution. We usually think that healing something means going back to our old ways. However, when we give the body quality nutritional augmentation, for example, then the recovery process accelerates, and if we stick with this new way of eating we are at less risk of falling back into AFS. In addition, stress dissipates when we live in line with our physical and emotional limitations.

To prevent or to fully heal from Adrenal Fatigue Syndrome, we need to believe and internalize the following mental framework:

- Our life cannot remain in a complex state beyond what it can handle; we all have limited nutritional reserves and energy to sustain this state.

- The more complex our life, the greater the internal energy demand on a day-to-day basis.

- Adrenal Fatigue Syndrome is a warning that we have exceeded the capacity threshold, and this is unlikely to be restored successfully long term if we base our approach on suppressing symptoms or on further stimulating the body.

- If we continue a path of complexity, we need ever increasing energy, which causes the marginal return to decline. In other words, our productivity becomes physically destructive to our body.

- Continual marginal decline ultimately leads to a net energy loss and depletion of internal resources. If this does not abate, our body progresses to crash and then failure.

- The best hope for sustained recovery involves a return to lifestyle simplicity that incorporates the vital nurturing of nutritional supplementation.

- We always recommend seeking a personalized approach from an experienced practitioner, because the wide variety of symptoms and the convoluted clinical picture of AFS often defy conventional medical logic. Unless the condition is very mild, we don't recommend self-navigation.

Tips for a Simple Life

- Identify the top four to five most important things to you and realign your commitment to these priorities. Say no to everything else.

- Downsize and reduce clutter in your surroundings to a comfortable level for you, and be happy about it. Adopt a minimalist approach to your home, acquiring and keeping only the necessary items and not much else. This kind of home is extremely peaceful to live in and easy to clean.

- Simplify your budget and financial life. Do not compare yourself with others. Be thankful for what you have and put aside greed.

- Eat simple foods, prepared simply. Avoid sugar. Drink water.

- Evaluate your time, and as necessary, redesign your day in line with simplifying your work and home tasks as much as possible.

- Limit your communications, such as email, Twitter, and Facebook, to certain times of the day and for a limited time; we seldom realize how draining social media can be, and not every email demands immediate attention.

- Use your time to be with people and things you love, but also spend time alone.

- Learn to recognize stress, and also learn to decompress. Find an outlet for self-expression, whether it be painting, reading, or walking.

- Consistently fortify your body with the needed nutrients every day in order to rebuild your internal nutritional reserves.

- Recognize that it is more important to be pleasant to everyone around you than to be right or in control.

- Finally, consider this simple nondenominational and universal prayer to guide your day.

The Simplicity Prayer

I surrender this day to you, dear God
The desires of my heart, for you to lead
The desires of my mind, for you to control

On your shoulders I place all burden
In your hands I place all questions
At your feet, I place all worries

I pray for faith when answers are not clear
I pray for release of complexity
To be replaced by the simplicity beneath

May we return to love as the only reality
May we return to simplicity as the only path
May our body be healed as we follow your way

Key Points to Remember

- Adrenal Fatigue Syndrome is ultimately the collapse of a body unable to handle the complexity of life. It is the body, in its wisdom, returning us to a simpler form of living. Those who heed this mandate will find recovery a learning process.

- A new approach to daily life is needed for most of us who have had busy lives. We should focus on balance and equilibrium.

- Returning to simplicity, while to many, it is psychologically unwelcome, it is a gift, not a curse.

- We need to return to the level that matches our body's capacity to handle stress and complex tasks.

- The best hope for sustained recovery involves a return to a simple lifestyle that incorporates the vital nurturing of nutritional supplementation.

Chapter 33

Looking to the Future

Now that you have read *Adrenal Fatigue Syndrome*, we hope you see, as we have, that it is part of the body's complex neuroendocrine stress response that merits our attention. While the adrenal glands may be at the forefront of attention in terms of symptomatology, the broader picture points to a continuum of systematic activation at first and eventual dysregulation of our neuroendocrine stress response system when pushed to the limit. *The autonomic nervous system is also dysregulated in addition to the adrenal glands in advance stages. The entire continuum is best termed Stress-induced Neuroendocrine Syndrome* (SINS). Therefore, full attention needs to be paid to the entire neuroendocrine system if we are to get to the bottom of this condition physiologically. At the deeper mental level, it reflects our body's inability to handle the complexity of modern life and the body's wise desire to return to simplicity for survival. No organ system is spared as the body forces us to deal with survival in the most rudimentary terms.

Currently, most conventionally trained doctors simply are not educated about AFS in medical school and postgraduate training. The quest in scientific medicine for complete understanding through modern scientific methods has advantages and could even be considered noble. However, a lack of complete understanding of a condition should never stand in the way of using natural therapies that achieve consistent and reproducible, positive, clinical results—and without negative consequences.

Intellectual arrogance has no place in the healing arts and can lead to a loss of practical wisdom. In order to truly understand Adrenal Fatigue Syndrome, we first need to humbly commit to filling in the gaps in our knowledge of neuroendocrinology. Educating ourselves is the first step toward healing. This is our biggest task. That is why we present with great detail the science behind this condition—to dispel any myth that this condition is not real. If you are a sufferer, no one can tell you your fatigue is not real when you are bedridden. Your body does not lie. As far as AFS sufferers are concerned, all they want is to get better. Although we have tried to explain the physiology and psychology involved in AFS, we know that most sufferers are less concerned about every pathological and physiological pathway than they are about therapies that will help them restore their health.

For clinicians, a lack of understanding can never negate positive clinical results, especially when patient evidence-based results are overwhelmingly positive. Fortunately, more forward looking health practitioners are now taking this seriously.

Common sense needs to prevail. We are at the crest of an information explosion on the neuroendocrine basis of how our body handles stress and its clinical ramification, Adrenal Fatigue Syndrome. This book is part of that movement, as we endeavor to educate the world about this condition. By now, you know why we have chosen to become part of this movement to educate and help. *Too many women and men are afflicted and have nowhere to turn.*

We have described the experience of many sufferers, and they enter choppy waters indeed. Their well meaning efforts at self care and healing often seem so logical at first, but end up detrimental in the long run. They deserve better.

The tide toward a more holistic approach in medicine is well on its way. Consider:

- 90 percent of Americans believe in natural medicine, and 70 percent have tried some form of alternative medicine sometime in their life.

- 40 percent report that vitamins and herbs are first choice therapies. Massage followed at 29 percent as the second most common therapy, followed by aromatherapy, yoga, and homeopathic products.

- About 74 percent of women and 57 percent of men take vitamins on a daily basis.

- 69 percent reported having used alternative medicine during the past year.

- In total, the number of visits to natural medicine health practitioners exceeds the number of visits to traditional MDs.

You are not alone if you feel helpless and lost in your quest to better health. Like many of our colleagues, we also are western trained and educated. We consider ourselves privileged to have discovered Adrenal Fatigue Syndrome and to have taken it seriously, because we believe in two vital principles:

- First, the body never lies;
- Second, just because something isn't within our body of knowledge, doesn't mean it does not exist.

In fact, our lack of knowledge was exactly what propelled us to pursue information about this complex condition over the years.

This book reflects, then, the product of our academic knowledge and clinical experience with Adrenal Fatigue Syndrome in the real world. We need much more research to more completely understand AFS in it social, physiological, and psychological context. We are excited and grateful to be in the forefront of clinical neuroendocrinological and AFS research and pass on our findings and experience to those who suffer from this condition and to our colleagues in healthcare who want to learn more. In the end, knowledge is the best prescription for healing, but our knowledge of the body and its workings are still far from complete. The more we know, the more we know how much we don't know. For example, with close to a century of research, we have yet to find a cure for the common cold or prevent hypertension at its root. We hope this book has given you a comprehensive view of the clinical profile of Adrenal Fatigue Syndrome, from its many physical, mind-body, and constitutional components. It is a complicated condition, and we make no apologies for saying so.

Our hope is that you are encouraged by knowing that recovery is at hand if you embark on a proper and comprehensive recovery program. We know recovery is possible because many have done so under our guidance. We also pledge to help you stay current on this dynamic, exciting field. The most effective way to stay current is through our website, *www.DrLam.com*.

Sign up for our free newsletter and watch for news and updates as more research comes online.

Thank you for joining us on this journey.

Michael Lam, M.D., M.P.H.
Dorine Lam, R.D., M.S., M.P.H.

Finding the Right Practitioner

The right healthcare practitioner can change your life. In the case of Adrenal Fatigue Syndrome, this is usually the most critical piece of the puzzle. Why? Because the vast majority of those with AFS experience myriad convoluted symptoms that confuse all but the most astute clinicians trained in this condition. It's essential to know what each symptom means, along with its significance. As you can see from the case studies, the right professional guidance can mean the difference between successful recovery and persistent failure.

Due to the general lack of Adrenal Fatigue Syndrome expertise among conventional and even alternative health practitioners, finding the right practitioner is easier said than done. Those with advanced Adrenal Fatigue Syndrome face the greatest challenges, as many have already been abandoned by conventional medicine and left to self-navigate.

It's worth spending the time to find the right clinician. Generally speaking, he or she should be an open minded and nutritionally oriented health professional. Additional clinical experience in endocrinology, cardiology, psychiatry, and neurology is beneficial, along with knowledge of using natural compounds in a holistic setting.

Insist on someone who can individualize your care, and look for someone who can examine diagnostic tests but also see beyond them to discern how you feel. Seek the clinician who believes that managing your adrenals requires a comprehensive approach, including modifying your diet, lifestyle, and exercise; this person's approach to natural compounds is both gentle and systematic and non-stimulating. Remember that a wrong approach can worsen your condition over time. In today's managed care and specialized environment, this is not an easy task, but neither is it impossible.

The Doctor Interview

You are entitled to ask a doctor key questions before making an initial appointment, and then based on the answers, ask yourself if this person is receptive to new ideas. What is his or her philosophy on how stress can affect the body? This will give you clues as to whether this doctor is holistic or conventional.

Later, when you talk with this doctor, does he or she clearly communicate the reasons you feel the way you do? An experienced doctor will generally have little problem tying in your various symptoms and giving you a comprehensive explanation. You should be able to receive direct answers to your questions in a way you can understand. This is part of being patient-oriented.

You can also ask about the doctor's philosophy of the adrenal glands as a key to the body's overall well-being and your symptoms of fatigue, along with other organ systems associated with your complaints, during the investigation. These questions help you indirectly gauge not only the doctor's knowledge of the adrenal system, but the more subtle understanding of adrenal function and Adrenal Fatigue Syndrome.

How to Best Communicate With Your Doctor

A good relationship is a two-way street, so the more clearly you communicate your problems, the easier it is for the doctor to address the issues. Here are simple tips to facilitate good communication:

- Have confidence in yourself, but do not show either an overly aggressive or passive attitude.

- Keep a journal of your health-related events and symptoms, noting when they come on (time of day or relating to an event or the menstrual cycle, for example), how they affect you, how you feel, and how and when you recover.

- Write down questions ahead of your appointment, so you can ask good questions and make the most of your appointment time.

- Trust your instincts. Your body is always right. Persist in finding the care you deserve. Don't settle for less.

Although we realize many doctors do not welcome patient-generated research, and some even become annoyed when patients bring them information, we recommend that you help your doctor stay informed. Print out articles relevant to your condition that you believe may help your doctor understand your situation, and submit these to your doctor for perusal ahead of time. Our Adrenal Fatigue Center at *www.DrLam.com* contains numerous articles that we constantly update. You can direct your doctor to our website. Forward thinking doctors, the real visionaries, thank us for providing this information online so they can learn and better serve their patients.

You have also benefitted from this book and other articles. You can better explain and describe your symptoms when you know more about your body and various conditions. This in turn helps your doctor help you.

If your doctor does not understand or cannot explain to you what is happening with clear confidence, chances are you need to consider finding another healthcare professional.

Investigate Other Options

Here are several tips if you cannot find the right practitioner:

- Connect with others who've had similar symptoms and investigate what they did to overcome their dysfunction. Do be careful not to draw conclusions too quickly, however. What works for one person may not work for another. You may be able to find a doctor through those who have been helped.

- Use the Internet. Search Adrenal Fatigue Syndrome and study relevant sites. Focus on educational sites that offer scientifically based information. Our site *www.DrLam.com* is a public educational website that contains the most easily searchable complete library of material on Adrenal Fatigue Syndrome on the web. Many articles on Adrenal Fatigue Syndrome not present in this book are available online, along with the latest news, FAQs (frequently asked questions), and an archive of questions many have asked through the years. You'll also find video and audio presentations of lectures on Adrenal Fatigue Syndrome. Those who like to be kept up to date on the latest news on this topic can sign up for our free electronic newsletter.

- Be wary of Internet forums because views expressed are often skewed and not objective in nature. What works for one person can in fact be toxic for another. Be skeptical of anyone who purports to have simple, quick fix or breakthrough solutions. Watch out for those who post angry messages or who are overly active online. These individuals may have hidden agendas or unresolved psychological or undisclosed physical issues well beyond AFS. Finally, be careful of one-size-fits-all approaches; these seldom work except for the mildest cases.

- If you are not sure whether you have Adrenal Fatigue Syndrome, or if you would like an assessment on the degree of your adrenal function, take our Three Minute Test in this book (Appendix F) or online at *www.DrLam.com.*

- If you have specific questions about your symptoms or condition, write to us directly from our website at *www.DrLam.com.* Each question is individually answered privately and in confidence.

Fortunately, travelling is not usually required in order to seek help. We serve clients all over the world. If you cannot find a practitioner with whom you are comfortable, or if you have no one to turn to, call us. (For details see our website.) Our telephone-based nutritional coaching program is an individualized one-on-one program designed to facilitate the fastest possible recovery using natural measures. It incorporates many principles and techniques discussed in this book.

Glycemic Index Table

The glycemic index (GI) is a measure of how much blood sugar stress a food creates. Controlling blood sugar is one of the pillars in a successful anti-aging diet, and high blood sugar is a direct reflection of high sugar intake. Therefore, it's important to know what foods are low in sugar.

Below is a table of common foods and their glycemic index. To reduce blood sugar stress, concentrate on foods with an index at or below 70. This will help create a more even flow of glucose into the blood. If you are eating high glycemic index food like white bread, always try to pair it with a low glycemic index food. If foods are mixed, the resulting index will be between the high and low values.

> Table 4, Glycemic Index Table, below lists common food products and their actual GI values. These numbers use glucose as a baseline, which is given a GI of 100. All the other values are relative to glucose.
>
> Recommended: GI <70; Avoid: GI >70; If Diabetic or hypoglycemic: avoid GI >60

Legumes		Grains		Pastas		Bread Products	
Baked Beans, canned	68	Barley, pearled	25	Angel Hair	45	Bagel	72
Black Beans	30	Buckwheat (kasha)	54	Bean Threads	26	French Bread	96
Black Eyed Peas	42	Bulgar	47	Gnocchi	67	Kaiser Roll	73
Butter Beans	31	Couscous	65	Pastas, brown rice	92	Melba Toast	71
Chick Peas	33	Cornmeal	68	Pastas, refined	65	Pita Bread	58

Legumes		Grains		Pastas		Bread Products	
Chick Peas, canned	42	Millet	71	Pastas, whole grain	45	Pumpernickel Bread	49
Fava Beans	80	Rice, brown	56	Star Pastina	38	Rye Bread	64
Kidney Beans	30	Rice, instant	85 –	Vermicelli	35	Rye Bread, whole	50
Kidney Beans, canned	52	Rice, white	70	**Snacks, Misc.**		Stuffing	75
Lentils, green	30	**Crackers**		Corn Chips	70	Tortilla, corn	70
Lentils, red	25	Graham Crackers	74	Fried Pork Rinds	OK	Waffles	76
Lima, baby, frozen	32	Rice Cakes	77	Olives	OK	White Bread	95
Pinto Beans	39	Rye Crispbread	67	Peanuts	10	Whole Wheat Bread	75
Soy Beans	18	Stoned Wheat Thins	68	Peanut M&M's	32	**Fruits**	
Split Peas	32	Water Crackers	72	Popcorn	56	Apple	39
Dairy Products		**Cereals**		Potato Chips	55	Apple Juice	41
Ice Cream, regular	61	All Bran	43	Pretzels	82	Apricots, dried	35
Ice Cream, low-fat	50	Bran Chex	59	Rice Cakes	77	Bananas, ripe	60
Milk, regular	27	Cheerios	75	Rich Tea	56	Cantaloupe	65
Milk, skim	32	Corn Bran	75	Vanilla Wafers	77	Cherries	23
Yogurt, sugar	33	Corn Chex	83	**Vegetables**		Grapefruit	25
Yogurt, aspartame	14	Cornflakes	84	All Green Vegetables	0 - 30	Grapefruit Juice	49

Legumes	Grains		Pastas		Bread Products	
	Cornflakes	84	All Green Vegetables	0 - 30	Grapefruit Juice	49
	Cream of Wheat	71	Bean Sprouts	<50	Grapes	46
	Grapenuts	68	Beets	64	Kiwi	52
	Life	66	Carrots	71 - 92	Mango	56
	Mueslix	60	Cauliflower	<50	Orange	42
	Nutri Grain	66	Corn	58	Orange Juice	51
	Oat Bran	55	Eggplant	<50	Papaya	58
	Oatmeal, regular	53	All onions	<50	Peach	35
	Oatmeal, quick	66	Parsnips	97	Pear	35
	Puffed Wheat	74	Peppers	<50	Pineapple	66
	Puffed Rice	90	Potato, russet (baked)	90	Pineapple Juice	43
	Rice Chex	89	Potato, instant mashed	83	Plum	29
	Rice Krispies	82	Potato, fresh mashed	73	Raisins	64
	Shredded Wheat	69	Potato, new, boiled	57	Strawberries	32
	Special K	54	Potato, french fries	75	Watermelon	74
	Total	76	Radishes	<50		
			Sauerkraut	<50		
			Sweet Potato	54		
			Tomato	38		
			Water Chestnuts	<50		
			Yams	51		
			Yellow Squash	<50		

Adapted from D.J.A. Jenkins et al., American Journal of Clinical Nutrition, Volume 34, 1981.

For Glycemic Index of 1200 foods, here is the link: *http://www.mendosa.com/gilists.htm.*

Appendix C

Liposomal Encapsulation Technology

In existence since the early 1970s, liposomal encapsulation technology (LET) is the newest delivery method used by medical researchers to transfer drugs that act as healing promoters to specific organs. In other words, LET offers targeted delivery of vital compounds to the body. The excellent transference capability of LET has led some manufacturers to use it in their topical moisturizers and other cosmetic products.

The astounding effects and advantages derived from LET are the reason that a number of nutritional companies use this technique in the oral delivery of dietary supplements.

The advantage of LET is its ability to carry power packed and non-decomposed natural compounds to pinpointed tissues and organs. Even if doses are 5 to 15 times less than normal supplemental intake, the delivery system's effectiveness remains unchanged. This reduction is both medically and economically significant.

Tablets, capsules, and topical nutritional products are affected by environmental conditions such as moisture, oxygen, and other unfavorable factors. For example, nutrients are likely degraded by enzymes and esophageal digestive juices prior to being absorbed into the body. In addition, binders, fillers, gelatins, and sugar are food additives that affect the absorption process. This partial assimilation caused by the incomplete disintegration of the tablet or capsule is a serious problem. LET shields substances from these negative properties, which are likely to take place within the gastrointestinal passage.

Liposomal encapsulation employs a phospholipid liposome (see the definition below) to construct a defense that repels the negative activities of the digestive juices, alkaline solutions, salts, and free radicals of the body. The duration of this protection lasts from the moment the nutrients are on their way toward the gastrointestinal tract, until the contents have reached the target tissue and are immediately taken in by the cellular structure and transferred into the intra-cellular space.

A majority of the liposomes in LET are composed of phospholipids. All bodily cells contain a protective membrane consisting of phospholipids. This substance is required by the body to grow and function.

Phospholipid Structure

Phospholipids are the main building blocks of cell membranes in the human body. The three major portions of the molecule consist of one head and two tails. The three molecular parts of the head are: glycerol, phosphate, and choline. The *hydrophilic* character of the head makes it captivating to water while the long tail is composed of saturated fatty acids. The *hydrophobic* trait of the fatty acids makes them repelled by water. The heads of the phospholipid line up side-by-side next to each other when placed in a water-based solution. Due to the hydrophobic tails, another phospholipid will line up tail-to-tail in response to this similar environment; they form an identical image of each other, thus making a natural environment of dual rows of closely packed phospholipid molecules called the *phospholipid bi-layer*. These bi-layers surround all the cells. The size of one bi-layer is equivalent to 1/1000th the thickness of one book page. Nutrients are ably directed in and out of the cells by different combinations of proteins found in the bi-layer of the phospholipid. Just imagine, we have 70 trillion cells in the body and 1,000 phospholipids are found in every single cell. Without the phospholipids, the body ceases to work properly because, as stated, they are the basic building blocks of the body. Various types of phospholipids are classified based on the type of fatty acids connected to the head of the choline phosphate.

The essential polysaturated fatty acids make *phosphatidylcholines (PC)*, essential phospholipids. Liposomal capsules are created by using these PC fatty acid phospholipids. Phospholipids and PC are both essential to life and the body requires them.

Benefits of Phospholipids

We derive many benefits from phospholipids. The most essential is its astounding anti-aging effect. For example, phospholipids can decrease total serum lipid (fat) and LDL (the bad cholesterol), increase HDL (the good cholesterol), decrease triglyceride and platelet aggregation, amplify red blood cell fluidity, heighten coronary circulation, expand exercise tolerance, increase quality of memory, increase immunity, and improve liver protection and rejuvenation.

Countless research studies have been conducted on the benefits of phosphatidyl-choline, and 500 human studies have proven that PC guards and improves the health of lipids.

Of all bodily organs, the liver performs the most essential activity. Nowadays, the liver is exposed to the highest level of toxic pollutants, such as gasoline, exhaust fumes, paint, pesticides, contaminated water, and many others. As the biggest organ, the liver is the front line of the body's defense against these toxins. The main work of body lipids is to detoxify and bring nourishment, including vitamins A, E, and D, and glycogen, to the whole body.

The liver absorbs and combines all the 100 essential enzymes needed for assimilating nutrients. The function of the liver is enormous: It filters one half gallon of blood every minute and every day it breaks down and detoxifies over 10,000 compounds like poisons, hormones, toxins, and enzymes. PC guards the liver from the toxins; every day, it takes 1000 to 2000 mg of PC to guard the liver from injuries just caused by alcohol. We also know that taking PC one day before exposure to radiation can protect the body against its harmful effects.

The heart, blood, and entire cardiovascular system are greatly improved by PC because of its ability to decrease LDL cholesterol and amplify HDL cholesterol. By taking in 1500 mg of PC every day for a month, studies show a 12-14percent increase of HDL ratio over the LDL ratio among diabetic patients. PC also lowers serum triglyceride and overall cholesterol levels, but the degree of reduction depends on the amount of the dosage and length of time it's taken. For example, we can see a 4.9 percent decrease in serum triglyceride after taking a 1500 mg PC dosage over a four week period. Taking in 3000 mg daily over an eight week period will reduce cholesterol by 44 percent. PC intake can bring about a maximum decrease in serum triglyceride, increase exercise tolerance, and improve cardiovascular system function.

Taking 1800 mg of PC daily for a month resulted in a significant improvement in the muscular and leg blood flow in a group of heart patients; these patients were able to walk, without any kind of chest pain, more than 100 times further by taking only PC.

PC protects cells in several ways. First, it lessens lipid peroxidation brought about by an increase in HDL and a decrease of serum lipid. (Peroxidation is a process that results in free radicals stealing electrons from the lipids in the membranes of the cells, thus causing cell damage.) Second, oxidized low-density lipids in cell membranes are replaced by PC. Third, oxidized cholesterol is eliminated by PC. PC conducts an overall cell repair of the lipid peroxidation. Several clinical instances have demonstrated the ability of PC to limit and prevent the reverse of the peroxidation process.

PC liposomes are the essential parts of LET and serve as the areas wherein the encapsulated supplements are delivered. Liposomes vary in size, which are determined by the process they were made. The measurement can range from hundreds of micrometers (one millionth of a meter) to under 100 nanometers (one billionth of a meter) and the structures are unilamellar (single layer), bilamellar (double layer), or mutlilamellar (multi layer). A variety of methods exist to prepare a liposome. To orally deliver nutrients, the main device is the mechanical method.

When categorizing the mechanical preparation process, we have three major classifications: extrusion, micro-fluidization, and sonification. The maximum state of liposomal technology should use a liposome below 200 nanometers with a bi-layer structure and phosphatidylcholine. Eggs and soy are the most common sources and must be stored at room temperature above freezing.

LET at Work

Glutathione and vitamin C represent an excellent example of LET's application. A majority of animals produce vitamin C in their livers and kidneys. The exceptions include humans, apes, and guinea pigs. Goats produce as much as 13,000 milligrams of vitamin C in a day, but can exceed 100,000 milligrams in the presence of pathogens and toxins.

In its traditional form, oral vitamin C had a slow rate of assimilation at high dose, yet vitamin C is called the super-antioxidant because of its ability to neutralize free radicals. If a high dosage is needed, it is advisable to take vitamin C intravenously because of superior blood and tissue absorption. When taken by mouth in high dose, only 10-15 percent of high dose vitamin C is absorbed. Using LET technology has greatly improved and updated the transfer of vitamin C into the cells, making it by far the best way for vitamin C to enter the hepatic (pertaining to the liver) system in its pure condition.

Vitamin C is guarded by PC liposomes from injury done by the enzyme and gastric juices in the digestive system. Once they enter the body, PC liposomes pass through the small intestine smoothly without expending any energy. The liposomes are carried by the system to the liver in complete form and are prepared to give off their content. The PC liposomes in the liver are scattered. The polyunsaturated PC is ingested by the liver cells as it frees the encapsulated vitamin C.

Common side effects of oral vitamin C (powder, capsule, and tablet forms) include diarrhea and gastric discomfort. Oral liposomal encapsulated vitamin C increases the supply of vitamin C into the cellular system much more effectively and without negative effects such as gastric distress, and extra load on the liver.

While liposomal encapsulation technology represents an excellent delivery system, it is important to note that normal routes of delivery (such as tablets, capsules, and powder forms) are still useful in that they offer different and complimentary forms of nutrient bioavailability to ensure a steady blood level throughout the day as desired.

Designing a comprehensive program combining various forms of delivery systems to ensure consistent nutrient delivery throughout the day requires extensive clinical experience. If done properly, one can see dramatic clinical results, and this is a hallmark of clinical excellence.

Several reputable brands are currently available on the market. LipoNano® C comes in a liquid form and offers a high potency form of liposomalized vitamin C. More vitamin C per unit dose means less has to be taken to get the same effect. Make sure you read the label carefully. Avoid products that contain alcohol which is taxing on the liver and, therefore, not recommended. Those in advanced AFS or who have compromised liver clearance are particularly vulnerable.

A Word about Preservatives

Preservatives are used in most liquid nutritional formulas. They serve to increase the shelf life of a product by preventing (or delaying, at least) spoiling. Commonly used preservatives include sodium benzoate, potassium sorbate and alcohol. Alcohol in particular has been long used by the pharmaceutical industry as a solvent, penetration-enhancer, disinfectant and preservative. A 7 to 12 percent alcohol content is commonly used in many skin-care products, a concentration that can be significantly toxic to skin cells. The skin, like liver, is one of the few organs capable of metabolizing alcohol to another cytotoxic chemical acetaldehyde.

In the case of advanced AFS, where liver function is often compromised at the subclinical level, intake of alcohol from such a preservative only adds further burden to the already weak and low clearance capability of the liver. Alcohol may therefore deter the healing process, and in extreme cases, precipitate adrenal crashes. Look for formulas that are non-alcoholic and have as little preservatives as possible.

The Neuroendocrine Basis of Adrenal Fatigue Syndrome

Stress enters our sphere through a small area of the brain stem called the locus coeruleus (LC) (also spelled locus caeruleus). Discovered in the eighteenth century, this area of the brain stem deals with physiological responses to stress and panic.

As an important homeostatic control center of the body, the LC receives input signals from a variety of sources, including the hypothalamus, amygdala, cerebellum, and prefrontal cortex. Emotional pain and stressors from the outside enter our inner world through these pathways. Once arrived, excitatory signals trigger production and release of norepinephrine from the LC. Norepinephrine has dual functions. In the brain, it acts as a neurotransmitter and keeps us aroused. Norepinephrine released from the LC also increases the sympathetic discharge/inhibit parasympathetic tone in the peripheral nervous system, exerting its excitatory effects directly on the target organ concerned, such as the heart. As a result, both the force of the heartbeat as well as the heart rate go up. Aside from being the principal production site of brain norepinephrine, the LC is also connected to many other parts of the CNS on the output side, including the spinal cord, brain stem, cerebellum, hypothalamus, amygdala, and cerebral cortex.

Collectively, the LC and the areas of the CNS affected by the norepinephrine it produces are described as the locus coeruleus-noradrenergic system, or LC-NA system. Distribution is ubiquitous and consistent with a prominent role for norepinephrine (also called noradrenaline or NA) in a variety of CNS functions and behaviors that include loco motor control, cognition, motivation, and attention.

Activation of the LC-NA system may be responsible for much of the psychological effect we see in Adrenal Fatigue Syndrome, including fear, anxiety, alertness, memory changes, and REM sleep dysregulation. Psychiatric research has documented that the role the LC plays in cognitive function in relation to stress is complex and multimodal. Once activated by stress, the LC responds by increasing norepinephrine secretion, which in turn activates the HPA axis, starting at the hypothalamus. The body goes on alert and prepares for impending danger.

The hypothalamus is an area of the brain located below the thalamus, just above the brain stem. By its various influences, the hypothalamus plays a key role in controlling hunger, sleep, thirst, circadian cycles, and body temperature. It is the beginning of the hypothalamic-pituitary-adrenal (HPA) hormonal axis. About the size of an almond, it produces and secretes certain neurohormones, one of which we call the corticotropin-releasing hormone (CRH). CRH is released from the hypothalamus when stimulated by norepinephrine from the LC. CRH travels to the pituitary gland and serves as a bridge to link the nervous system to the endocrine system. The neuroendocrine connection is established.

The pituitary gland is an endocrine gland about the size of a pea and is a protrusion off the bottom of the hypothalamus at the base of the brain. It secretes nine hormones that keep the body in homeostasis. Upon arrival to the anterior pituitary gland, CRH triggers and induces the formation and release of adrenocorticotropic hormone (ACTH). ACTH travels to the adrenal cortex and is responsible for orchestrating the synthesis of a family of steroids including cortisol, the master anti-stress hormone.

The HPA axis works concurrently and alongside the LC-NA system. The HPA axis goes into action when the LC-NA system is activated. While the LC-NA system's effect tends to localize to the CNS, the HPA axis effect, more diffused, affects the entire body, mediated by cortisol and other stress response hormones. This is graphically illustrated as follows:

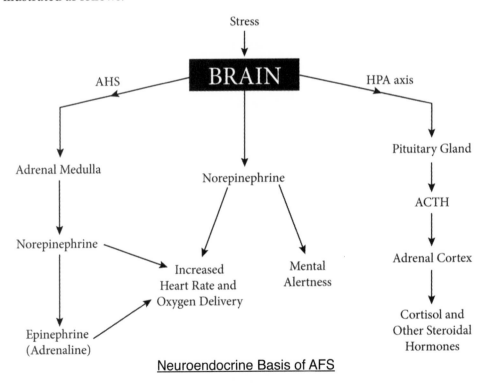

Neuroendocrine Basis of AFS

Therefore, the body has three, well designed anti-stress mechanisms in place to protect us: brain norepinephrine keeps us alert in the CNS, systemic norepinephrine keeps our cardiovascular system ready to take action physically by way of the sympathetic nervous system (SNS), and a family of steroids from the adrenal cortex helps generate energy and reduce inflammation. Activating any or all of these three systems in varying degrees is enough to help us deal with unwelcomed stress under most normal circumstances and ensure that our daily living is smooth.

The SNS is part of the autonomic nervous system (ANS), which has five branches. Working together in unison, these five branches regulate the internal housekeeping functions of the body at rest and in emergency. The sympathetic nervous system is responsible for up- and down-regulating many homeostatic mechanisms in living organisms. Fibers from the SNS innervate tissues in almost every organ system, providing at least some regulatory function to things as diverse as urinary output, pupil diameter, and gastrointestinal motility.

The other four branches of the ANS are:

- the parasympathetic nervous system (PNS),
- the adrenomedullary hormonal system (AHS),
- the enteric nervous system (ENS), and
- the sympathetic cholinergic system (SCS)

Normal bodily housekeeping functions of daily living are regulated by a perfect balance primarily by the PNS (and its chemical messenger acetylcholine) and the SNS (and its chemical messenger norepinephrine). The nervous system is illustrated in the following diagram:

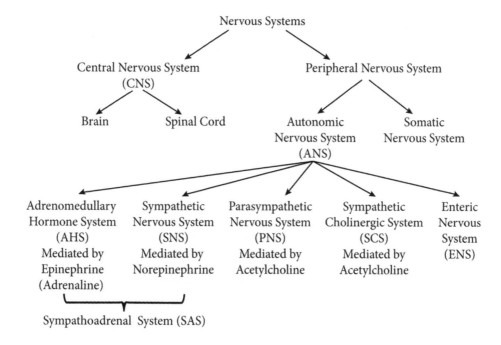

It is absolutely necessary for the SNS to be involved in regulating even small stressors such as standing up or exercise in order for daily living to be seamless. Messages travel through the SNS in a bidirectional flow. Incoming signals carry sensations such as heat, cold, or pain.

Outgoing messages can trigger changes in different parts of the body simultaneously. For example, they can increase peristalsis in the esophagus; piloerection (goose bumps) and perspiration (sweating); widen passages of the bronchi; decrease motility of the large bowel; constrict blood vessels; and raise blood pressure. Thanks to the SNS, LC-NA system, and HPA axis working together each time stressors arrive, individuals in early stages of AFS may experience stress, but seldom notice any significant clinical dysfunction. Working behind the scenes, they help us deal with stress without us knowing about it.

Adrenomedullary Hormone System (AHS) to the Rescue

When stress becomes extreme, the *adrenomedullary hormonal system* (AHS), also known as the sympathetic adrenergic system, is activated. What makes the AHS physiologically unique is the way the synaptic pathways are structured. Synapses occur between pre- and post-ganglionic neurons of the AHS within the adrenal medulla instead of outside the adrenal glands as is the case with the SNS. Because the adrenal medulla develops in tandem with the SNS, it therefore acts as a modified sympathetic ganglion.

The incoming nerve fibers come directly from cell bodies in the spinal cord. The fibers pass through the para-vetebral ganglia by way of splanchnic nerves without stopping or relaying their signals via cells in the ganglia. This is a direct link highway to the adrenal medulla. The speed of transmission is extraordinarily fast as a result. Furthermore, the post-ganglionic neurons do not leave the medulla. Instead, they directly release a large amount of epinephrine and a proportionally smaller amount of norepinephrine into the bloodstream.

Epinephrine, the most potent catecholamine, serves as an emergency hormone largely responsible for executing the fight-or-flight response, with norepinephrine as a helper. Upon release, epinephrine is carried to the cardiovascular system and other parts of the body. It increases blood glucose levels, increases pulse rate and blood pressure, quiets the gut, stimulates metabolism, and dilates blood vessels in skeletal muscle. At the heart, we see the rate and force of contractions increased. Key organs responsible for getting us out of physical danger, such as the heart, therefore receive excitatory stimuli from norepinephrine directly transmitted through the SNS, as well as both epinephrine and norepinephrine secreted from the adrenal medulla through the AHS. This double protection maximizes our chances of survival in times of danger.

A Gang of Four

From a neuroendocrine perspective, we have four stress response systems well in place within the body from the moment we are born. They are the LC-NA system, HPA axis, SNS, and AHS. In varying degrees, all four systems work constantly around the clock and they balance each other to ensure homeostasis and help us with stress. Multiple feedback loops are in place to help accomplish this mission.

There is a clear and logical pattern of the activation sequence that defines how the body decides which system to activate, to what degree, and under what circumstances. Perceived stress, for example, may be handled differently hormonally than actual stress. Therefore, this gang of four serves an ongoing function to protect and serve our survival needs.

Any one of these systems can be overtaxed and dysregulated. The causes range from toxins, chronic stress, medications, and hereditary factors, just to name a few. Out of these, chronic stress is perhaps the biggest culprit. Overtaxed systems invariably lead to dysregulation and breakdown as a function of time. Symptoms of AFS are merely reflections of such stress response activation, burden, dysregulation, breakdown, compensatory effect, and ultimately collapse of this process over time. For example, we see classic signs of hypoglycemia and low blood pressure, both reflective of HPA axis dysregulation, in early Adrenal Exhaustion. Dysregulation of the AHS with epinephrine overload tends to occur later on.

The Neuroendocrine Cascade in AFS

Now that you know the various chemical messengers involved, let's take another look at the stress response from a neuroendocrine perspective as AFS advances through its various stages. From this cascade, you will see how the body systematically handles different levels of stress with different response systems, all logically. When stress enters the body, the immediate central command of the stress response lies in the brain. Controlled by the LC, mediated through the LC-NA system by the brain neurotransmitter norepinephrine, the body is aroused and put on alert when stress arrives at its doorstep. This action is immediate and localized to the CNS.

The HPA axis also activates and serves as the messenger chain that ultimately controls the field command center located in the adrenal cortex, where various hormones are produced, including cortisol. These hormones have a diffusive effect throughout the body, increasing energy and glucose, and reducing inflammation.

In addition, the SNS is called into action as part of the readiness drill.

The sum of all three systems forms a complex structure and is likely to be involved early on with AFS, though the degree in which each of the systems participates is highly variable and not known. Great overlap is expected, and that signifies a well designed system with multiple control points. Successful deployment of the three systems of stress control in early stages of AFS returns the body to a normal state. Thus, no symptoms are reported by those suffering from Stage 1 and 2 AFS.

If stress is unrelenting, HPA axis signaling is increased. The adrenal cortex workload is put on overdrive. Cortisol output rises. This is Stage 2 of AFS. A persistent high cortisol level has many unintended consequences, the most prominent of which is dyslipidemia and central obesity; both are forerunners of metabolic syndrome. As Stage 2 progresses, persistent HPA axis over- stimulation and burn out may reach a point where dysregulation is on the horizon.

This point is reached when we enter Stage 3A of Adrenal Exhaustion. Cortisol output is compromised at the adrenal glands by this time. Independently, excessive norepinephrine peripherally may overwhelm the body's other organs, such as the heart. Slight cardiac palpitations may surface. The LC-NA system may be over-stimulated as well if stress is unresolved. With constant brain arousal, a growing sense of being irritable and anxious is common. We also start seeing clinical and subclinical signs of HPA axis dysregulation, including hypoglycemia and low blood pressure. Anxiety, brain fog, and a cognitive toll also increase as the LC-NA system stretches to the limit.

If left unresolved, further deterioration of the HPA axis dysregulation may arise as Stage 3A progresses, triggering other downstream hormonal axes dysregulation as we enter Stage 3B. The dysfunction of one organ system, such as the adrenal gland, can trigger a domino effect, leading to dysfunction of other organ systems. An example of this is the ovarian-adrenal-thyroid (OAT) axis imbalance in women, and the adrenal-thyroid (AT) axis imbalance in men. Multiple glands are now involved. The fire now spreads to involve multiple hormonal imbalances, with concurrently low cortisol, low progesterone, and low thyroid. With the HPA dysregulated and OAT axis imbalanced, the sympathetic nervous system (SNS), already activated before, is now put in overdrive as a compensatory reaction as we enter Stage 3C. Excessive norepinephrine, the key hormone of the SNS, builds up. This can lead to heart palpitations, increased fatigue, and panic attacks. This hormone, normally playing a low key homeostatic regulation function of daily living, now becomes part of the emergency anti-stress team. It is now also responsible for some of the fight-or-flight responses to get the body ready for impending doom and for priming other hormones for action.

If stressors are still not resolved after the above three systems are well deployed, the body, in its final attempt to overcome stress, puts the adrenomedullary hormonal system (AHS) on overdrive. The AHS is already on alert and working behind the scenes as needed from earlier phases. As the body enters late Stage 3C and 3D of Adrenal Exhaustion, the AHS goes on full throttle. A large amount of epinephrine and a smaller amount of norepinephrine are released from the adrenal medulla directly into the blood stream, flooding the body. This ensures that the vital organs, such as the brain and heart, get the necessary blood flow and thus oxygen for survival. Other less important systems for survival sacrifice temporarily, such as the re-production and gastric systems. The AHS is designed to be a temporary emergency stress response of last resort. Long term stimulation without adequate rest may lead to AHS dysfunction, putting the body into a state of further disequilibrium, and at the end, disarray. This frequently appears in sufferers who take metabolic stimulants to keep up their energy when faced with fatigue, not knowing that this strategy can be harmful to the AHS.

If not reversed on a timely basis, the overall anti-stress hormonal supply chain continues to deteriorate. Cortisol and other hormones become grossly dysregulated and severely depleted. This generally occurs in advanced phases of Adrenal Exhaustion. In its last ditch attempt to increase production of hormones, undesirable and destabilizing positive feedback loops may be activated in the process. Crashes are common. If not reversed, the body has no choice but to continue to down-regulate to conserve energy concurrently.

Over time, it draws nearer to failure as it runs out of necessary basic reserve to prime the hormonal pump for normal basic function. To conserve energy, the body admits defeat, surrenders and turns to activating what reserve is left standing as it enters a basic survival mode. This is accomplished by further down-regulation of essentially all bodily functions, the last of which to be sacrificed is the brain. This effectively reduces energy output to a level close to a vegetative state as the final preparation for impending collapse. It comes as no surprise that those with advanced AFS are invariably incapacitated and bedridden.

Who is in Control?

From a neuroendocrinological perspective, it is clear that the body's multiple stress response pathways offer redundancy systems to handle stress the vast majority of the time. It has ensured the survival of our species for quite some time. What is confusing clinically in AFS, is that these pathways can be activated a few at a time, or all at once, and quickly or slowly, as the body sees appropriate for that moment in time. The body is truly in control, despite what appears to be total confusion from a conventional medical logic perspective.

> **To fully appreciate the body's heroic effort to rescue us from stress, it is important to understand first that our brain is in control of our body through the neuroendocrine system. What one person perceives as stressful may not be for another. Based on the perceived level of stress by the mind, the body automatically activates any or all of the anti-stress mechanisms in place by way of hormones and neurotransmitters.**

In order for us to fully grasp the big picture, clinicians and sufferers alike need to take a step back, because it is easy to be confused from a closer or subjective perspective. The picture from afar is crystal clear: that of a body in trouble, unable to maintain homeostasis; and trying all its ways and means to recover on its own with the only method it knows—activating any or all of the built in stress response systems modulated by the neurological and endocrine systems working in tandem. The more severe the stress, the more other systems, such as the musculoskeletal, psychiatric, cardiac, and immune, are also affected adversely.

The body is a closed system. Severe dysregulation of one system invariably impacts other systems. This is inescapable. Despite this clinical chaos, one can see a controlled collapse that is logical and systematic from the body's point of view. Symptoms are simply the messages or signs the body sends us as warnings of impending danger, thereby alerting us to take appropriate action. Despite a losing battle if stressors are not removed, the mind continues to be ultimately in charge throughout this ordeal through various neuroendocrinological stress response pathways.

The neuroendocrine basis of AFS is solid and clear. Evidence based scientific research has proven beyond a doubt that stress can and does kill.

Suggested Reading and Resources on the Adrenal Fatigue Syndrome

In addition to the books, CDs and DVDs listed in the front of *Adrenal Fatigue Syndrome*, here are additional free readings and resources from our website, *www.DrLam.com/afs/*. When on the site, just click on the topic of interest. Each will help you understand the scientific basis of our approach to Adrenal Fatigue Syndrome we take throughout this book.

Acidosis

Aging Brain

Andropause

Atrial Fibrillation

Beef, Chicken, or Fish

Blood Thinners and
    Nutritional Supplements

Chelation

Cholesterol

Dehydration

Detoxification

DHEA

Diabetes

Eggs—Good for your body?

Endometriosis

Nutritional Supplements—
    To Take or Not?

Omega 3 Fatty Acid

Oral Health

Progesterone

The Big Fat Lie

Estrogen Dominance

Fibroids

Heart Disease Prevention—
    A Complete Nutritional Approach

Hypothyroidism

Insulin and Aging:

Magnesium and Aging

Menopause

Metabolic Syndrome

Milk—The Perfect Food?

My Doctor Is Killing Me

New Markers of Cardiovascular Disease

Nutritional Medicine

Upper Limits Vitamin C and E Intake

Water

Where to Buy Supplements

Why Conventional Medicine Rejects
    Adrenal Fatigue Syndrome

After Recovery

After your recovery from Adrenal Fatigue Syndrome, the natural progression is to embark on an anti-aging program where you begin to reverse the biological clock naturally, while keeping AFS at bay. We have a complete library on this in our website. The following articles are helpful and found also on *www.DrLam.com/afs/*.

Anti-aging Program	Dr. Lam's Smoothie Recipe
Anti-aging Strategies	Customized Exercise Routine
Blood Type Diet	Links to Various Health Centers
Osteoporosis	Calories That Count
Woman's Optimal Daily Allowance	Men's Optimal Daily Allowance
Links to Natural Protocols for Common Health Conditions	

For the Avid Reader in Natural Health

You can download our free online ebooks from our home page at *www.DrLam.com*: *Beating Cancer with Natural Medicine*
5 Proven Secrets to Longevity

Other Useful Links

New information and links on natural health and Adrenal Fatigue Syndrome are regularly added to our website library. These include many nonprofit educational organizations, links to scientific journals, periodicals, and additional recommended books.

Here is the link: *http://www.DrLam.com/links.asp*

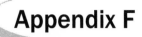

3 Minute Adrenal Fatigue Syndrome Test

Here is a checklist of common symptoms associated with Adrenal Fatigue Syndrome. Check the boxes that are applicable. See your score below and find out what you can do about it.

☐ Tendency to gain weight especially at the waist and inability to lose it.

☐ High frequency of getting the flu and other respiratory diseases that tend to last longer than usual.

☐ Reduced sex drive.

☐ Lightheaded when rising from a supine position.

☐ Unable to remember things and unclear thinking.

☐ Lack of energy in the mornings and also in the afternoon between 3-5:00 PM.

☐ Feel better suddenly for a brief period after a meal.

☐ Need coffee or stimulants to get going in the morning.

☐ Crave for salty, fatty, and high protein food such as meat and cheese.

☐ Increased symptoms of PMS for women; periods are heavy and then stop, or almost stop on the 4th day, only to start to flow again on the 5th or 6th day.

☐ Pain in the upper back or neck for no apparent reasons.

☐ Easily startled.

☐ Decreased ability to handle stress and responsibilities.

☐ Body temperature is off balance; hands and feet feel cold, face feels warm, or hot flashes.

☐ Unexplained hair loss.

☐ Tendency to tremble when under pressure.

☐ Multiple allergies such as asthma, hay fever, skin rashes, eczema, hives, and food sensitivity.

Enter the number of checkmarks you have made: _____

What does your score mean?

If your score is 4 or below, chances are you do not have Adrenal Fatigue Syndrome unless your symptoms are quite severe. There may be other dysfunction in place. Adrenal Fatigue Syndrome is unlikely to be significantly involved, although we can't be sure without a detailed history. You can adopt many of the dietary and lifestyle recommendations in this book as they are generally conducive to good health. Group 1 and 2 nutritional supplementations (Chapters 20, *First Line of Defense—Gentle Nutrients*, and Chapter 21, *Second Line of Defense—Glandulars and Herbs*) are generally well tolerated if your doctor approves. If you do not improve within a reasonable amount of time, write to us through our website with your score and what you did. We will give you our thoughts in confidence.

If your score is 5-9, you may or may not have Adrenal Fatigue Syndrome. Many conditions mimic AFS, so if you have not already done so, visit your doctor for further medical investigation. If you are given a clean bill of health but remain symptomatic, consider Adrenal Fatigue Syndrome. The higher your score on the test, the higher your risk of Adrenal Fatigue Syndrome. You also can adopt many of the dietary and lifestyle recommendations mentioned in this book, but be cautious when it comes to nutritional supplementation, as they can worsen the condition if not properly used. If you are not sure where you stand or what to do, then write directly and privately to us online through our website (*www.DrLam.com*) with your score and a brief history. We'll give you our assessment and suggestions in confidence.

If your score is 10 or above, it is imperative that you become fully educated about Adrenal Fatigue Syndrome and alert your doctor about this condition. The more severe your symptoms, the more dysfunctional your adrenal glands likely are. We *do not* recommend self-navigation as it often makes the condition worse over time. If you cannot find someone knowledgeable to help you, if you fail to improve on your recovery plan, and are not sure where you stand or what to do next, then write to us directly and privately through our website (*www.DrLam.com*). Let us know your score, a detailed medical history, and your main complaints. We will reply to you in confidence and give you some guidance.

This free test is also available online at our website *www.DrLam.com*.

Appendix G

Nutritional Supplement Blends for AFS

Not all supplements are created the same. Quality varies greatly, depending on ingredients and the manufacturing process. Inferior quality supplements can deter the recovery process and actually make things worse. Buying supplements based on price alone is a common recovery mistake.

To ensure the highest quality and consistency based on latest research, we have formulated our own line (Dr.Lam) of dietary supplements. They are made specifically for those with AFS and those who believe in using nutritionals to deter the aging process. Most people with AFS are highly sensitive. We have to be very careful about what we recommend. Knowing the exact blend and ingredients of each formulation gives us great insight and advantage on how to match each person's nutritional need with their body state during each step of their recovery. These products are made in the United States under strict manufacturing standards.

The complete line is available at *SupplementClinic.com*, the most complete online dietary supplement retailer dedicated to AFS, providing everything from supplements to books, video and saliva test kits. In addition to having reasonable price and excellent service, they ship worldwide. Royalties received go to support the ongoing mission of *DrLam.com*.

Some of the most popular of Dr. Lam's nutritional formulations designed for Adrenal Fatigue Syndrome are:

Quantamax®: Quantamax is a technologically advanced health drink formulated in a special matrix of mineral ascorbates, amino acids, co-factors, and immune-enhancing nutrients. This support provides the nutrients necessary to help rebuild and rejuvenate the important adrenal and cardiovascular collagen network in our bodies, leading to healthier adrenals, skin and decreased risk of cardiovascular disease. This blend formula provides for quick and gentle energy boosts without the over-stimulatory, spiky side-effect of ascorbic acid.

C-Support: C-Support is a cutting-edge blend of four different sources of Vitamin C including ascobyl palmitate, the fat soluable form. This formula provides a precise balanced ratio designed for sustained release to achieve optimal biological activity of Vitamin C in the body.

Pandrenal®: Pantethine, along with pantothenic Acid (Vitamin B5), forms a powerful blend in supporting adrenal glands and normal cholesterol levels in the body. Both are needed, and having the right ratio of each is important to harvest the synergistic effect. It is manufactured in a hermetically sealed soft-gel to deliver the purest and most potent combination possible.

Adreno-Blast™: The formula contains a blend of adrenal glandular, adaptogenic herbs, and four types of ascorbates designed to increase overall body energy, while decreasing exhaustion and fatigue. This is particularly useful for those in mild or recovering AFS when the body is stable.

LipoNano® C: LipoNano C represents a major breakthrough in the therapeutic nutrient delivery system of Vitamin C, with several key characteristics. First, Liposomal Encapsulation Technology (LET) is used. It combines nano-technology and bio-technology in a powerful way to take advantage of characteristics of liposomes similar to that made by Mother Nature, using natural ingredients such as essential fatty acids and phospholipids. Second, these liposomes are naturally strong and sized perfectly for maximum stability during transport and easy penetration at the cellular level, just as Mother Nature intended. Third, the liposomes contain nutrients and synergistic co-factors in a micro-bubble. Cellular bioavailability is significantly enhanced. Due to the high potency of this formula, always start a with small amount.

LipoNano® Glutathione: Glutathione, an antioxidant produced by the body that fastens to and gets rid of toxins, is necessary to help purge the body of poisonous metabolic waste and to maintain the immune system. When exposed to aging and stress, our glutathione levels drop. Synergistic co-factors, such as Vitamin E and B12, are important elements that enhance clinical outcome. Replenishment is critical to enhance AFS recovery.

Chapter Notes

Chapter 1

Addison, T. *On the Constitutional and Local Effects of Diseases of the Supra-renal Capsules.* Special ed. (Birmingham, Ala: Classics of Medicine Library, 1980). Originally published: Samuel Highley, London, 1855.

Arlt, W., Allolio, B. "Adrenal insufficiency." Lancet 361 (2003): 1881-93.

Betterle, C., Dal Pra, C., Mantero, F., Zanchetta, R. "Autoimmune adrenal insufficiency and autoimmune polyendocrine syndromes: autoantibodies, autoantigens, and their applicability in diagnosis and disease prediction." *Endocr. Rev. 23* (2002): 327-364.

Dorin, R., Qualls, C., Crapo, L. "Diagnosis of adrenal insufficiency." *Annals of Internal Medicine,* 139(3) (2003): 194–204.

Juliano, L. M., Griffiths, R. R. "A critical review of caffeine withdrawal: empirical validation of symptoms and signs, incidence, severity, and associated features." *Psychopharmacology 176* (2004): 1–29.

Kong, M. F., Jeffcoate, W. "Eighty-six cases of Addison's disease." *Clin. Endocrinol.* (Oxf.) 41 (1994): 757-761.

Karling, P., et al. "Gastrointestinal Symptoms Are Associated with Hypothalamic-Pituitary-Adrenal Axis Suppression in Healthy Individuals." *Scandinavian Journal of Gastroenterology 42,* no. 11 (November 2007): 1294–1301.

Chapter 2

Arlt, W., Callies, F., Koehler, I., et al. « Dehydroepiandrosterone supplementation in healthy men with an age-related decline of dehydroepiandrosterone secretion." *J Clin Endocrinol Metab 86* (2001):4686–4692.

Arvat, E., Di Vito, L., Laffranco, F., et al. "Stimulatory effect of adrenocorticotropin on cortisol, aldosterone, and dehydroepiandrosterone secretion in normal humans: dose-response study." *J. Clin. Endocrinol. Metab. 88* (2000): 3141-3146.

Bachmann, G., et al. "Female androgen insufficiency: The Princeton Consensus Statement on definition, classification and assessment." *Fertil Steril 77* (2002): 660-665.

Baulieu, E. E., Thomas, G., Legrain, S., et al. « Dehydroepiandrosterone (DHEA), DHEA sulfate, and aging: Contribution of the DHEA study to a sociobiomedical issue." *Proc Natl Acad Sci USA 97* (2000):4279–4284.

Charmandari, E., Tsigos, C., Chrousos, G. P. "Neuroendocrinology of stress." *Ann. Rev. Physiol. 67* (2005): 259–284.

Chrousos, G. P, Kino, T. "Glucocorticoid action networks and complex psychiatric and/or somatic disorders." *Stress 10* (2007): 213–219.

Chrousos, G. P., Loriaux, D. L, Gold, P. W., (eds). "Mechanisms of Physical and Emotional Stress" *Advances in Experimental Medicine and Biology*, Vol. 245 (Plenum Press, New York, 1988).

Crofford, L. J., Pillemer, S. R., Kalogeras, K. T., et al "Hypothalamic-pituitary-adrenal axis perturbations in patients with fibromyalgia." *Arthritis Rheum.37*(11) (1994): 1583-92.

Epel, E. S., McEwen, B., Seemanm T., et al. "Stress and body shape: stress-induced cortisol secretion is consistently greater among women with central fat." *Psychosomatic Medicine, 62* (2000): 623–632.

Farag, N. H., Moore, W. E., Lovallo, W. R. et al. "Hypothalamic–pituitary–adrenal axis function: relative contributions of perceived stress and obesity in women." *Journal of Women's Health 17* (2008): 1647–1655.

Fuller, R. W. "The involvement of serotonin in regulation of pituitary-adrenocortical function." *Front Neuroendocrinol.* 13(3) (1992):250-70.

Griep, E. N., Boersma, J. W., de Kloet, E. R. "Altered reactivity of the hypothalamic-pituitary-adrenal axis in the primary fibromyalgia syndrome." *J Rheumatol*, 20 (1993):469-474.

Guyton, A. C., Hall, J. E. "Textbook of medical physiology, 10th ed. Philadelphia: WB Saunders Company (2000):869-83.

Hartzband, P. I., Van Herle, A. J., Sorger, L., et al. "Assessment of the hypothalamic-pituitary-adrenal (HPA) axis function: comparison of the ACTH stimulation, insulin-hypoglycemia and metyrapone tests." *J Endocrinol Invest* 11 (1988):769-76.

Heim,C., Ehlert, U., Dirk, H., Helhammer, H. "The potential role of hypocortisolism in the pathophysiology of stress-related bodily disorders." *Psychoneuroendocrinology* 25 (2000):1-35.

Lundberg, U. "Stress hormones in health and illness: the roles of work and gender." *Psychoneuroendocrinology* 30 (2005): 1017-21.

Petrides, J. S., Gold, P. W., Mueller, G. P., et al. Marked differences in functioning of the hypothalamic–pituitary–adrenal axis between groups of men." *Journal of Applied Physiology*, 82 (1979–1988).

Qi, D., Rodrigues, B. "Glucocorticoids produce whole body insulin resistance with changes in cardiac metabolism. American Journal of Physiology." *Endocrinology and Metabolism* 292 (2007) : E654–E667.

Rasmuson, S., Olsson, T., Hagg, E. "A low-dose ACTH test to assess the function of the hypothalamic-pituitary-adrenal axis." *Clin Endocrinol* (Oxf) 44 (1996):151-6.

Wren, B. G., Day, R. O., McLachlan, A. J., Williams, K. M. "Pharmacokinetics of estradiol, progesterone, testosterone and dehydroepiandrosterone after transbuccal administration to postmenopausal women." *Climacteric* 6(2) (2003): 104-111.

Yehuda, R., Resnick, H., Kahana, B., et al. "Persistent hormonal alterations following extreme stress in humans: Adaptive or maladaptive?" *Psychosom Med* 55 (1993): 287-297.

Lupien, S. J., et al. 'Stress Hormones and Human Memory Function across the Lifespan. *Psychoneuroendocrinology* 30, no. 3 (April 2005): 225–242.

Demitrack, M. A., et al. 'Evidence for Impaired Activation of the Hypothalamic-Pituitary-Adrenal Axis in Patients with Chronic Fatigue Syndrome." *Journal of Clinical Endocrinology & Metabolism* 73, no. 6 (December 1991): 1224–1234.

Chapter 5

Chrousos, G. P. "The hypothalamic-pituitary-adrenal axis and immune-mediated inflammation." *N. Engl. J. Med.* 332 (1995): 1351–1362.

Chrousos, G. P. "The role of stress and the hypothalamic–pituitary–adrenal axis in the pathogenesis of the metabolic syndrome: neuro-endocrine and target tissue-related causes." *Int. J. Obes.* (London) 24 (2000): S50f–S55f.

Duclos, M., Marquez Pereira, P., Barat, P. et al. "Increased cortisol bioavailability, abdominal obesity, and the metabolic syndrome in obese women." *Obesity Research* 13 (2005): 1157–1166.

Kern, S., et al. "Glucose Metabolic Changes in the Prefrontal Cortex Are Associated with HPA Axis Response to a Psychosocial Stressor." *Psychoneuroendocrinology* 33, no. 4 (May 2008):517–529.

Chapter 6

Aaron, L. A., Buchwald, D. "Chronic diffuse musculoskeletal pain, fibromyalgia and co-morbid unexplained clinical conditions." *Best Pract Res Clin Rheumatol.*17(4) (2003):563-74.

Adler, G. K., Manfredsdottir, V. F., Creskoff, K. W. "Neuroendocrine abnormalities in fibromyalgia." *Curr Pain Headache Rep.* 6(4) (2002): 289-98.

Akkus, S., Delibas, N., Tamer, M. N. "Do sex hormones play a role in fibromyalgia?" *Rheumatology* 39 (2000): 1161-1163.

Anderson, R. A. "Nutritional factors influencing the glucose/insulin system: chromium." *J Am Coll Nutr.* 16 (1997): 404-410.

Arnold, L. M., Keck, P.E., Welge Jr., J. A. "Antidepressant treatment of fibromyalgia. A meta-analysis and review." *Psychosomatics.* 41(2) (2000):104-13.

Catena, C., Lapenna, R., Baroselli, S., et al. "Insulin sensitivity in patients with primary aldosteronism: a follow-up study." *Journal of Clinical Endocrinology and Metabolism* 91 (2006): 3457–3463.

Chrousos, G. P. "The stress response and immune function: clinical implications; the 1999 Novera H. Spector lecture." *Ann. NY Acad. Sci.* 917 (2000): 38–67.

Eisinger, J., Plantamura, A., Ayavou, T. "Glycolysis abnormalities in fibromyalgia." *J Am Coll Nutr* 13 (1994):144-148.

Fallo, F., lLa Mea, P., Sonino, N. et al. "Adiponectin and insulin sensitivity in primary aldosteronism." *American Journal of Hypertension* 20 (2007): 855–861.

Fallo, F., Veglio, F., Bertello, C., et al. "Prevalence and characteristics of the metabolic syndrome in primary aldosteronism." *Journal of Clinical Endocrinology and Metabolism* 91 (2006): 454–459.

Geenen, R., Jacobs, J. W., Bijlsma, J. W. "Evaluation and management of endocrine dysfunction in fibromyalgia. *Rheum Dis Clin North Am.* 28(2) (2002):389-404.

Giacchetti, G., Sechi, L. A., Rilli, S., et al. "The rennin–angiotensin–aldosterone system, glucose metabolism and diabetes. *Trends in Endocrinology and Metabolism* 16 (2005): 120–126.

Gran, J. T. "The epidemiology of chronic generalized musculoskeletal pain." *Best Pract Res Clin Rheumatol.* 17(4) (2003): 547-61.

Henquin, J. C. "Triggering and amplifying pathways of regulation of insulin secretion by glucose. *Diabetes* 49 (2000): 1751–1760.

Stechmesser, E., Scherbaum, W. A., Grossman, T., Berg, P. A. "An ELISA method for the detection of autoantibodies to adrenal cortex." *J. Immunol. Methods* 80 (1985): 67-76.

Lupien, S. J. et al. "Cortisol Levels During Human Aging Predict Hippocampal Atrophy and Memory Deficits." *Nature Neuroscience* 1, no. 1 (May 1998): 69–73.

Chapter 7

ACOG Committee on Gynecologic Practice. ACOG committee opinion number 322. "Compounded bioidentical hormones." *Obstet. Gynecol.* 106(5) (2005): 1139-1140.

Andersen, S., Bruun, N. H., Pedersen, K. M., Laurberg, P. "Biologic variation is important for interpretation of thyroid function tests." *Thyroid.* 13 (2003):1069-1078.

Bachman, G. A., Schaefers, M., Uddin, A., Utian, W. F. "Lowest effective transdermal 17ß-estradiol dose for relief of hot flushes in postmenopausal women." *Obstet. Gynecol.* 110(4) (2007): 771-779.

Bagchi, N., Brown, T. R,, Parish, R. F. "Thyroid dysfunction in adults over age 55 years. A study in an urban US community." *Archives of Internal Medicine* 150 (1990): 785-787.

Ballweg, M. L., and the Endometriosis Association. *The Endometriosis Sourcebook: The Definitive Guide to Current Treatment Options, the Latest Research, Common Myths About the Disease, and Coping Strategies – Both Physical and Emotional.* (Chicago, Ill: Contemporary Books, 1995).

Barbieri, R. L. "Hormonal therapy of endometriosis." *Infertil Reprod Med Clin North Am.* 3 (1992): 187-200.

Barnett, A. H., Donald, R. A., Espiner, E. A. "High concentrations of thyroid-stimulating hormone in untreated glucocorticoid deficiency: indication of primary hypothyroidism?" *Br Med J* (Clin Res Ed) 285 (1982): 172-173.

Boothby, L. A., Doering, P. L., Kipersztok, S. "Bioidentical hormone therapy: a review." *Menopause* 11(3), 356-467 (2004).

Chrousos, G. P., Torpy, D., Gold, P. W. "Interactions between the hypothalamic–pituitary–adrenal axis and the female reproductive system: clinical implications." *Ann. Intern. Med.* 129 (1998): 229–240.

Chu, J. W., Crapo, L. M. "The treatment of subclinical hypothyroidism is seldom necessary." *J Clin Endocrinol Metab.* 86 (2001):4591-4599.

Cirigliano, M. "Bioidentical hormone therapy: a review of the evidence." *J. Womens Health* 16(5) (2007): 600-631.

Kudielka, B. M., Kirschbaum, C. "Sex differences in HPA axis responses to stress: a review." *Biological Psychology,* 69 (1) (2005): 113-32.

Chapter 9

Adler, G. K., Kinsley, B. T., Hurwitz, S., Mossey, C. J., Goldenberg, D. L. "Reduced hypothalamic-pituitary and sympathoadrenal responses to hypoglycemia in women with fibromyalgia syndrome." *Am J Med.*106(5) (1999):534-43.

Alavi, A., Hirsch, L. J. "Studies of central nervous system disorders with single photon emission computed tomography and positron emission tomography: evolution over the past 2 decades." *Semin Nucl Med.* 21(1) (1991):58-81.

Blackburn-Munro, G., Blackburn-Munro, R. E. "Chronic pain, chronic stress and depression: coincidence or consequence?" *J Neuroendocrinol.*; 13(12) (2001):1009-23.

Bunney, W. E. Jr., Davis, J. M. "Norepinephrine in depressive reactions: A review." *Arch Gen Psychiatry* 13 (1965): 483-494.

Cahill, D. J., Wardle, P. G., Maile, L. A., et al. "Ovarian dysfunction in endometriosis-associated and unexplained infertility." *J Assist Reprod Genet.* 14 (1997):554-7.

Epstein, S. E., Stampfer, M., Beiser, G. P. "Role of capacitance and resistance vessels in vasovagal syncope. *Circulation* 37 (1988): 524–533.

Faber, J., Petersen, L., Wiinberg, N., et al. "Hemodynamic changes after levothyroxine treatment in subclinical hypothyroidism. *Thyroid*, 12 (2002): 319-324.

Flaa, A., Sandvik, L., Kjeldsen, S. E., Eide, I. K., Rostrup, M. "Does sympathoadrenal activity predict changes in body fat? An 18 year follow up study." *Am J Clin Nutr.* 87(6) (2008): 1596–601.

Hammond, C. B., Maxson, W. S. "Current status of estrogen therapy for the menopause." *Fertil Steril.* 37 (1982):5-25.

Hollowell, J. G., Staehling, N. W., Flanders, W.D., et al. "Serum TSH, T(4), and thyroid antibodies in the United States population (1988-94): National Health and Nutrition Examination Survey (NHANES III). *Journal of Clinical Endocrinology and Metabolism*, 87 (2002): 489-499.

Kahaly, G. J., Dillmann, W. H. "Thyroid hormone action in the heart. *Endocrine Review*, 26 (2005): 704-728.

Kakucska, I., Qi, Y., Lechan, R. M. "Changes in adrenal status affect hypothalamic thyrotropin-releasing hormone gene expression in parallel with corticotropin-releasing hormone." Endocrinology136 (1995): 2795-2802.

Kjaer, M., Sécher, N. H., Galbo, H. "Physical stress and catecholamine release." *Baillieres Clin Endocrinol Metab.* I(2) (1987):279–98.

Ljung, T., Holm, G., Friberg, P., et al. "The activity of the hypothalamic–pituitary–adrenal axis and the sympathetic nervous system in relation to waist/hip circumference ratio in men." *Obesity Research*, 8 (2000): 487–495.

Lombardi, F., Sandrone, G., Pernpruner, S., et al. "Heart rate variability as an index of sympathovagal interaction after acute myocardial infarction." *Am J Cardiol* 60 (1987): 1239–1245.

McHardy-Young, S., Lessof, M. H., Maisey, M. N. "Serum TSH and thyroid studies in Addison's disease." *Clin. Endocrinol.* (Oxf.) 1 (1974): 45-56.

Mircioiu, C., Perju, A., Griu, E., et al. "Pharmacokinetics of progesterone in postmenopausal women: 2. Pharmacokinetics following percutaneous administration." *Eur. J. Drug Metab. Pharmacokinet.* 23(3) (1998): 397-402.

Sneddon, J. F., Counihan, P. J., Bashir, Y. "Assessment of autonomic function in patients with neurally mediated syncope: Augmented cardiopulmonary baroreceptor responses to graded orthostatic stress." *J Am Coll Cardiol* 21 (1993): 1193–1198.

Thiedke, C. "Alopecia in women." *American Family Physician* 67(5) (2003): 1007–1014.

Weinstein, L. "Hormonal therapy in the patient with surgical menopause." *Obstet Gynecol.* 75 (1990): 47S-50S.

Valentino, R., et al. "Unusual Association of Thyroiditis, Addison's Disease, Ovarian Failure and Celiac Disease in a Young Woman." *Journal of Endocrinological Investigation* 22, no. 5 (May 1999):390–394.

Van Den Eede, F., Moorkens, G. "HPA-Axis Dysfunction in Chronic Fatigue Syndrome: Clinical Implications." *Psychosomatics* 49, no. 5 (September–October 2008):450.

Chapter 10

Beishuizen, A., Thijs, L. G. "Relative adrenal failure in intensive care: an identifying problem requiring treatment?" *Best Pract Res Clin Endocrinol Metab* 15 (2001): 513-31.

Bloomfield, D., Maurer, M., Bigger, J. T. "Effects of age on outcome of tilt-table testing." *Am J Cardiol* 83 (1999): 1055–1058.

Boscaro, M., Betterle, C., Volpato, M., et al. "Hormonal responses during various phases of autoimmune adrenal failure: no evidence for 21-hydroxylase enzyme activity block in vivo." *J. Clin. Endocrinol. Metab.* 81 (1996): 2801-2804

Bouachour, G., Tirot, P., Varache, N., Gouello, J. P., Harry, P., Alquier, P. "Hemodynamic changes in acute adrenal insufficiency." *Intensive Care Medicine,* 20(2), (1994): 138–141.

Chosy, J. J., Graham, D. T. "Catecholamines in vasovagal fainting." *J Psychosom Res* 9 (1965): 189–194.

Drucker, D., McLaughlin, J. "Adrenocortical dysfunction in acute illness." *Crit Care Med* 14 (1986):789-91.

Liu, B., Mittmann, N., Knowles, S. R., Shear, N. H. "Hyponatremia and the syndrome of inappropriate secretion of antidiuretic hormone associated with the use of selective serotonin reuptake inhibitors: a re-view of spontaneous reports." *CMAJ* 155 (1996): 519-27.

Tsigos, C., Chrousos, G. P. "Hypothalamic-pituitary-adrenal axis, neuroendocrine factors and stress." *J Psychosom Res.* 53(4) (2002): 865-71.

Chapter 11

Fischer, H. P., Eich, W., Russell, I. J. "A possible role for saliva as a diagnostic fluid in patients with chronic pain. *Semin Arthritis Rheum.* 27(6) (1998): 348-59.

Putignano, P., Dubini, A., Toja, P., et al. "Salivary cortisol measurement in normal-weight, obese and anorexic women: comparison with plasma cortisol." *European Journal of Endocrinology* 145 (2001): 165–171.

Wood, B., Wessely, S., Papadopoulos, A., Poon, L., Checkley, S. "Salivary cortisol profiles in chronic fatigue syndrome." *Neuropsychobiology* 37 (1998): 1-4.

Kudielka, M. J., Broderick, E., and Kirschbaum, C. "Compliance with Saliva Sampling Protocols: Electronic Monitoring Reveals Invalid Cortisol Daytime Profiles in Noncompliant Subjects." *Psychosomatic Medicine* 65 (2003): 313–319.

Taruim H., Nakamura, A. "Saliva Cortisol. A Good Indicator for Acceleration Stress. *Aviation, Space and Environmental Medicine* 58, no. 6 (June 1987): 573–575.

Bigert, C., Bluhm, G., Theorell, T. "Saliva Cortisol—a New Approach in Noise Research to Study Stress Effects." *International Journal of Hygiene and Environmental Health* 208, no. 3 (2005): 227–230.

Raff, H. "Utility of Salivary Cortisol Measurements in Cushing's Syndrome and Adrenal Insufficiency." *Journal of Clinical Endocrinology and Metabolism* 94, no. 10 (October 2009): 3647–3655.

Nicolson, N. A., Van Diest, R. "Salivary Cortisol Patterns in Vital Exhaustion." *Journal of Psychosomatic Research* 49, no. 5 (2000):335–342.

Chapter 15

Alesci, S., et al. "Major depression is associated with significant diurnal elevations in plasma IL-6 levels, a shift of its circadian rhythm, and loss of physiologic complexity in its secretion: clinical implications." *J. Clin. Endocrinol. Metab.* 90 (2005): 2522–2530

American Psychiatric A. "Diagnostic and Statistical Manual of Mental Disorders." (American Psychiatric Press, Washington DC. 1994).

Baillie, A. J., Rapee, R. M. "Predicting who benefits from psychoeducation and self help for panic attacks. *Behav. Res. Ther.* 42(5) (2004): 513–527.

Ballweg, M. L. "Blaming the victim: The psychologizing of endometriosis." *Obstet Gynecol Clin North Am.* 24 (1997): 441-53

Barden, N., Reul, J. M., Holsboer, F. "Do antidepressants stabilize mood through actions on the hypothalamic-pituitary-adrenocortical system? *Trends Neurosci* 18 (1995): 6-11.

Brady, L. S., Whitfield, H. J. J., Fox, R. J., et al. "Long term antidepressant administration alters corticotropin-releasing hormone, tyrosine hydroxylase, and mineralocorticoid receptor gene expression in rat brain." *J Clin Invest* 87 (1991): 831-837.

Brown, G. R., Anderson, B. "Psychiatric morbidity in adult in patients with childhood histories of sexual and physical abuse." *Am. J. Psychiatry* 148 (1991): 55–61.

Chrousos, G. P., Gold, P. W. "The concepts of stress and stress system disorders: overview of physical and behavioral homeostasis." *JAMA* 267 (1992): 1244–1252.

Felitti, V. J., et al. "Relationship of childhood abuse and household dysfunction to many of the leading causes of death in adults." *Am. J. Prevent. Med.* 14 (1998): 245–258.

Maes, M., Meltzer, H. Y. "The serotonin hypothesis of major depression," in Bloom, F. E., and Kupfer, D. J. (eds): *Psychopharmacology: The Fourth Generation of Progress.* (New York: Raven Press, 1995), 933-944.

Simms, R. W. "Fibromyalgia is not a muscle disorder." Am J Med Sci. 315(6) (1998): 346-50. VanItallie, B. "Stress: A Risk Factor for Serious Illness." *Metabolism* 51, no. 6, Supplement 1 (June 2002):40–45.

Chapter 16

Flocke, S. A., Miller, W. L., Crabtree, B. F. "Relationships between physician practice style, patient satisfaction, and attributes of primary care." *J Fam Pract.* 51(10) (2002): 835–840.

Chapter 20

Afkhami-Ardekani, M., Shojaoddiny-Ardekani, A. "Effect of vitamin C on blood glucose, serum lipids & serum insulin in type 2 diabetes patients." *Indian J Med Res.*126(5) (2007): 471-4.

Audera, C., Patulny, R. V., Sander, B. H, "Douglas RM. Mega-dose vitamin C in treatment of the common cold: a randomised controlled trial." *Med J Aust.* 175(7) (2001): 359-362.

Berandi, J. M., Ziegenfuss, T. N. "Effects of ribose supplementation on repeated sprint performance in men." *J Strength Cond Res* 17 (2003):47-52.

Bounous, G., Molson, J. "Competition for glutathione precursors between the immune system and the skeletal muscle: Pathogenesis of chronic fatigue syndrome." *Med Hypotheses.* 53(4) (Oct. 1999): 347–9.

Bruno, R. S., Leonard, S. W., Atkinson, J., et al. "Faster plasma vitamin E disappearance in smokers is normalized by vitamin C supplementation" [Discussion: 2007; 42: 578–80]. *Free Radic Biol Med* 40 (2006): 689–97.

Covens, A. L., Christopher, P., Casper, R. F. "The effect of dietary supplementation with fish oil fatty acids on surgically induced endometriosis in the rabbit." *Fertil Steril.* 49(4) (1988): 698-703.

Drive, C., Georgeou, A. "Variable effects of vitamin E on Drosophila longevity." *Biogerontology* 4 (2003): 91–5.

Enlander, Derek. "CFS Treatment using Glutathione in Immunoprop." *The CFS Handbook* (2002): 58–62.

Falk, D. J., Heelan, K. A., Thyfault, J. P., Koch, A. J. "Effects of effervescent creatine, ribose, and glutamine supplementation on muscular strength, muscular endurance, and body composition." *J Strength Cond Res* 17 (2003): 810-16.

Gandini, S., Merzenich, H., Robertson, C., Boyle, P. "Meta-analysis of studies on breast cancer risk and diet: the role of fruit and vegetable consumption and the intake of associated micronutrients." *Eur J Cancer.* 36 (2000): 636-646.

Hornig, D., et al. "Ascorbic acid." In: *Modern Nutrition in Health and Disease.* (Philadelphia, PA: Lea and Febiger, 1988), 417.

Hsieh, C. C., Lin, B. F. "Opposite effects of low and high dose supplementation of vitamin E on survival of MRL/lpr mice." *Nutrition* 21 (2005): 940–8.

Institute of Medicine. "Dietary Reference Intakes for Vitamin C, Vitamin E, Selenium, and Carotenoids." (Washington, DC: National Academy of Sciences, 2002). Accessed Sept. 14, 2007.

Kompauer, I., Heinrich, J., Wolfram, G., Linseisen, J. "Association of carotenoids, tocopherols, and vitamin C in plasma with allergic rhinitis and allergic sensitization in adults." *Public Health Nutr.* 9 (2006): 472-9.

Laight, D. W., Carrier, M. J., Anggard, E. E. "Antioxidants, diabetes and endothelial dysfunction." *Cardiovasc Res.* 47 (2000): 457-464.

Levine, G. N., Frei, B., Koulouris, S. N. "Ascorbic acid reverses endothelial vasomotor dysfunction in patients with coronary artery disease. *Circulation* 93 (1996): 1107-1113.

Lipman, R. D., Bronson, R. T., Wu, D. et al. "Disease incidence and longevity are unaltered by dietary antioxidant supplementation initiated during middle age in C57BL/6 mice. *Mech Ageing Dev* 103 (1998): 269–84.

Liu, J. F., Lee, Y. W. "Vitamin C supplementation restores the impaired vitamin E status of guinea pigs fed oxidized frying oil." *J Nutr* 128 (1998): 116–22.

Masaki, K. H., Losonczy, K. G., Izmirlian, G. "Association of vitamin E and C supplement use with cognitive function and dementia in elderly men." *Neurology.* 54 (2000): 1265-1272.

Massie, H. R., Aiello, V. R., Doherty, T. J. "Dietary vitamin C improves the survival of mice. *Gerontology* 30 (1984): 371–5.

"Nutrients and Nutritional Agents." In: Kastrup, E. K., Hines, Burnham T., Short, R. M., et al, eds. *Drug Facts and Comparisons* (St. Louis, Mo: Facts and Comparisons, (2000), 4-5.

Padayatty, S. J., Levine, M. "Vitamin C and coronary microcirculation," *Circulation* 103 (2001): E117.

Pompella, A., Visvikis, A., Paolicchi, A., De Tata, V., Casini, A. F. "The changing faces of glutathione, a cellular protagonist." *Biochemical Pharmacology* 66 (8) (2003): 1499–503.

Raitakari, O. T., Adams, M. R., McCredie, R. J. "Oral vitamin C and endothelial function in smokers: short term improvement, but no sustained beneficial effect." *J Am Coll Cardiol* 35 (2000):1616-1621.

Richards, R. S,, Roberts, T. K. "Blood parameters indicative of oxidative stress are associated with symptom expression in chronic fatigue syndrome. *Redox Rep.* 1 (5) (2000): 35–41.

Sharma, M. K., Buettner, G. R. "Interaction of vitamin C and vitamin E during free radical stress in plasma: an ESR study." *Free Radic Biol Med* 14 (1993): 649–53.

Thomas, R. J. "Excitatory amino acids in health and disease." *J Am Geriatr Soc.* 43(11) (1995): 1279-89.

Zimme, H. G. "Normalization of depressed heart function in rats by ribose." *Science* 220 (1983): 81-2.

Sanders, M. E,, Klaenhammer, T. R. "The Scientific Basis of Lactobacillus Acidophilus NCFM Functionality as a Probiotic." *Journal of Dairy Science* 84, no. 2 (February 2001): 319–331.

Scholz, R. W., Graham, K., Gumpricht, Reddy C., C. "Mechanism of interaction of vitamin E and glutathione in the protection against membrane lipid peroxidation." *Ann NY Acad Sci* 570 (1989):514-7.

Chapter 21

Chong, S. K. F. "Ginseng: is there a use in clinical medicine?" *Postgrad Med.* 64 (1988): 841-846.

Fessenden, J. M., Wittenborn, W., Clarke, L. "Gingko biloba: case report of herbal medicine and bleeding postoperatively from a laparoscopic cholecystectomy." *Am Surg.* 67 (2001): 33-35.

Shintani, S., Murase, H., Tsukagoshi, H., et al. "Glycyrrhizin (licorice) induced hypokalemic myopathy: report of 2 cases and review of literature." *Eur Neurol.* 32 (1992): 44-51.

Stickel, F., Egerer, G., Seitz, H. K. "Hepatotoxicity of botanicals." *Public Health Nutr.* 3 (2000):113-124.

Grandhi, A., Mujumdar, A., Patwardhan, B. "A Comparative Pharmacological Investigation of Ashwagandha and Ginseng. *Journal of Ethnopharmacology* 44, no. 3 (December 1994):131–135.

Bhattacharya, S. K., Muruganandam, A.V. "Adaptogenic Activity of Withania Somnifera: An Experimental Study Using a Rat Model of Chronic Stress." *Pharmacology, Biochemistry and Behavior* 75, no. 3 (June 2003):547–555.

Chapter 22

Albert, S. G., Deleon, M. J., Silverberg, A. B. "Possible association between high-dose fluconazole and adrenal insufficiency in critically ill patients." *Crit Care Med* 29 (2001):668-70.

Annane, D., Sèbille, V., Charpentier, C., et al. "Effect of treatment with low doses of hydrocortisone and fludrocortisone on mortality in patients with septic shock." *JAMA* 288 (2002):862-71.

Coursin, B. D., Wood, K. E. "Corticosteroid supplementation for adrenal insufficiency." *JAMA* 287 (2002):236-40.

Davison, S. L., Bell, R., Donath, S. et al. "Androgen levels in adult females: changes with age, menopause, and oophorectomy." *Journal of Clinical Endocrinology and Metabolism* 90 (2005): 3847–3853.

Demling, R., DeSanti, L. "Oxandrolone, an anabolic steroid, significantly increases the rate of weight gain in the recovery phase after major burns." *J Trauma* 43 (1997):47-50.

Dixon, R. B., Christy, N. P. "On the various forms of corticosteroid withdrawal syndrome." *Am J Med* 68 (1980): 224-230.

Kimball, C. P. "Psychological dependency on steroids?" *Ann Intern Med* 75 (1971):111-113.

Ling, M. H. M., Perry, P. J., Tsuang, M. T. "Side effects of corticosteroid therapy." *Arch Gen Psychiatry* 38 (1981): 471-477.

Nair, K. S., Rizza, R. A. "O'Brien P et al. DHEA in elderly women and DHEA or testosterone in elderly men." *N Engl J Med* 355 (2006):1647–1659.

North American Menopause Society: "Estrogen and progestogen use in peri- and post menopausal women: March 2007 position statement of the North American Menopause Society." *Menopause* 14(2) (2007): 168-182.

O'Dwyer, A. M, "Lightman SL, Marks MN et al. Treatment of major depression with metyrapone and hydrocortisone." *J Affect Disord* 33 (1995): 123-128.

Oppert, M., Reinicke, A., Graf, K. J., et al. "Plasma cortisol levels before and during 'low-dose' hydrocortisone therapy and their relationship to hemodynamic improvement in patients with septic shock." *Intensive Care Med* 26 (2000):1747-55.

Streck, W. F., Lockwood, D. H. "Pituitary adrenal recovery following short-term suppression with glucocorticoids." *Am J Med* 66 (1979):910-14.

Walker, C. R. "Bioidentical hormone replacement therapy. A natural option for perimenopause and beyond." *Adv. Nurse Pract.* 9(5) (2001): 39-42.

Wolkowitz, O., Reus, V., Roberts, E., et al. "Dehydroepiandrosterone (DHEA) treatment of depression." *Biol Psychiatry* 41 (1997): 311-318.

Wolkowitz, O. M., Reus, V. I., Weingartner, H. et al. "Cognitive effects of corticosteroids." *Am J Psychiatry* 147 (1990): 1297-1303.

Wren, B. G., McFarland, K., Edwards, L. "Micronised transdermal progesterone and endometrial response." *Lancet* 354, no. 9188 (1999): 1447-1448.

Bellingrath, S., Weigl, T., Kudielka, B. M. "Cortisol Dysregulation in School Teachers in Relation to Burnout, Vital Exhaustion, and Effort-Reward-Imbalance." *Biological Psychology* 78, no. 1 (April 2008):104–113.

Chapter 23

Adam, T. C., Epel, E. S. "Stress, eating and the reward system." *Physiology & Behavior* 91(2007): 449–458.

Baker, P. G., Barry, R. E., Read, A. E. "Detection of continuing gluten ingestion in treated celiac patients." *BMJ* 1 (1975): 486-8.

Ciclitira, P. J., Ellis, H. J., Fagg, N. L. "Evaluation of a gluten free product containing wheat gluten in patients with celiac disease." *BMJ* 289 (1984): 83.

Ciclitira, P. J. "Gluten-free diet - what is toxic?" *Best Pract Res Clin Gastroenterol* 19 (2005): 359-71.

Chapter 25

Kaukinen, K., Collin, P., Holm, K., et al. "Wheat starch-containing gluten free flour products in the treatment of celiac disease and dermatitis herpetiformis. A long term follow-up study." *Scand J Gastroenterol* 34 (1999): 163-9.

Peraaho, M., Kaukinen, K., Paasikivi, K., et al. "Wheat-starch-based gluten-free products in the treatment of newly detected celiac disease: prospective and randomized study." *Aliment Pharmacol Ther* 17 (2003): 587-94.

Johnston, S. D., Smye, M., Watson, R. P. "Intestinal Permeability Tests in Coeliac Disease." *Lancet* 359, no. 9314 (April 13, 2002): 1352.

Chapter 26

Almeida, J. C., Grimsley, E. W. "Coma from the health food store: interaction between kava and alprazolam [letter]." *Ann Intern Med.* 125 (1996): 940-941.

Attarian, H. P. "Helping patients who say they cannot sleep. Practical ways to evaluate and treat insomnia." *Postgrad Med.* 107 (2000): 127-142.

Bain, K. T. "Management of chronic insomnia in elderly persons." *Am J Geriatr Pharmacother. 52 (1973): 307-308; 35 (2001): 1449-1457; 4 (2006): 168-192.*

Branco, J., Atalaia, A., Paiva, T. "Sleep cycles and alpha-delta sleep in fibromyalgia syndrome." *J Rheumatol.* 21(6) (1994): 1113-7.

Citera, G., Arias, M. A. Maldonado-Cocco JA et al. "The effect of melatonin in patients with fibromyalgia: a pilot study." *Clin Rheumatol.* 19(1) (2000): 9-13.

Drewes, A. M., Andreasen, A., Jennum, P, Nielsen, K. D. "Zopiclone in the treatment of sleep abnormalities in fibromyalgia." *Scand J Rheumatol.* 20(4) (1991): 288-93.

Escher, M., Desmeules, J., Giostra, E., et al. "Hepatitis associated with kava, a herbal remedy." *BMJ.* 322 (2001): 139.

Garfinkel, D., Laudon, M., Nof, D., Zisapel, N. "Improvement of sleep quality in elderly people by controlled-release melatonin." *Lancet.* 346 (1995): 541-544.

Garfinkel, D., Zisapel, N., Wainstein, J., Laudon, M. "Facilitation of benzodiazepine discontinuation by melatonin: a new clinical approach." *Arch Intern Med.* 159 (1999): 2456-2460.

Kaplan, Z., Amir, M., Swartz, M., Levine, J. "Inositol treatment of post-traumatic stress disorder. *Anxiety* 2(1) (1996): 51–52.

Webb, S. M. "Fibromyalgia and melatonin: are they related?" *Clin Endocrinol* (Oxf). 49(2) (1998):161-2.

Zhdanova, I. V., Wurtman, R. J., Regan, M. M., et al. "Melatonin treatment for age-related insomnia." *J Clin Endocrinol Metab.* 86 (2001): 4727-4730.

Richards, K., et al. "Use of Complementary and Alternative Therapies to Promote Sleep in Critically Ill Patients." *Critical Care Nursing Clinics of North America* 15, no. 3 (September 2003): 329–340.

Baskett, J. J., et al. "Does Melatonin Improve Sleep in Older People? A Randomised Crossover Trial." *Age and Ageing* 32, no. 2 (March 2003): 164–170.

Chapter 27

Broocks, A., Bandelow, B., Pekrun, G., et al. "Comparison of aerobic exercise, clomipramine, and placebo in the treatment of panic disorder." *Am. J. Psychiatry* 155(5) (1998): 603–609.

Galbo, H., Holst, J. J., Christensen, N. J. "Glucagon and plasma catecholamine responses to graded and prolonged exercise in man." *J Appl Physiol.* 38(1) (1975):70–6.

Kjaer, M. "Adrenal medulla and exercise training." E*ur J Appl Physiol Occup Physiol.* 77(3) (1998): 195–9.

Kjaer, M. "Epinephrine and some other hormonal responses to exercise in man: with special reference to physical training." *Int J Sports Med.* 10(1) (1989): 2–15.

Mannerkorpi, K., Iversen, M.D. "Physical exercise in fibromyalgia and related syndromes." *Best Pract Res Clin Rheumatol.* 17(4) (2003): 629-47.

McMurray, R. G., Hackney, A. C. "Interactions of metabolic hormones, adipose tissue and exercise." Sports Med. 35(5) (2005): 393–412.

Moldofsky H. "Management of sleep disorders in fibromyalgia." *Rheum Dis Clin North Am.* 2002;28(2):353-65.

Chapter 28

Audin, K., Bekker, H. L., Barkham, M., Foster, J. "Self-help in primary care mental health: a survey of counsellors' and psychotherapists' views and current practice." *Primary Care Mental Health* 1 (2003): 89–100.

Bartels, A., Zeki, S. "The neural basis of romantic love." Neuroreport,11 (2000): 3829-34.

Bartels, A., Zeki, S. "The neural correlates of maternal and romantic love." *Neuroimage,* 21 (2004): 1155-66.

Chapter 32

Asbring, P., Narvanan, A. L. "Patient power and control: a study of women with uncertain illness trajectories." *Qualitative Health Research* 14 (2004):226–240.

Asbring, P., Narvanan, A. L. "Women's experiences of stigma in relation to chronic fatigue syndrome and fibromyalgia." *Qualitative Health Research* 12 (2002): 148–160.

Index

5-HTP 207, 282, 342-4

A

acid
  alpha-lipoic 253, 260
  hydrochloric 305
  malic 246, 269
  pantothenic 236, 254-5, 261, 266, 272
acid reflux 305
acidophilus 262-3, 305
ACTH 11, 19, 22-4, 30, 57, 79, 147, 428
activities
  stressful 391, 393
  sympathoadrenal 446
adaptogen 33, 278, 280-1
adaptogenic properties 238, 273, 278, 282-3
  good adrenal 240
addiction 52, 56, 192, 241, 282, 286, 290
Addison's disease 6, 10-11, 15, 22, 62, 67,
  82, 146-7, 178, 278, 291, 441, 446-7
adrenal
  burnout 8, 349
  health 74, 77, 105, 271, 344
  hormones 23-4, 108, 133, 146-7, 285, 291
    anti-stress 8
    key 20, 140, 147, 226
  recovery 85, 108, 138, 163, 183, 282, 311,
    349, 382, 385
Adrenal Breathing 200, 339, 347, 349-50,
  353-4, 356, 367
  advanced 355
  Exercises 49, 200-1, 319, 339-40, 350-1,
    353-4, 367, 380, 393, 396-8
adrenal cortex 21-2, 30, 51, 79, 88, 99, 101,
  127, 149, 289, 428-9, 431, 444
adrenal cortisol, baseline functions 149
adrenal cortisol level 71
adrenal crash intensity, levels of 160
adrenal crash phase 382
adrenal crash symptoms 159, 170

adrenal crashes 128, 134-5, 137-8, 153-4,
  156-60, 164-5, 167-8, 224-5, 286, 290,
  294-5, 345-6, 356-7, 369, 379-85, 387-8
  experience 153, 259
  major 167, 169
  precipitate 324, 425
adrenal dysfunction 9, 15, 86, 89, 91, 109,
  204
adrenal exhaustion 8, 11, 13, 15, 25, 61-2,
  67-8, 86, 88-91, 93, 117-18, 120-1, 124-5,
  127, 129-30, 432-3
  advanced 67, 81, 170, 257, 261
  early 87, 113, 431
adrenal extracts 274
adrenal failure 11, 15, 35, 44, 51, 61-2, 69,
  154, 165, 226-7, 229, 232
  autoimmune 447
  risk 227, 232
adrenal fatigue 6, 9, 12, 52, 161, 191, 235,
  237, 239, 241, 313
  very mild 252
Adrenal Fatigue Center 414
Adrenal Fatigue Syndrome
  advanced 49, 61, 78, 83, 90, 108, 143, 151,
    200-1, 203, 207, 214, 240, 259-60, 345,
    349
    stages of 23, 48, 63, 65, 67, 69, 83, 165,
      286-7, 386
    symptoms of 201, 207
  diet 313
  early stages of 18, 51, 53, 55, 57, 59, 79, 99,
    157, 173
  mild 204, 230, 240, 273, 337
  stages 29, 154, 160, 162, 164, 171, 229, 232
  sufferer, typical 171
  sufferers
    advanced 260
    most 157
  symptoms of 3-4, 9, 19, 47, 102, 115, 126,
    128, 143, 165, 192, 201, 203, 205, 207,
    214

P

About the Authors

Michael Lam, M.D., M.P.H., A.B.A.A.M., is a western trained physician specializing in nutritional and anti-aging medicine. Dr. Lam received his Bachelor of Science degree from Oregon State University, and his Doctor of Medicine degree from the Loma Linda University School of Medicine in California. He also holds a Master's degree in Public Health. He is board certified by the American Board of Anti-Aging Medicine where he has also served as a board examiner. Dr. Lam is a pioneer in using nontoxic, natural compounds to promote the healing of many age-related degenerative conditions. He utilizes optimum blends of nutritional supplementation that manipulate food, vitamins, natural hormones, herbs, enzymes, and minerals into specific protocols to rejuvenate cellular function.

Dr. Lam was first to coin the term, *ovarian-adrenal-thyroid (OAT)* hormone axis, and to describe its imbalances. He was first to scientifically tie in Adrenal Fatigue Syndrome (AFS) as part of the overall neuroendocrine stress response continuum of the body. He systematized the clinical significance and coined the various phases of Adrenal Exhaustion. He has written four books: *The Five Proven Secrets to Longevity, Beating Cancer with Natural Medicine, How to Stay Young and Live Longer, and Estrogen Dominance*. In 2001, Dr. Lam established *www.DrLam.com* as a free, educational website on evidence-based alternative medicine for the public and for health professionals. It featured the world's most comprehensive library on AFS. Provided free as a public service, he has answered countless questions through the website on alternative health and AFS. His personal, telephone-based nutritional coaching services have enabled many around the world to regain control of their health using natural therapies.

Dorine Lam, R.D., M.S., M.P.H., is a registered dietitian and holistic clinical nutritionist specializing in Adrenal Fatigue Syndrome and natural hormonal balancing. She received her Bachelor of Science degree in Dietetics, holds a Master's Degree in Public Health in Nutrition, and a Master of Science degree in Nutrition from Loma Linda University, in Loma Linda, California. She is also a board-certified, Anti-Aging Health Practitioner by the American Academy of Anti-Aging Medicine. She coauthored with Michael Lam, M.D., the book *Estrogen Dominance* and numerous articles on Adrenal Fatigue Syndrome. Her personal research and writing focuses on the metabolic aspect of Adrenal Fatigue Syndrome. She is married to Michael Lam and is an integral part of the telephone-based nutritional coaching team helping people overcome Adrenal Fatigue Syndrome.

Dr. Lam's Adrenal Recovery Series

Dr. Lam has created a Mini-series of books as well as Singles for your use to aid in your recovery. *Adrenal Fatigue Syndrome* is comprehensive guidebook ... the Mini and Singles series allows you to have "select" sections that support and enhance your education and recovery. They are easier to carry with you for reference, allowing you to bookmark specific sections during your recovery program.

The Mini Series of paperback and ebooks include:

Psychology of Adrenal Fatigue Syndrome:
How the Mind-Body Connection Affects Your Recovery

Anatomy of Adrenal Fatigue Syndrome: Clinical Stages 1 – 4

Natural Therapeutics to Adrenal Fatigue Syndrome:
Proper Use of Vitamins, Glandulars, Herbs, and Hormones

Dietary and Lifestyle Therapeutics to Adrenal Fatigue Syndrome:
Your Personal Recovery Toolbox

Estrogen Dominance: Hormonal Imbalance of the 21st Century
(Expanded Version)

The Singles Series of ebooks include:

Neuroendocrine Basis of Adrenal Fatigue Syndrome:
The Physiology of Fatigue

Adrenal Crashes: How to Prevent and Recover Quickly

Diagnostic Testing for Adrenal Fatigue Syndrome:
Everything You Need to Know

Adrenal Fatigue Syndrome Progression and Case Study:
What is Coming Ahead

Your Constitution and Adrenal Fatigue Syndrome:
How Your Genetic Makeup Can Affect Your Recovery

Travel Tips and Adrenal Fatigue Syndrome: How to Avoid Adrenal Crashes

Ovarian-Adrenal-Thyroid Axis Imbalance:
Why Your Thyroid Medications May Not Be Working

7 Adrenal Recovery Mistakes: What Successful Recovery Avoid

Anti-aging and Adrenal Fatigue Syndrome:
Incorporating an Anti-aging Program Into Your Recovery

Myths of Adrenal Fatigue Syndrome: Separating the Facts from the Fiction

Individual copies can be ordered from *www.DrLam.com*
as well as through online retailers.

Notes

Notes